T0093977

Blood in Motion

Abraham Noordergraaf

Blood in Motion

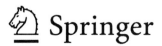 Springer

Abraham Noordergraaf, Ph.D.
Bioengineering Department
University of Pennsylvania
Philadelphia, PA 19104, USA
anoor@seas.upenn.edu

ISBN 978-1-4614-0004-2   e-ISBN 978-1-4614-0005-9
DOI 10.1007/978-1-4614-0005-9
Springer New York Dordrecht Heidelberg London

Library of Congress Control Number: 2011932431

© Springer Science+Business Media, LLC 2011
All rights reserved. This work may not be translated or copied in whole or in part without the written
permission of the publisher (Springer Science+Business Media, LLC, 233 Spring Street, New York,
NY 10013, USA), except for brief excerpts in connection with reviews or scholarly analysis.
Use in connection with any form of information storage and retrieval, electronic adaptation, computer
software, or by similar or dissimilar methodology now known or hereafter developed is forbidden.
The use in this publication of trade names, trademarks, service marks, and similar terms, even if they are
not identified as such, is not to be taken as an expression of opinion as to whether or not they are subject
to proprietary rights.

Printed on acid-free paper

Springer is part of Springer Science+Business Media (www.springer.com)

*This book reflects a lifetime of scientific
endeavor and personal discovery
and is dedicated to all those whose role
is indelibly imprinted on these pages.*

Preface

Blood in Motion is a textbook on cardiovascular science. It sets out to introduce, entice, and explain the cardiovascular system to the reader using a classical system in teaching: anatomy, physiology, general operation, and specific systems. It is specifically designed to support the interests of students and experienced physiologists and clinicians.

This book is subdivided into three parts which comprise a total of 11 chapters. Part I, including the first two chapters, presents a historical perspective of cardiovascular knowledge and complements that with Chap. 2 which deals with current insights into the physiology of the cardiovascular system. Part II explores sections of the circulatory loop, starting with an in-depth treatment of the veins, and including the lymphatic, the microcirculation, the arterial system, and the heart. Part III incorporates approaches to the cardiovascular system as a whole, both in physiology and in science, such as modeling. This part introduces impedance-defined flow and offers the reader its application in mathematical modeling.

The design is such that each chapter can be read or studied as an independent unit.

Each chapter begins with a citation, in its original form, focusing on the topic to be addressed, a digest of the material in the chapter, and ends with a conclusion dealing with the message the reader may have found in the chapter.

The questions at the end of each chapter lean toward intellectual integration more so than factual reproduction. They are diverse in difficulty while asking the reader to apply multiple facts, suggestions, and concepts offered in the text. The answers given are in line with the text, and include motivation for the choices made.

Illustrations selected are distinctive with respect to their nature as well as in their utilization. Major points in thinking or in the discussion of a point are supported by illustrations to help the reader in visualizing. The intention is to support the rationale in the text more than to supply evidence for the purpose of conviction. The captions are self-explanatory and together with the figure will offer information independent of the text. As much as possible, cross referencing has been avoided.

While presented as a whole, *Blood in Motion* includes thinking, rethinking of countless scientists over many years. References have been used extensively, but not exhaustively, to offer the reader the opportunity to return to the original text allowing analysis of the work and the original authors' conclusions as opposed to modern reviews of that work. While this involves more work, the understanding which returning to the original work offers may itself unravel conflicting data or findings.

The reader beware, *Blood in Motion* presents facts in evidence and supportive thinking as well as suppositions not in evidence. It is intrinsically biased as it does not attempt or purport to be a review of cardiovascular science. The philosophy underlying the book allows for choices between main-line thinking and visions perhaps still deemed to be approaching the "fringes" of accepted science. These choices are identified in the text, allowing and stimulating the reader to explore for themselves which avenue appeals.

Philadelphia, PA, USA   Abraham Noordergraaf

Acknowledgments

The writing of a book such as this, in which reflection, facts, and suppositions are brought together to form a united and seemingly logical unit, involves a great deal of reading, as well as interactions and suggestions from others. Without this, the writing would have been neither fun nor fruitful.

Science is a continuum and this is reflected in the form and content of this book. When I was a young assistant to Professor Burger at the University of Utrecht, he approached me and informed me, indignantly, that a German paper had claimed that mammalian cardiac values were unnecessary: the heart could move blood around the cardiovascular circuit without them. He charged me to look into the feasibility of what seemed to him to be a preposterous claim. However, this potentially intriguing query lost priority and only resurfaced decennia later when the modeling of cardiac values was an issue. Searches in libraries and computers as well as interviews turned up only benevolent smiles, until Professor and Mrs. Thomas Kenner were able to provide the link. The former was able to supply the Proceedings of a symposium during which the subject was discussed. With the Proceedings, edited by Pestel and Liebau (in German), I was finally able to return to the initial assignment, which resulted in a generalization of William Harvey's teachings.

Besides recognizing the instigator of a focus in *Blood in Motion*, the above also explains the philosophy underlying the book: patience, critical analysis by an open mind, a willingness to provisionally accept an idea until it can factually be repudiated, and wide-ranging discussions are core aspects which can be recognized.

In doing this, I am indebted to many individuals and organizations:

It is my pleasure to offer my thanks to members of my family, who evolved in surprising roles:

To Alexander A. Noordergraaf for filling the demanding positions of being my computer system teacher, administrator, and Helpdesk. To Jeske I. Noordergraaf V.M.D. and Jim McCarthy M.S. for providing access to antiquarians and for exposure to the conduct of equine veterinary practice.

To Lt. Colonel (R) Gerrit J. Noordergraaf M.D. Ph.D and Cathy Noordergraaf M.S. for the innumerable, lively, discussions about the roles and hierarchy in fundamental and clinical science, about what could be meant as opposed to what was stated, about cardiopulmonary resuscitation (CPR) as a science within circulatory sciences in general, and of course for their abiding hospitality.

To their daughter Jeske, who when challenged showed convincingly that even in the minds of today's High School students, mathematics and the interest in understanding what it means is alive and well. I am also indebted to her for her exceptional help in working through the manuscript formula by formula and figure by figure, when the computer became subversive. To their son Tristan, who decided that a "good, old" copy could not be as great as a "better, new" digital version, my thanks for the persistence in helping with the figures. In this regard, appreciation is also due to Igor Paulussen M.Sc., a people person and technical wizard.

To Annemiek and Jim Young, Esqs., for their help in understanding the legalities in Science, in and outside its and my Ivory Tower, as well as for the many pleasant dinners required to enlighten me in the legal mindset.

I would also like to specifically recognize:

The late Professor Herman C. Burger Ph.D. for setting me on the high road which, finally, led to the style in the writing of this book.

Professor Mohamad N. Itani D.M.D. for help in sorting out texts in Arabic, while attending to my dental needs.

Professor Johnny T. Ottesen Ph.D. for contributing to the exposure of a previously unknown cardiac property induced by the respiratory system.

Professor Stig Andur Pedersen for providing insights into the philosophy in René Descartes' teaching.

Professor Chris Quick for providing extensive documentation about the lymphatic system, including some of his own research.

The numerous students at the Universities of Utrecht, NL, and Pennsylvania, USA, who through course work or project analyses posed creative questions.

Listed in chronological order of graduation, especially inspiring were former Ph.D. students Gerard Jager, Ernst Attinger M.D., Ed Kresch, Jerry Pollack, Nico Westerhof, Lee Huntsman, Piet Verdouw, Jules Melbin V.M.D., Ron Brower, Jan Baan, Tatsuo Iwazumi, Franco Peluso, Harvey Mayrovitz, Joel Greenburg, Dennis Silage, Bill Hunter, Ashok Ranada, John Li, Bob McNally, Gary Drzewiecki, Jurg Jaggi, Larry Muscarella, Joe Palladino, Sina Rabbany, David Berger, Allison Hoydu, Fred Frasch, Jan Mulier M.D., Michael Danielsin, Chris Quick, Bojan Knap M.D., and LtCol (R.) Gerrit (Tan) Noordergraaf M.D. Ph.D.

The enduring and generous financial support by both the Federal Aviation Agency through the late William R. (Bill) Scarborough M.D. and the National Heart, Lung, and Blood Institute of the National Institutes of Health, at their conception strongly stimulated by the late Samuel A. Talbot Ph.D., facilitated the execution of these studies meaningfully.

I would like to express my appreciation to Charles Greifenstein, Curator of Archives and Manuscripts at the Historical Library of the College of Physicians of Philadelphia, for his willingness and ability to produce classical documents for inspection and inspiration. Christopher Stanwood and Erin McLeary, Historical

Reference Librarians in the same organization, for prompt and accurate responses to sometimes unusual requests. For Godelieve Engelbers and Sjors Clements, Chief Librarians at the St. Elisabeth Hospital and Brabant Medical School, my admiration for rising to each challenge I presented, both large and small, to delineate, find, and produce materials.

For the use of figures I would like to thank all the colleagues and publishers who allowed me to use or adapt their original work and the Publisher at Springer, for their attention and care in the preparation of this book.

Abraham Noordergraaf

Contents

Part I
Synoptic Reviews of Thinking in
Circulatory Physiology

Chapter 1
Synoptic Reviews of Cardiovascular Science from Different Approaches

In the time of Socrates a nearer approach was made to the method. But at this period man gave up inquiring into the works of nature, and philosophers diverted their attention to political science and to the virtues which benefit mankind

— Aristoteles. From Ogle's rendition of the original Greek text of De Partibus Animalium (1882).

Digest: Aristoteles details the method of studying nature, the need of which was originally argued by Socrates. Its two parts were specified, centuries later, by Descartes as mathematical and experimental. In current times the method may be viewed as consisting of a series of foci that require balanced judgment. The method used in this book is outlined.

It has long been argued that experiment and theory are natural twins (though they have not always been on amicable terms).

1.1 Cardiovascular Science from a Chronological Approach

During the period ca. 3000 BCE–1600 BCE, the Egyptian culture generated anatomical information from victims of regional battles and from accidents occurring during the construction of the pyramids (Table 1.1). The Mesopotamian civilization, during that time, developed early concepts in mathematics and took tentative steps in the development of biomathematics. Hammurabi's code introduced the distinction between invasive and noninvasive procedures and established medical liability. Neither culture dealt with ideas about a cardiovascular system.

The oldest known effort to organize available information into a system emerged much later as the Greek civilization matured. Erasistratos presented the first cardiovascular theory around 200 BCE. Galenos, ca. 200 CE, familiarized himself with it and modified it. Subsequently, the relevant documents, reported to have been written by Erasistratos, were lost.

A. Noordergraaf, *Blood in Motion*, DOI 10.1007/978-1-4614-0005-9_1,
© Springer Science+Business Media, LLC 2011

Table 1.1 Selected giants in the field of days long past

	Egypt	Mesopotamia	Greece	UK	Others
3000 BCE	Imhotep (deified Egyptian physician)				
Old Kingdom 2000 BCE		*Babylonia* Hammurabi and medical code			
		Assyria/Neo-Assyria King Assurbanipal Sumerian pictograms (peak performance ca. 1600)			
1000 BCE			*Beginning ca. 600*		
			Development of first steps into biomath		
			Hippocrates (Corpus)		
			Socrates/Plato		
			Aristoteles		
			Alexander the Great		
		Ptolemeus I & II	Erasistratos		
			Tertullianos		
0			Galenos		
400 CE					
1000 CE					Ibn an-Nafîs
1400 CE					Caesalpinus
				Harvey	Malphigi
					Servetus
					Descartes
1700 CE					Vesalius

BCE denotes Before Current Era

According to Galenos, blood is formed in the liver, where it is also provided with natural spirit. The blood is then distributed to all organs through the veins. He also assumed the presence of pores in the ventricular septum. The pores would permit blood flow from the right ventricle to the left ventricle. Major criticism of this concept was presented by Ibn an-Nafîs ca. 1270 and again by Servetus in 1553 (Servetus 1553). The critics could not find the pores.

Caesalpinus (1593) and Harvey (1628), respectively introduced on theoretical grounds and on experimental grounds, the concept of circulation of the same blood in a closed loop, now including the pulmonary circulation. The heart alone was thought to provide the motive force that sustains the circulation. Although incorporation of the pulmonary vascular bed resolved the issue of the septal pores, Harvey found it obligatory to introduce peripheral pores to connect the smallest arteries to the smallest veins.

Malpighi, an early microscopist, discovered in (1661) that capillary vessels actually connect the arterial vasculature to the venous vascular beds, which eliminated the need for Harvey's assumption of peripheral pores. New problems arose, however.

During the 1800s, a number of scientists raised doubts about the validity of Harvey's proposal that the heart alone is capable of driving the blood around the closed circuit. Their concerns focused in particular on venous return. Donders nominated the respiratory system as a candidate for providing support to the circulation. The issue whether such a mechanism could actually be operational went unresolved for well over a century.

Liebau demonstrated that in closed loop fluid-mechanical models, comprising tubes with different properties and free of valves, steady flow could be generated by compressing one tube periodically at some point (illustrated in Fig. 9.4). This observation led him to speculate that cardiac and venous valves might be superfluous (1956), thereby contradicting prevailing teaching.

In 1960, Kouwenhoven et al. introduced noninvasive cardiopulmonary resuscitation (CPR) for the treatment of victims of a heart attack serious enough to cause the heart to stop pumping and the respiration to fail as a consequence. The method, periodic chest compression, interrupted by artificial respiration, proved to induce a significantly lower survival rate than its invasive precursor, which it was supposed to duplicate. The earlier procedure required surgical opening of the chest, insertion of a hand, and massaging the ventricles directly. The lower survival rate raised an additional barrage of questions concerning the operation of the cardiovascular system, for only few of which reliable answers became available readily.

Solutions to the problems identified in the last three paragraphs above began to emerge as late as the end of the twentieth century. First, Liebau's observations on steady flow proved to be due to the nonuniform distribution of the impedances of his tubes. The realization that the cardiovascular system is strongly nonuniform along any longitudinal pathway resulted in the formulation of the concept of impedance-defined flow. Impedance-defined flow, which is often bidirectional, offers a generalization of Harvey's unidirectional flow imposed by the heart (Moser et al. 1998). Second, the concept identified a large number of additional pumps, distributed throughout the cardiovascular system, which expanded the range of control features governing the magnitude of cardiac output, especially during exercise.

It has been reported that the cardiac valves may all be open in total heart failure. If alterations in CPR-induced shape of vessels are assumed to be negligible, impedance-defined flow considerations then predict that most or all regular flow is supplanted by sloshing, i.e., little or no transport of oxygen, metabolites, etc.

takes place, hence Liebau's speculation about the superfluity of cardiac and venous valves was exaggerated. If changes in shape are taken into account, high pressures administered during CPR tend to collapse large veins, reducing blood flow, which, recent computer studies suggest, require more time to refill than allotted by conventional massage, thereby continuing seriously reduced blood flow.

Application of impedance-defined flow considerations to Donders' nomination of the respiratory system as aiding the cardiovascular system, confirmed not only that Donders' idea was proper, but that it constitutes only one example of several systems, such as the neural system, that can exert significant positive or negative influence on cardiac output (Noordergraaf GJ et al. 2006).

1.2 Cardiovascular Science from an Ideological Point of View

Aristoteles (384–322 BCE) argued elaborately that the study of nature requires investigators to follow a specific method. He described this Method as consisting of at least two parts, referred to as causes, namely necessity and final end or final object. Thus of a phenomenon observed in nature (e.g., respiration), it must be shown that it takes place for such and such a final object; it must also be shown that this or that part of the process is necessitated by this or that other stage of it. Necessity will sometimes mean hypothetical necessity, the necessity, i.e., that the requisite antecedents shall be there, if the final end is to be reached; and sometimes absolute necessity, such necessity as that between substances and their inherent properties and characters.

Democritus, regarded as the founder of atomistic natural philosophy and a contemporary of Socrates (c. 470–399 BCE), was, in the judgment of Aristoteles, the first to come close to using the method and that in spite of himself.

Over the centuries, interest in cardiovascular science continued to wax and wane, until eventually the Western Renaissance inspired a long and sustained era of progress. Thus, in his Discourse on the Method, Descartes (1596–1650) could expand upon Aristoteles' view by reasoning that, to him, mathematics should provide the starting point for explaining what is observed in nature.[1] Adherence to his own teaching proved difficult: In part five of the Discourse, where he discusses the movement of blood, he agrees with Harvey that blood is in perpetual motion around a circuit, but disagrees about the cause of the motion. Here, Descartes harks back to much older ideas by claiming that it is the heat from the heart, as described in more detail in his letter to Van Beverwijck (1672).

---

[1]Descartes had come a long way from the view of Guy Patin (1601–1672), like himself a contemporary of William Harvey. Patin, an ardent and vocal supporter of the Galenus theory, when Doyen de la Faculté de Mèdecine de Paris, is reported to have declared that the circulation of blood is "paradoxale, impossible, inintelligible, absurde, nuisible à la vie de l'homme" (Bordas edition of Le Discourse).

Aristoteles' original method, as well as Descartes' Method, can be expanded further. They recognized two classes of activities: design of experiments and observation on the one hand and mathematical analysis on the other. These interactions can be formulated and extended to a novel and contemporary approach, which consist of some seven levels of organization while continuing to incorporate the original concepts.

These levels are:

Level 1. Design of an experiment, followed by collection and reporting of experimental data on the subject of interest. Statistical analysis may be helpful in evaluating whether differences observed are likely to have significance. In many instances, this level remained the final one for a long period. In particular, clinicians have produced numerous examples at this level, likely induced by their training institutions.

Level 2. A tentative interpretation as to the cause of the observations may be conceived and formulated. This then expresses an initial theory in words, i.e., in a qualitative form.

Level 3. The qualitative theory should give rise to additional questions, which require additional experimental data. These may or may not modify the tentative interpretation. In other words, level 3 may require iteration of levels 1 and 2. Sir George Pickering (1964) offered an incisive analysis of the differences, real or imagined, between practicing physicians and experimental scientists.

Level 4. Replacement of the qualitative theory by a quantitative one, which entails devising a set of equations based on natural laws, which duplicate, in whole or in part, the experimental data that gave rise to them. If successful, this set of equations represents the investigator's quantitative interpretation embodied in the form of an analytical model. Such a comprehensive model compactly summarizes the measured system's behavior through characterization of the properties of its components and their interaction.

The experimental data has only now been "understood," and the parameters that govern the behavior of the system, rather than the variables observed, have been identified. The parameters should have biological meaning instead of furnishing a supply of convenient constants. This has, in the past, often been the end stage of a study.

In fact, investigators have occasionally been known to pay scant attention to the preceding levels even when accessible. The models they formulated have a tendency to live their own lives, often in splendid isolation and free of practical utilization. Bioscientists have left traces of such isolated activities, potentially causing other investigators to be misdirected or confused by what seemed to be parallel or unique thinking, but offering only a dead end.

Level 5. The solution of the equations should expose unknown mechanisms, thereby raising new questions, which require new experiments; the model now carries a message.

Level 6. Expansion of the level 4 model to incorporate any new discoveries.

Level 7. The level 6 model may be reduced by weeding out minor effects, then used as a building block, after appropriate validation against well-established experimental data, for analysis of phenomena in situations where experimental access is not achievable or unethical, as well as for a building block to proceed to a higher level of organization. The need for reduction applies especially to models of such complexity as to overwhelm potential users.

Validation raises its own questions. Since a given model will rarely require validation against a complete biological system, the investigator must decide what features should carry the main focus, how accurate the agreement between experiment and theory should be in the face of the variability of data extracted from a living system, etc.

Biological systems contain many subsystems with individual, specialized responsibilities, all of which together sustain system operation. Owing to its complexity, subsystem responsibilities tend to impose competing or even contradictory requirements in certain areas. It appears that nature has straightened out conflicts to a level that is "good enough," rather than perfect, though it may have tried, but found the results less satisfactory. Nature leads investigators into making approximations, though it does not volunteer where and to what extent such approximations may be applied. This challenges even the scholar's insight.

A danger for any researcher is to become riveted to one side of a conflict area. The attraction may also become to bypass the original procedure of quantitative biological research by concentrating entirely on either the modeling aspects, such as striving to duplicate nature in precious perfection, or the experimental challenges, distractions that should be resisted vigorously. When a suitable balance is not achieved, the cross fertilization by experimental and mathematical studies may be lost. This tends to inhibit the process of insight development. Telling the full story from detailed experiments or from sophisticated modeling of such a one-sided approach tends to be disappointing. Even an occasional infusion of a view from the opposite side can have a surprisingly clarifying effect.

The expansion of the number of scientific fields has complicated adherence to the structure proposed by Aristoteles and Descartes, as the introduction of mathematics may lag far behind, or may appear too strict to apply.

The term "model" is used in several other meanings, such as the animal model, and the fluid-mechanical and electrical models, the latter being generally superseded by the mathematical model with respect to flexibility. All of these models, including the animal model, have their own restrictions. It may be challenging to compare the virtues of experiments on humans, with their allure of studying reality, with those of mathematical models, supported by a computer. In the former, most, or all, of nature's complexities are included, many unknown to the experimenter. In the mathematical model, as a result of simplifications made by the investigator, many of nature's complexities are absent. However, the investigator knows in detail what aspects are included in the model.

In the idealistic discussion of the various levels above, experimental results are implicitly assumed to be trustworthy. This is not necessarily the case as has been demonstrated frequently by intense debates among experimentalists who reached opposite conclusions from supposedly identical studies in which boundary conditions or parameter values were different, though unknown to the investigators, but possibly influencing reproducibility negatively. The material in this book offers examples of a few such instances. Such difficulties complicate adherence to the philosophy laid down by Socrates, Aristoteles, and Descartes.

This textbook deals with the circulation of blood through the closed system consisting of the heart, the arteries, the microcirculation, and the veins which return the propelled blood to the heart. It consists of three parts. The first part concentrates on the long historic studies to understand how the system works starting with the Mesopotamian and Egyptian eras.

The second part focusing on the properties and behavior of the vital subsystems puts the subsystems together to form the closed circuit. In it, Harvey's concept of a simple blood pump, the heart, is expanded to a multitude of pumps with the aid of a new fluid-mechanical concept denoted impedance-defined flow, which responds to major criticism on Harvey's ideas. A list of questions appears at the end of each of these chapters tending to identity errors in older works while promoting novel perceptions. The third part deals with the normal and the abnormal closed loop.

1.3   Conclusions

The succession of high and low points in the chronological summation exposes long time interruptions between successive high points. Though this can be attributed, in part, to the small number of people really committed to the field and to the distractions offered by discussion of popular topics that eventually proved to offer little. One wonders, however whether nature resists the development of new ideas by allowing investigators to make the same mistakes over and over again.

Socrates made an impressive effort to create order in scientific endeavors, a topic that continues to attract the attention of philosophers and researchers.

1.4   Summary

Chapter 1 opens with synoptic reviews. The chronological approach offers an overview of the high and low points in the development of concepts about the cardiovascular system, starting with the Mesopotamian and Egyptian era and tracing through to current times. This is followed by an ideological approach which is primarily philosophical in nature and deals with performing experiments while interacting, at seven levels, with analytical considerations.

References

Beverwijck Joh van.: Wercken der Geneeskonste. Schipper, Amsterdam, 1672.

Caesalpinus A.: Quaestionum Medicarum, Liber secundus, p. 234, Venice, 1593

Duomarco J.L. and Rimini R.: Energy and hydraulic gradients along systemic veins. Am. J. Physiol. 178: 215–220, 1954.

Harvey G.: Exercitatio Anatomica, De Motu Cordis et Sanguinis in Animalibus, Frankford, 1628.

Kresch E., Granelli M. and Melbin J.: Wave Experiments in Collapsible Tubes. Ch. 26 in: Cardiovascular System Dynamics, J. Baan et al. (eds.), MIT Press, Cambridge, 1978.

Liebau G.: Möglichkeit der Förderung des Blutes im Herz- und Gefäszsystem ohne Herz- und Venenklappenfunktion. Verh. deutschen ges. Kreislauff., 22. Tagung. Seite 354–359, 1956.

Malpighi M.: De Pulmonibus Observatio Anatomica. Epistolae printed by G.B. Ferroni, Bologna, 1661.

Moreno A.H.: Dynamics of Pressure in the Central Veins. Ch. 28 in: Cardiovascular System Dynamics, J. Baan et al. (eds.), MIT Press, Cambridge, 1978.

Moser M., Huang J.W., Schwarz G.S., Kenner T., Noordergraaf A.: Impedance defined flow. Generalisation of William Harvey's concept of the circulation - 370 years later. Int. J. Cardiov. Med. and Science 1: 205–211, 1998.

Noordergraaf G.J., Ottesen J.T., Kortsmit W.J.P.M., Schilders W.H.A., Scheffer G.J. and Noordergraaf A.: The Donders model of the circulation in normo- and pathophysiology. Cardiov. Eng. 6: 53–72, 2006.

Pickering G.: Physician and scientist. Brit. Med. J. 2: 1615–1619, 1964.

Servetus M.: Christianismi Restitutio. Published anonymously in 1553.

Appendix

Questions

1.1 If model making ever reaches the level at which the properties of a biological object become indistinguishable from those of its model, such a model becomes superfluous. Is this conclusion valid?

1.2 Is there a difference between validation of a model and its application for interpretation of observed phenomena?

1.3 Provide an example in which experimentalists reached opposite conclusions from supposedly identical studies.

Answers

1.1 No, the variations among normals would still have to be explained, for one reason, proneness to acquisition of abnormalities, for another.

1.2 Yes, validations concern an argument about the level of accuracy of a model compared to the experimental data on which it is built. Interpretations deal with why the experimental data have the observed qualities.

1.3 Upstream wave propagations through central veins, due to atrial contraction, was observed by Duomarco and Rimini (1954) and by Kresch et al. (1978) to be restricted to just outside the heart, though Moreno (1978) observed that the pulse travels all the way to the feet (Chap. 3), offers just one example.

Chapter 2
The Cardiovascular System and Its Modes of Operation

ὅμοιον γὰρ τό τ᾽ ἐν τῇ δεξιᾷ κοιλίᾳ τῆς
χαρδίας αἷμα καὶ τὸ κατὰ πάσας τὰς
φλέβας ὅλῳ τῷ ξῴῳ. καθάπερ γε καὶ τὸ
κατὰ τὰς ἀρτηρίας ἁπάσας ὅμοιόν ἐστι
τῷ κατὰ τὴν ἀριστερὰν κοιλίαν.

— Galenus (ca. 131–ca. 201, first name unclear).
From Kühn, vol. v, p. 537, 1823.

Digest: The oldest known symbols for the heart are reproduced. K ng Hammurabi's code introduces legal liability, which makes Mesopotamian medicine literally superficial and stimulates development of mathematical and astronomical studies instead, unlike concurrent Egyptian developments in medicine. After a long interlude, Greek civilization takes over and Hippocrates assembles his Corpus, which assimilates old Egyptian knowledge, but does not offer a comprehensive concept for the operation of the cardiovascular system. Erasistratos subsequently develops such a concept, which is only known through Galenós after the modifications he introduces in it. The Galenic concept survives until Caesalpinus and Harvey replace it by proposing that the same blood circulates in a closed loop. The heart becomes the central and only pump to sustain this circulation, though a number of researchers become convinced that it is too weak to assume that responsibility alone and suggest that other mechanisms must be existent to provide support. Liebau shows empirically that steady flow can be induced in a closed circuit free of valves and ventures to suggest that cardiac valves may be superfluous. This eventually leads to the concept of impedance-defined flow and offers a quantitative mathematics based interpretation of flow phenomena not considered possible at the time.

The cardiovascular system continues to reveal additional flexibility.

A. Noordergraaf, *Blood in Motion*, DOI 10.1007/978-1-4614-0005-9_2,
© Springer Science+Business Media, LLC 2011

2.1 Antiquity

2.1.1 Introduction

In the civilizations that developed in major river valleys such as the fertile Euphrates-Tigris and Nile regions, curiosity and training of the human mind led to the formation of cultures. The dawn of Western science and thinking may be traced to these valleys. Some of what these people knew and thought may have roots in even older centers of civilization (Table 1.1).

In the centers of cultural activity in Mesopotamia and Egypt, awareness of the beating heart may well have preceded the development of script, because pictograms of the heart appear in the oldest known forms of writing. Figure 2.1 shows the development of the Sumerian pictogram (about 2500 BCE) to late Assyrian and Babylonian (around 500 BCE) cuneiform. Likewise, during the earliest Egyptian dynasties (2900–2700 BCE) hieroglyphs for the heart were employed; they display their own development. In both river valleys, the peripheral arterial pulse was palpated, indicating factual knowledge of at least a few of the locations where the pulse can be felt.

2.2 Mesopotamia

No evidence has been found of any Mesopotamian concept of the circulation: the heart beat and the appearance of the peripheral arterial pulse were not perceived in a cause and effect relation. Instead, the peripheral pulse was used to help identify the nature of the sickness and the likelihood of the patient's recovery. Information from the venous system was also utilized since the color, degree of filling, and the distribution of superficial veins were noted in pregnant women as well as on

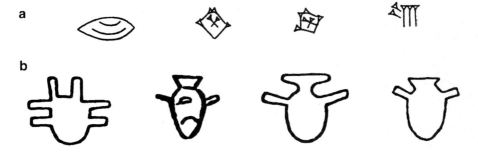

Fig. 2.1 (**a**) The heart from Sumerian pictogram (at *left*) to late Assyrian and Babylonian cuneiform. (**b**) Hieroglyphs for the heart during the first two Egyptian dynasties (2900–2700 BCE) (Reprinted by permission of the publisher from Majno. Copyright @ 1975 by the President and Fellows of Harvard College)

swollen feet. Instead of considering the heart as a pump, it was viewed as the seat of intelligence (Majno 1975).

In Nineveh, tablets have been found which claim that King Assurbanipal registered the three ways available to people who fall sick: healing with drugs, surgery with a brass knife, and prescriptions by sorcerers (Majno 1975). If treatments were recorded, virtually all were anonymous (Leichty 1988). Much of this dealt with superficial wounds, nothing with major surgery. As a consequence, it is not surprising that insight in the anatomy and operation of the cardiovascular system hardly evolved.

The reason for being circumspect about surgical intervention is found in the code assembled by the Babylonian King Hammurabi. This code contains 282 laws, chiseled in a large black stone of diorite around 1700 BCE. The separate laws are traditionally referred to as paragraphs.

Figure 2.2a shows a reproduction of a small part of the original text (Harper 1904), while Fig. 2.2b reproduces Harper's transliteration and translation of paragraph 215. This paragraph is just one example of where the law sets the physician's fee for performing a specific, successful, operation. Ten shekels have been estimated as covering the labor cost of building a substantial house (Majno 1975). The risk of performing surgery is defined in paragraph 218 (Fig. 2.2c). Hammurabi's code tends to mete out severe penalties for failure. There was no liability involved in the administration of drugs or with prescriptions ordered by a physician or a sorcerer. Taking no action at all was not considered malpractice. This may represent the first instance of an effort to distinguish between invasive and noninvasive treatment (Noordergraaf A 1998).

Mesopotamian medicine comes across as restrictive. Little progress appears to have been made over a period of many centuries after their civilization peaked during the period of around 1800–1600 BCE.

The same period of peak activity witnessed rapid progress in mathematics and activity in astronomy. In mathematics, a simple number theory, based on the sexagesimal system (base 60) was developed. The Pythagorian theorem became known. Squares and cubes could be calculated as well as the corresponding roots. The precursor of the logarithm became available. Consequently, the areas and volumes of simple shapes could be calculated. This facility was used to solve irrigation problems, subdivide land, figure the number of bricks required for a given construction project, etc. Under restricted conditions, linear and quadratic equations could be solved, e.g., the relative growth predicted for two flocks of sheep comprising different numbers, and having different birthrates (Neugebauer and Sachs 1945).

Hence, mathematical considerations entered the life sciences very early. Such was not the case with astronomy. Dating of tablets, much extended and refined over the last century, indicates that early Babylonian astronomy was restricted to crude observations of the stars, the planets, and the moon; this information was applied to calculate time (e.g., of the seasons) and in astrology. Although a few tablets appear to suggest a concept of a universe of eight spheres, one of the moon, it took about ten centuries before astronomy acquired a consistent mathematical theory (Neugebauer 1957).

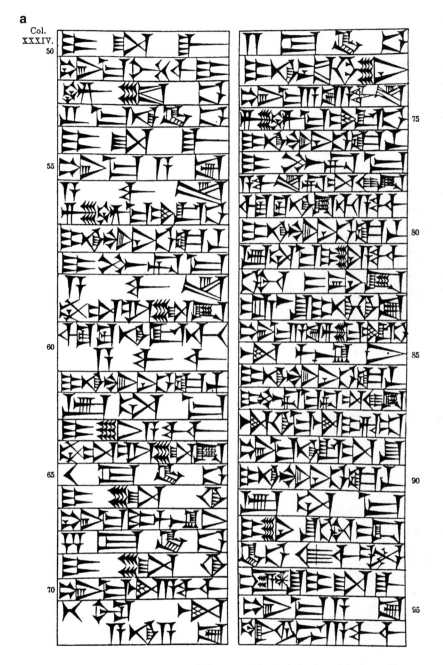

Fig. 2.2 (**a**) Lines 50–96 of column 34 of Hammurabi's Code in the original cuneiform script. This text reads from *left to right* and from *top to bottom*. (Reproduced by permission from Harper (1904).) (**b**) Harper's transliteration and translation of paragraph 215 (lines 55–66 in the *left hand column* of Fig. 2.2a). In the transliteration, *lower case* letters indicate Akkadian words, *upper case* Sumerian words. (Reproduced by permission from Harper (1904).) (**c**) Transliteration and translation of paragraph 218 (lines 74–83 in the *right hand column* of Fig. 2.2a) (Reproduced by permission from Harper (1904))

b   § 215—XXXIV, 54–65.

55 šum-ma A.ZU 56 a-wi-lam ᵇzi-im-ma-am kab-
tam 57 i-na GIR.NI siparrim 58 ᵕ-bu-uš-ma 59
a-wi-lam ᵇub-ta-al-li-iṭ 60 u lu na-ɡab-ti ᵇa-wi-lim
61 i-na GIR.NI siparrim 62 ip-te-mᴙ 63 i-in a-wi-
lim 64 ub-ta-al-li-iṭ 65 X šiḳil kaᴇpim 66 i-li-ḳi

§ 215.

❰ If a physician operate on a man for a severe wound (or make
a severe wound upon a man) with a bronze lancet and save the
man's life; or if he open an abscess (in the eye) of a man with
a bronze lancet and save that man's eye, he shall receive ten
shekels of silver (as his fee).

c   § 218.—XXXIV, 73–82.

74 šum-ma A.ZU a-wi-lam 75 ᴤi-im-ma-am kab-
tam 76 i-na GIR.NI siparrim 77 i-bu-uš-ma 78
a-wi-lam uš-ta-mi-it 79 u lu na-gab-ti a-wi-lim 80
i-na GIR.NI siparrim 81 ip-te-ma i-in a-wi-lim 82
uḫ-tab-bi-it 83 rittê-šu i-na-ki-su

§ 218.

❰ If a physician operate on a man for a severe wound with a
bronze lancet and cause the man's death; or open an abscess (in
the eye) of a man with a bronze lancet and destroy the man's
eye, they shall cut off his fingers.

Fig. 2.2 (continued)

2.3 Egypt

Unencumbered by a bureaucracy surrounding their legal system, and active in
embalming and mummification, the Egyptians of the Old Kingdom had
ample opportunity to observe the body's internal anatomy. In addition, treatment
of battle victims and victims suffering from accidents occurring during the
construction of the pyramids provided frequent opportunities for observation of
the living. The combination, as became clear from the study of Egyptian papyri
(Breasted 1930; Bardinet 1995), generated insights superior to that of their
Babylonian counterparts during roughly the same era.

The brain as an organ appeared for the first time. Neural control of movement was
assigned to the brain and the spinal cord, though their connection was not appreciated.
The heart was recognized as the center of distributed vessels (cf. Fig. 2.1). To evaluate

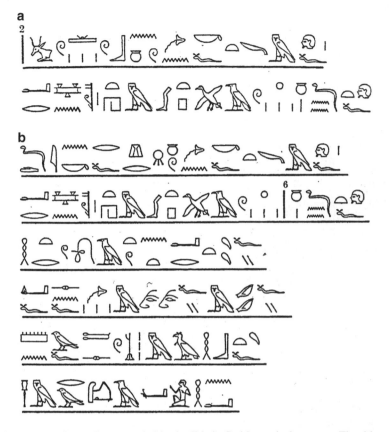

Fig. 2.3 (a) Part of case 7 as recorded in the Edwin Smith surgical papyrus: The title, and an announcement of the instructions. The translation reads: Instructions concerning a gaping wound in his head, penetrating to the bone, (and) perforating the sutures of his skull. (Adapted from Breasted (1930)). (b) The patient's examination, and the first diagnosis. The original text is written in hieratic, a cursive, much more difficult to read form of hieroglyphic writing. The figure displays the conversion into hieroglyphics. (By permission from Breasted (1930)). (c) Examination after the first treatment. Conclusion: treatment is not to be continued (Adapted from Breasted (1930))

a patient's condition, the action of the heart beat was observed peripherally including on the surface of the brain, expressed as "the heart speaks in all the limbs of the body" (Oppenheim 1962; Bardinet 1995), but blood vessels and nerves were not distinguished. Two main vessels were known in the thorax, one to the lungs and one to the heart. Blood was conceived to play an active role. Blood in the lobes of the lungs was thought to receive life spirit (i.e., air). The distinction between "vessels" filled with blood or with air remained vague.

Figure 2.3a–c reproduces part of Case 7 (of 48) as described in the Edwin Smith Surgical Papyrus and addresses evaluation, diagnosis, and treatment of a gaping head wound. In this particular example, the heart's activity enters into the physician's examination.

The Smith papyrus is dated to the seventeenth century BCE. It is written in the form of a document for instruction. This papyrus is considered to be a (an edited)

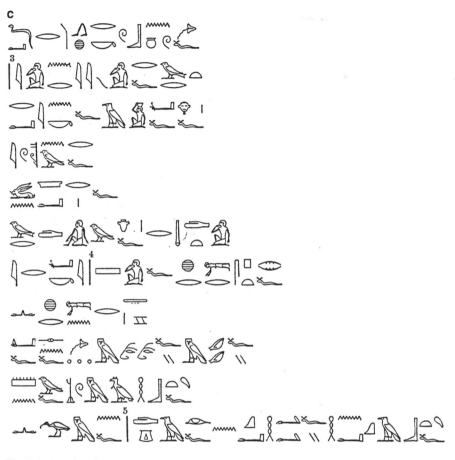

Fig. 2.3 (continued)

copy of a much older document, perhaps going back to Imhotep (thirtieth century BCE) the deified Egyptian physician. The Greek and Roman gods of medicine Asklepios and Aesculapius possibly identify with him.

No evidence has been found in support of Old Kingdom contributions to the development of mathematics. Its computational system remained a primitive additive procedure. In astronomy, the most significant contributions were the introduction of the "Egyptian year," consisting of 365 days (Neugebauer 1975) and the division of the day and the night in 12 h each (Wells 1996).

2.4 Mesopotamia and Egypt After 1600 BCE

After the cultures passed their respective zeniths in the development of mathematics and in biomedicine, in both areas around the same time (circa 1600 BCE), a long period prevailed of editing and copying tablets and papyri for linguistic adaptation and preservation of traditional knowledge and wisdom (Oppenheim 1962). It appears that the decline in conceiving new material was more pronounced in Mesopotamia than in Egypt. In Egypt, this activity was primarily in the hands of physician-priests (Breasted 1930).

2.4.1 Classic

The early stirrings of the Greek Empire may be placed around 600 BCE when Egypt lived under its 26th dynasty with Sais in the Nile delta as its capital. A new era of growth in medical science, in mathematics and in astronomy was about to manifest itself.

Hippocrates of Cos (460 – ca. 370 BCE) assembled his famous Corpus, a collection of works by a range of authors, which in Littré's Greek/French edition comprises nine volumes (Littré 1839–1861). This work has been hailed as a work of Greek genius, based on the assumption that it resulted from spontaneous generation. The assumption is likely based on the fact that the key to reading hieroglyphics had been lost. Akerblad (1802), Young (1818), and especially Champollion (1822) contributed to its decipherment by analyzing the Rosetta stone (Budge 1976). It has since become evident that Hippocrates as well as other Greek intellectuals lived and studied in Egypt (Breasted 1930). The resulting close contacts facilitated the transition from Egyptian to Greek medicine: Hippocrates' practice of treating a dislocated mandible is identical to the one described in the Edwin Smith papyrus of some 20 centuries earlier (Breasted 1930). Iversen (1939) found that the Hippocrates treatise on gynecology follows its Egyptian precursor dating back at least 10 centuries. There is a broad array of additional examples in medicine available, as well as in a variety of other fields, including mathematics and astronomy, of straightforward transfer of knowledge and ideas from Egypt and Mesopotamia to Greek culture (Pirenne 1963; Steuer and de Saunders 1959). Supporting evidence is furnished by Plato, a younger contemporary of Hippocrates, in the Timaeus dialogue (Hamilton and Cairns 1987).

Ptolemeus (ca. 130 BCE) devised his geocentric system for the movement of the planets, though the heliocentric system had been formulated earlier. Recent analysis of Ptolemeus' work has cast a shadow on his scientific integrity (Newton 1977). Astrology became deemphasized.

It should not come as a surprise that the Hippocratic Corpus contains a diversity of opinions. This diversity is so wide that the debate on what really belongs to it and what is of later vintage has not been closed.

A number of common views in the Corpus may nevertheless be recognized. These views are that the body is totally irrigated by vessels. There are two major vessels in the thorax, one of which provides mechanical suspension for the heart. Arteries furnish suspension for the lungs and this term is sometimes used for vessels that carry blood through the legs. There is a generic term (phlebs) for all sorts of conduits, some of which are fluid filled and provide cooling. Blood nourishes the whole body. The source of nourishment is in the abdomen. Air is supplied to the entire body via breathing and transportation through vessels (Oppenheim 1962).

The teaching, in the Corpus as well as in general practice, on the heart varies enormously. Some authors view it as a respiratory organ with the lungs containing a reservoir of blood. Others allow that all blood carrying vessels may ultimately be connected to the heart, a view reflected by Plato: "the fountain of the blood which races through all the limbs." Arteries and veins by the modern definition were not distinguished (Hamilton and Cairns 1987). The Hippocratic Corpus does not recognize a circulatory system (Duminil 1983).

Alexander the Great made both Mesopotamia and Egypt part of the Greek empire which must have intensified intellectual contact between Mesopotamia and Egypt on the one hand and Greece on the other. After his death in 323 BCE, one of his generals proclaimed himself King of Egypt, as Ptolemeus I, Soter. Ptolemeus I founded the Museum in Alexandria to which he and his son, Ptolemeus II attracted a number of the prominent scientists of their time. Here, Greek intellectuals could draw on the ancient wells of knowledge. Alexandria, founded by Alexander, as a Greek city located in Egypt was ideally located for that function.

In the Museum, anatomical investigations were pursued in a consistent fashion under patronage of the rulers, uninhibited by religious prejudice. Two of the physicians who benefitted from this opportunity by settling in Alexandria in the third century BCE were Herophylos of Chalcedon and Erasistratos of Chios.

Herophylos is credited with the introduction of the distinction between arteries and veins, primarily by observing that the wall of arteries is at least six times as thick as that of veins. He taught that the heart pumps blood into the arteries and measured the heart's rhythm from the arterial pulse, probably using the Egyptian waterclock (*klepsydra*) as his time base (Duminil 1983). He also found the connection between the brain and the spinal cord.

Erasistratos, who studied in Athens before settling in Alexandria, is viewed as having contributed the distinction between nerves and vessels (Breasted 1930). He is the first known scientist who made an ambitious effort to synthesize several thousand years of observation into a comprehensive system that included transport through arteries, veins, and nerves. This work became known to, and strongly influenced the thinking of, Galenós of Pergamon (131–ca. 200 CE) about four centuries later.

Galenós became physician to the gladiators in Pergamos, then moved to Rome where he was appointed physician to the Roman Emperor Marcus Aurelius. After Latinizing his name, Galenus, a prolific writer, left a multitude of inconsistent statements, as had his predecessors. Being familiar with the heart valves, he modified the synthesis, written by Erasistratos at a few significant points.

The essence of the Galenic system, as distilled by Siegel (1968, Fig. 2.4), but not necessarily fully subscribed to by others (e.g., Harris 1973), may be summarized as follows. Blood is formed in the liver where it assimilates natural, i.e., nutritive spirit. This blood is distributed by the veins to nourish all parts of the body. The heart, which he distinguished from voluntary muscle, draws a fraction of this venous blood into the right ventricle through its active dilation. Some of this

Fig. 2.4 Diagram of
Galenus' description of the
operation of the
cardiovascular system in the
adult. Vena cava superior
(*VCS*), vena cava inferior
(*VCI*), right atrium (*RA*), left
atrium (*LA*), pulmonary vein
(*PV*), pulmonary artery (*PA*),
aorta (*Ao.*), portal vein (*Po.
V.*) (By permission from
Siegel (1968))

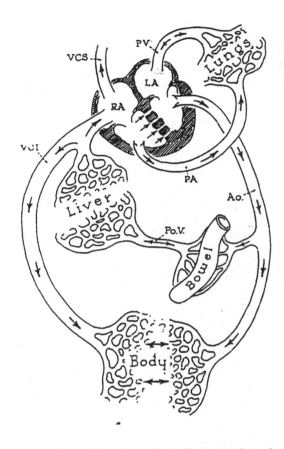

blood is forced into the pulmonary artery toward the lungs through contraction of
the thorax, and some penetrates into the left ventricle via pores in the interventricular septum.

The blood in the left ventricle acquires vital spirit with air from the lungs
transported via the pulmonary vein. Sooty residues (waste products) move through
the same vessel in the opposite direction, i.e., from the left chamber to the lung (two
arrows in the pulmonary vein in Fig. 2.4). Blood endowed with vital spirit is
distributed throughout the body by the arteries, it being drawn from the left
ventricle by the pulsatile properties of the arteries.

The brain, one recipient of vital spirit, transforms part of it into the third kind of
spirit, animal spirit. Animal spirit is distributed over the body through the hollow
nerves, thereby enabling the body's locomotion (Siegel 1968).

Although Galenus' exposition was found lucid, convincing, and flexible, it
became the subject of criticism during its long lifetime. The criticism tended to
focus on two aspects: two-way transport through the pulmonary vein, and the pores
in the interventricular septum.

Ibn an-Nafîs (1210–1288), an Arab physician and autodidactic commentator
on the Koran (Qur'an in modern transliteration, Abdel Haleem 2004), criticized

Avicenna. Galenus' translator into Arabic, by rejecting the presence of septal pores and by arguing that blood moves from the right ventricle via the pulmonary artery to the lungs, then via the pulmonary veins to the left ventricle (i.e., unidirectional transport). In the lungs the blood mixes with air and is purified (Meyerhof 1931). Ibn an-Nafîs' writing on the circulation remained unknown to the Western world until 1922.

In 1553, Michael Servetus, a physician and scholar with a broad interest who taught mathematics at the University of Paris, anonymously published a book that critically addressed two topics. In Chapter V he criticized the same two items in the teaching of Galenus as had, unbeknownst to him, Ibn an-Nafîs', while reaching similar conclusions. No one seems to have paid attention to this chapter for more than a century. In the other chapters, Servetus criticized the doctrine of the Holy Trinity, the first explicit formulation of which is attributed to Tertullianus, a contemporary of Galenus, though its root may lie in the monotheism of Egyptian origin (Kirsch 2004). These chapters received prompt attention. Servetus was accused and convicted of heresy and burned at the stake outside Geneva in the same year that his book appeared (Cournand 1964).

With the European Renaissance in full development, and the rise of interest in experimentally oriented investigations, e.g., how the mammalian body operates, more critical commentaries appeared in rapid succession. Vesalius, reportedly a fellow student of Servetus in a dissection course, expressed his doubts about the existence of the septal pores in 1543. Columbus described the pulmonary circulation once more in 1559. Canano as well as Vesalius announced their discovery of valves in certain veins in or around 1537, which Fabricius definitely established in his book published in 1603. Vesalius' book, published in 1543, is claimed to deviate from Galenus' teaching in more than 200 instances. Peripatetically, i.e., on theoretical grounds, Caesalpinus offered his view of the circulation as a closed circuit in 1593. These developments culminated in William Harvey's work which appeared in book form in 1628, well before Newton's Principia Mathematica (1687). All of this caused deep chagrin to Galenus' devotees.

In addition to the criticism on Galenus' teaching, there was also inspiration to modify and update his theory. Friedrich Hoffmann proposed a hydrodynamic machine: Three fluids circulate in the body, blood, lymph, and nerve spirit. They have to flow with appropriate relative magnitudes to prevent diseased states. Hoffmann's book appeared in 1695, i.e., more than 60 years after Harvey's.

2.4.2 Renaissance/Contemporary

Harvey's central consideration was that his experimental observations in conjunction with his calculations revealed that the heart ejects more blood in half an hour than the body contains. Hence, his conclusion that the same blood must continuously perform a circular motion. Since this contradicted basic tenets of the Galenic model, Harvey rejected formation of blood in the liver, cardiac suction of blood, the presence of septal pores and two-way transport through vessels. Instead, he made the heart the central blood moving organ, a consequence of the alternate contraction and relaxation of its muscular walls and the presence of valves.

Acknowledging the contributions made by Columbus and by a number of other predecessors, including his teacher Fabricius, but not by Caesalpinus, Harvey argued that blood moves through a wide open channel from the right ventricle through the pulmonary artery to the lungs, through pores in the lungs to the pulmonary veins on its way to the left auricle. Therefore, there was no need to assume invisible pores in the often thick septal wall. Then it moves from the left auricle to the left ventricle which forces blood into the aorta. Branches of the aorta provide channels to the peripheral organs, from where the blood reaches the veins through pores in the tissue. The veins return the blood to the right auricle, from where it moves to the right ventricle, thus completing a circular pathway. Harvey pointed out that the direction of opening of the valves in the heart fits this picture perfectly. This primarily descriptive interpretation will acquire causal features in Chap. 10.

The only part missing from the circular pathway was the connection between arteries and veins, the pores. He postulated their existence, thereby furnishing a heavy weapon to his many opponents, until Malpighi, born in the year Harvey's book was published, discovered the capillaries in 1661 by applying an improved version of the recently invented microscope. Together, Harvey and Malpighi established the paradigm closely resembling the currently accepted closed system (Fig. 2.5), the gross anatomy for the major vessels being essentially the same as that proposed by Galenus (Fig. 2.4).

Since normally there is fluid-mechanical separation, though incomplete functional separation, between the two sides, it is appropriate and has proven useful to regard the heart as two pumps, i.e., the left heart and the right heart, each consisting of two contractile chambers.

Considering the manner in which the vascular beds connect the pumps, the closed loop may be schematized as in Fig. 2.6. This diagram illustrates what Harvey had conceived when he spoke of the "circular" motion of blood (clockwise in Fig. 2.6). In Fig. 2.7, the heart itself and major circulatory structures are shown schematically in somewhat greater detail. The four cardiac chambers are indicated, as well as the four sets of leaflets that impose unidirectional flow. This gives rise to a condition of profound significance: average flow through the two pumps and the two vascular beds must be equal. It should be noted that the coronary circulation, i.e., the vascular bed of the heart itself, is a component of the systemic circulation.

The four valves lie in the plane which separates atria and ventricles (Fig. 2.8). Their names are, in the direction of flow, tricuspid (a) and pulmonary valve (b) (in the right heart), and mitral (c) (or bicuspid) and aortic valve (d) (in the left). The leaflets of the atrioventricular valves are supported by chordae tendineae and papillary muscle (Fig. 2.9).

The two vascular beds, designated "systemic" and "pulmonary" (Fig. 2.7), exhibit similarities in architectural pattern. In the direction of blood flow, the vessels first exhibit prolific branching such that the total cross-sectional area increases despite the fact that daughter vessels are narrower than mother vessels.

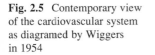

Fig. 2.5 Contemporary view
of the cardiovascular system
as diagramed by Wiggers
in 1954

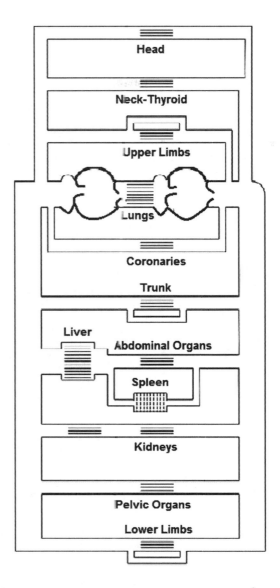

The number of capillaries, the smallest blood vessels. is estimated to exceed 10^9 in the human. Subsequently, beyond the capillary beds, the inverse occurs: small vessels combine to form larger vessels.

Galileo Galilei taught the heliocentric system of planetary motion, proposed (again) by Copernicus, at the University of Padua, Italy, at about the time that Harvey pursued his medical studies there. It has been suggested that Galilei's teaching of the circular movement of the planets around the sun, inspired Harvey to conceive his circular movement of blood.

Harvey reported that he had to overcome "evil criticism of his discovery of the circulation of the blood, such as a feeble infant as yet unworthy to have seen the

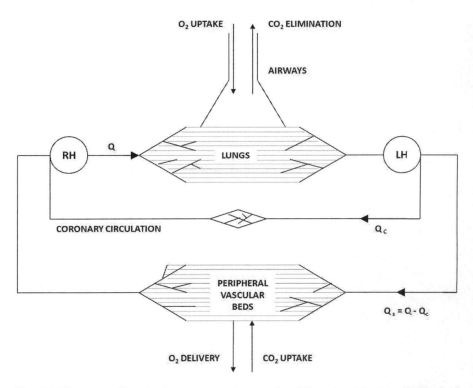

Fig. 2.6 The mammalian circulatory system forms a closed loop containing two sizable fluid pumps in series: the right heart (*RH*) and the left heart (*LH*). Q denotes total blood flow in the closed loop, Q_c flow through the coronary circulation, Q_s through the systemic peripheral beds

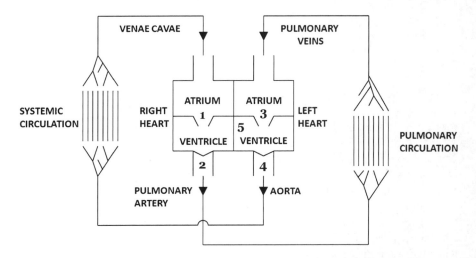

Fig. 2.7 Sketch of the circulatory system indicating the four chambers of the heart and its system of valves. In the normal case, complete fluid separation between the left and right sides of the heart is provided by the septum. *Arrows* indicate direction of positive flow, Q_s flow through the systemic vascular beds. (1) the tricuspid valve; (2) the pulmonary valve; (3) the mitral valve; (4) the aortic valve; (5) the septum separating the right and left heart

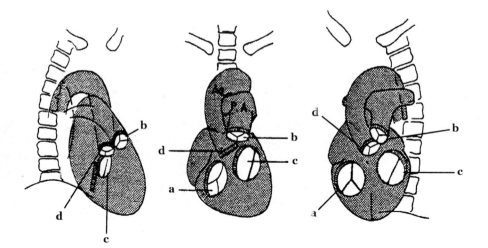

Fig. 2.8 Three views of the human heart with the valves drawn in. *Ao* denotes the aorta, *PA* the pulmonary artery, *a* the tricuspid valve, *b* the pulmonary valve, *c* the mitral valve, and *d* the aortic valve. The first heart sound coincides with the closure of the atrioventricular valves (*a* and *c*), the second with the closure of the pulmonary and aortic valves (*b* and *d*)

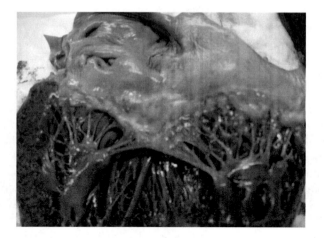

Fig. 2.9 Mitral valve apparatus of a human in the open position. The chordae run from the heads of the papillary muscle to the border as well as to other locations of the leaflets. The papillary muscles themselves are anchored in the ventricular wall

light" (Harvey 1952), but gradually, his concept of the circulation gained acceptance. His monumental work retained a number of features embodied in Galenus' theory such as the abdominal source of nutrition and gas exchange occurring in the lungs, while introducing new interpretations, such as one way transport of the same blood, abolition of the spirits, and rejection of suction. It opened the way for his followers to study the function of the respiratory system, the digestive system, etc. and the concurrent roles of the blood transport system in these and many other aspects of life-sustaining functions.

In his book, Harvey made the heart the exclusive pump that propels blood around the circle. Eventually, this idea was criticized, notably by Weber in 1834, who claimed that other (unspecified) forces help support the circulation; by Jones in 1852 who felt that "the supplementary force of rhythmical contraction of the veins [...] is called forth to promote the flow in the [bat's] wings, which [...] are, in a considerable degree, though not entirely, beyond the sphere of the heart's influence"; by Donders, who proposed in 1856 that the respiratory system assists the heart in its pumping effort by periodically increasing and decreasing the pressure around the thoracic vena cava; and by Ozanam in 1881 and 1886, who concluded from his experiments that pulsation of arteries modify flow to the heart in some of their companion veins.

Before the issue passed out of style temporarily, the proposal by Donders resulted in a vigorous debate between opponents and proponents flaring up inter-mittently for more than a century without achieving a satisfactory solution. The basic question remained why when blood, displaced by vessel compression and escaping in two directions, should not just return from those two directions in the exactly the same proportion, yielding no net forward flow (Chap. 8).

2.4.3 Contemporary/Future

The conversion of fluid flow, or electrical current, from unsteady to steady, or vice versa, has intrigued artists, physicians, physicists, and engineers of various specialties over time. A number of solutions have been found, of which placement of one or more valves, such as in the heart, is a relevant example for the generation of steady flow by a pulsatile source, as argued effectively by Harvey.

Commencing in 1954, and perpetuating his work for decades, the physician Liebau constructed hydraulic models, free of valves, to demonstrate the occurrence of steady flow in response to periodic compression at a particular site. Reconstruc-tion of one of his models confirmed Liebau's observations (Moser et al. 1998). His motivation was to show that similar compression of veins, free of valves, can aid blood flow around the cardiovascular circuit, even in the absence of cardiac valves (Liebau 1956). Despite support by contemporary fluid-dynamicists, he was unable to offer an interpretation why, and under what conditions, steady flow could be generated in such fluid-dynamic models. The issue continues to fascinate fluid-dynamicists, e.g., Manopoulos et al. (2006).

Taking a different approach, Moser et al. (1998) identified the mechanism as well as a set of conditions that must be satisfied for steady flow to occur. They also found that periodic compression is not the sole way to generate steady flow: periodic linear or rotational acceleration and deceleration of blood containing vessels may achieve the same purpose. Since one of the conditions is the presence of different impedances, steady flow so generated was called impedance-defined flow. Inasmuch as impedances are often frequency dependent, the magnitude of the steady flow achieved may depend on the frequency with which compression, or

acceleration, is applied. As a further consequence, the direction of the steady flow
may be in opposite directions for different frequencies.

The presence of a valve, if properly located, may increase the magnitude of the
steady flow or it may facilitate the provision of special features, such as the creation
of a high pressure reservoir as in the aorta and the pulmonary artery. Valves that
open and close periodically may make an impedance of time-varying interest,
thereby possibly introducing strong nonlinearities. As the mechanism behind
impedance-defined flow allows for the presence of valves, the heart's pumping,
as advocated by Harvey, is a special case of impedance-defined flow.

Figure 2.10 shows a closed loop in fluid-mechanical symbols as well as its
electrical equivalent utilizing electrical symbols to illustrate some of the key features
of impedance-defined flow. The circuits are reduced to their bare bones to prevent
distraction from the essential properties. Focusing on Fig. 2.10a, the circuit consists
of two elastic reservoirs, marked C_0 and C_1, connected by two rigid tubes, one of
which is narrow, the other wide. The system is fluid filled. Reservoir C_0 is compressed by an external force, then allowed to relax, in a periodic fashion. The narrow
tube is assumed to have a sufficiently small radius for the viscous effects to
dominate inertial effects of the fluid. In the wide tube, the conditions are assumed
to be reversed. These conditions appear more clearly in Fig. 2.10b. The cycle of
events may be separated into two parts: (a) the compression phase displaces fluid
from C_0 to C_1 via the narrow channel, or the wide channel, or both, and (b) during the
relaxation phase, a fraction of the fluid stored in C_1 will return to C_0, the fraction
depending on the duration of the time interval to the next compression.

Pressures $p_0(t)$, $p_1(t)$, flows $Q_0(t)$, $Q_1(t)$, $Q_2(t)$ and volumes $V_0(t)$, $V_1(t)$ prevailing
in the circuit may be computed from two sets of four simultaneous equations, one
set for phase (a), another for phase (b). They read:

Phase a

$$Q_0(t) = Q_1(t) + Q_2(t) \tag{2.1}$$

$$p_0(t) - p_1(t) = R_1 Q_1(t) \tag{2.2}$$

$$p_0(t) - p_1(t) = L_2 dQ_2/dt \tag{2.3}$$

$$Q_1(t) + Q_2(t) = C_1 dp_1/dt \tag{2.4}$$

Phase b

$$Q_1(t) + Q_2(t) = -C_0 dp_0/dt \tag{2.5}$$

$$p_0(t) - p_1(t) = R_1 Q_1(t) \tag{2.6}$$

$$p_0(t) - p_1(t) = L_2 dQ_2/dt \tag{2.7}$$

$$Q_1(t) + Q_2(t) = C_1 dp_1/dt \tag{2.8}$$

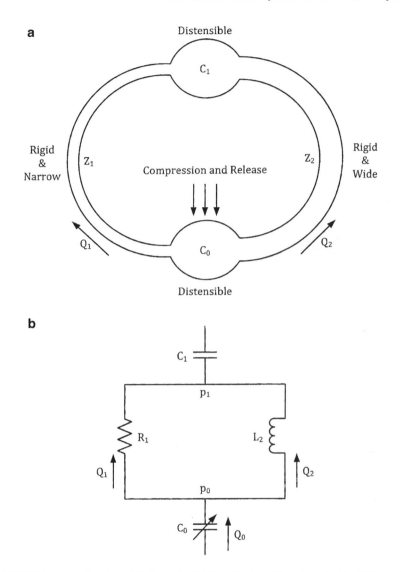

Fig. 2.10 This instructional model, drawn in fluid mechanical (**a**) and in electrical (**b**) symbols, consists of two compliant reservoirs C_0 and C_1, connected by two rigid pathways, one narrow and one wide. The flow impedance Z_1 of the *narrow* channel is R_1 (frequency independent), of the *wide* channel $j\omega L_2$ (frequency dependent) $j = \sqrt{-1}$ In (**a**) the single *arrows* mark Q_1 and Q_2 and define the positive direction of the flows Q_1 and Q_2; in (**b**) the *vertical arrows* define the positive direction of Q_0, Q_1, and Q_2

In these equations, R_1 denotes the viscous effect in the narrow channel, L_2 the inertial effect in the wide one. To keep the equations transparent, nonlinear elastic phenomena in reservoir C_0 were bypassed by setting $p_0 = 0$ at the onset of the relaxation phase, thereby introducing a simple discontinuity instead.

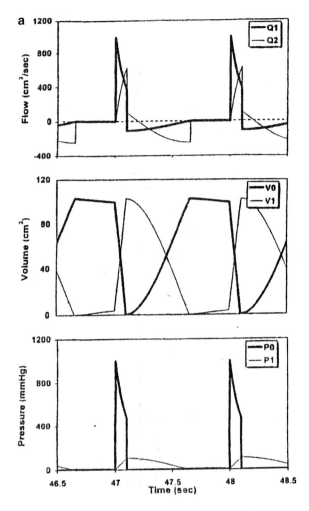

Fig. 2.11 (a) Pressures, flows, and reservoir volumes, V, as functions of time, calculated with the aid of Eqs. 2.1–2.8 for the valveless closed loop depicted in Fig. 2.10. (b) Same after placement of a valve that restricts flow Q_1 to nonnegative values. (c) Computed values of steady flow around the closed circuit of Fig. 2.10 for three cases: valveless (*dots*), with a valve that prevents Q_1 from going negative (*squares*), with a valve that keeps Q_2 from going negative (*triangles*). Positive values signify clockwise, negative values counterclockwise steady flow. Efficiency is defined as percentage of maximum possible flow. All graphs are displayed as a function of compression frequency (Adapted from Moser et al. (1998))

Figure 2.11a–c display results selected from the solution of Eqs. 2.1–2.8. In Fig. 2.11a the circuit is free of valves. During the compression phase, flow is seen to prefer the narrow channel, during the relaxation phase the wide channel. In Fig. 2.11b the solution is shown when a valve restricts Q_1 from going negative. Steady flow around the circuit,

$$\bar{Q}_1 = \bar{Q}_2 = \frac{1}{T} \int_0^T Q_1(t)\,\mathrm{d}t \qquad (2.9)$$

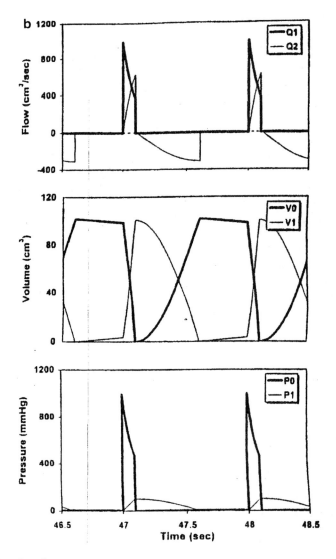

Fig. 2.11 (continued)

(*T* denotes the duration of one cycle) is reproduced in Fig. 2.11c for three conditions.

Figure 2.12 shows similar results for a more complex analysis of the same valveless condition as above in which introduction of the discontinuity was avoided by taking into account the compliant properties of the collapsed segment, using material presented in Chap. 3, Fig. 3.3, which impacts on Eqs. 2.5–2.8. Inspection disclosed that the magnitude of steady flow around the circuit is sensitive to the speed with which release is effected (Question 2.5; Patel 2004).

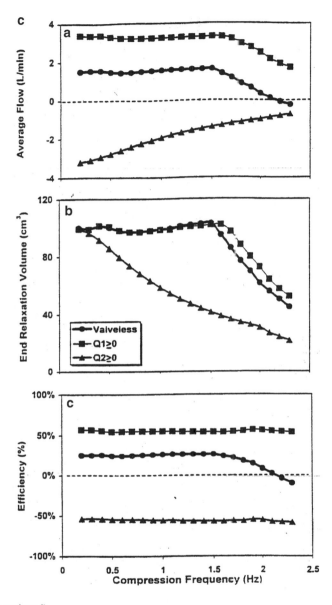

Fig. 2.11 (continued)

The key to understanding the origin of steady flow around the circuit is the presence of different impedances. When C_0 is compressed, outflow will be larger along the path with the smaller impedance, in casu the resistive pathway, which is frequency independent. During the relaxed phase the inductive path offers the smaller impedance, since its expression, $j\omega L_2$, contains $\omega = 2\pi f$, with f = frequency

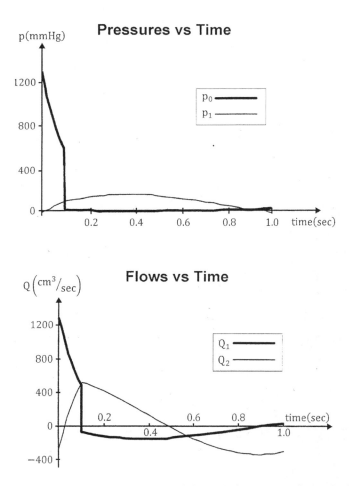

Fig. 2.12 Steady state results for pressures and flows during compression and release after elimination of the discontinuity in Fig. 2.10. Graphs computed by Patel (2004). See text for explanations for p_0, p_1, Q_1 and Q_2

of the components of the signal. As a consequence, rapid compression tends to generate more steady flow around the circuit than slow compression.

It is now possible to formulate general conditions that allow the generation of steady flow. These are: (1) Energy must be furnished to the system to move the fluid. $Q_1 = 0$ without compression of the passive vessel; (2) the circuit must contain a compliant reservoir to allow for storage of the displaced fluid; (3) The impedance of the two pathways must be different and at least one must be a complex number. If both are complex numbers, their phases must be different (Moser et al. 1998). Bovard et al. (2004) carried out flow measurements as a function of compression site in a fluid filled two tube model similar to one of Liebau's originals.

Chapter 8 addresses severe limits of applicability of this valveless closed loop to the mammalian cardiovascular system, such as its inability to generate or sustain high pressure arterial reservoirs (Sect. 5.1).

Harvey, in his book, advances three prime considerations in support of his view that the same blood performs a circular movement. The third of these deals with return, to the heart, of blood in the veins. In his argument, Harvey relies heavily on the abundance of valves in superficial arm veins. He apparently failed to observe that skeletal muscle contraction and relaxation promotes blood flow in the direction of the heart. Had he made this observation, he might have felt compelled to modify his statement that the heart alone is responsible for the circulation of blood; in everyday life, it clearly is not.

One is then forced to think in more general terms about what makes blood move. Blood can move in response to any one, or a combination of the following causes:

- A pressure gradient is created along a vessel, or along the vasculature, e.g., by the heart.
- Contraction and relaxation of a blood vessel, or a cardiac chamber, in response to pressure augmentation, or neural or metabolic stimuli.
- Compression, or expansion, and release of a blood vessel, or vessels, e.g., by the respiration, or by skeletal muscle contraction and relaxation.
- Acceleration and deceleration of part, or the whole, of the cardiovascular system, e.g., during walking (active) or shaking (passive).
- Alteration of the gravitational field with respect to the body, e.g., by changing body orientation (change in vector direction), or in space (change in vector magnitude).
- Conversion of steady flow to pulsatile flow, which affects load impedance.
- Compression, or expansion, and release by artificial means, e.g., by an intra-aortic balloon pump, or a foot pump.

In addition, for distribution purposes, the resistive and inertial effects of blood itself can be manipulated by control mechanisms. The applicability and utilization of these causes will form one of the major foci of this book, operating in the interest of many functions, including

- Transporting oxygen from the environment and delivering it to the body tissues
- Collecting carbon dioxide from the tissues and eliminating it from the body
- Performing many other transport functions, such as of metabolites, hormones, etc.
- Allowing for the control of many of these features

2.5 Conclusions

Despite ancient Mesopotamian and Egyptian scientific, factual, knowledge, even as late as Hippocrates' Corpus, the need to see the circulation as a system as opposed to loosely connected pieces, did not reach cognition. This contrasts with the development of a system for the protection of patients from inappropriate invasive care and the collection of factual anatomical information.

Retrospectively, one recognizes the pervasive tendency to collect and connect facts, adding convenient truths such as the "intraventricular pores" and "two way motion in vessels" to facilitate the chosen explanation. Further discussion then no longer focused on the base idea, but gravitated toward discussions of the distracting factors.

2.6   Summary

Covering history from antiquity, this chapter characterizes the major difference between Mesopotamian and Egyptian interest and activity, and identifies the birth of the concept that mammals possess a cardiovascular system, endowed with three spirits, during the classic Greek period. Since Egyptian documents were anonymous, with rare exceptions and their early translations into Greek were signed, the Western world interpreted them as Greek originals. It took a long time for this to be corrected, in particular, as Egyptian (hieroglyphic) script could not be read any longer until the Rosetta stone had become available (1799). Mesopotamian law introduced medical liability. Andreas Caesalpinus and William Harvey upgraded the classic ideas to the Renaissance level.

References

Abdel Haleem M.A.S.: The Qur'an. A new translation. Oxford Univ. Press, New York NY, 2004.

Bardinet T.: Les Papyrus Médicaux de l'Égypte Pharaonique. Fayard, Paris, 1995.

Bovard M.S., Connell W.R., Moore S.E., Palladino J.L.: Quantifying impedance defined flow. Proc. 30th IEEE Northeast Bioeng. Conf., Springfield MA, pp. 192–193, 2004.

Breasted J.H.: The Edwin Smith Surgical Papyrus. Univ. of Chicago Press, 1930.

Budge E.A.W.: Egyptian Language. Dover, New York NY, 1976.

Cournand A.: Air and Blood. Ch. 1 in: Circulation of the Blood. Men and Ideas. A.P. Fishman and D.W. Richards (eds.). Oxford Univ. Press, New York, 1964.

Donders F.C.: Physiologie des Menschen, Hirzel, Leipzig, 1856.

Duminil M.P.: Le Sang, Les Vaisseaux, Le Coeur dans la Collection Hippocratique. Paris: Societé d'Edition "Les Belles Lettres", 1983.

Hamilton E., Cairns H. (eds.): Plato: The Collected Dialogues. Bollinger Series 71, Princeton University Press, Princeton, 1987.

Harper R.F.: The Code of Hammurabi, King of Babylon About 2250 BCE. University of Chicago Press, Chicago, 1904. (Note: Later dating places Hammurabi's ascension to the throne at 1792 BCE.)

Harris C.R.S.: The Heart and the Vascular System in Ancient Greek Medicine. Clarendon Press, Oxford, 1973.

Harvey W.: On the Motion of the Heart and Blood in Animals (Translated by R. Willis). On the Circulation of the Blood. On the Generation of Animals. Encycl. Britannica, pp. 263–496, 1952.

Hoffmann F.J.: Fundamentae Medicinae ex Principiis Naturae Mechanicis in Usum Philiatrorum Succinte Propositu, Halle, 1695.

Iversen E.: Papyrus Carlsberg VIII with some remarks on the Egyptian origin of some particular birth prognons. Ac. Copenhagen 26: 5, 1939.

Kirsch J.: God against the gods. Penguin Group, New York NY, 2004.

Leichty E.: Guaranteed to cure. A Scientific Humanist, University of Pennsylvania Museum, Philadelphia 1988:9. Studies in memory of Abraham Sachs. Occasional publications of the Samuel Noah Kramer Fund.

Liebau G.: Möglichkeit der Förderung des Blutes im Herz- und Gefäszsystem ohne Herz- und Venenklappenfunktion. Verh. deutschen ges. Kreislauff., 22. Tagung. Seite 354–359, 1956.

Littré É. (ed.): Oeuvres Complètes d'Hippocrate. Ballière, Paris (9 volumes), 1839–1861.

Majno G.: The Healing Hand: Man and Wound in the Ancient World. Harvard University Press, Cambridge, 1975.

Malpighi M.: De Pulmonibus Observatio Anatomica. Epistolae printed by G.B. Ferroni, Bologna, 1661.

Manopoulos C.G., Mathioulakis D.S. and Tsangaris S.G.: One-dimensional model of valveless pumping in a closed loop and a numerical solution. Physics of Fluids 18: 017106, 2006.

Meyerhof M.: Der Lungenkreislauf nach el-Koraschi. Commentary on El-Tatawi's dissertation (Freiburg i. B., 1924). Mitteilungen zur Geschichte der Medizin und der Naturwissenschaften 30: 55–56, 1931.

Moser M., Huang J.W., Schwarz G.S., Kenner T., Noordergraaf A.: Impedance defined flow. Generalisation of William Harvey's concept of the circulation - 370 years later. Int. J. Cardiov. Med. and Science 1: 205–211, 1998.

Neugebauer O.: The Exact Sciences in Antiquity. Brown University Press, 1957

Neugebauer O.: A History of Mathematical Astronomy, Part ii. Book iii, Springer Verlag, Berlin, 1975

Neugebauer O. and Sachs A. (eds.): Mathematical Cuneiform Texts. Am. Oriental Soc. and Am. Schools of Oriental Res., 1945.

Newton R.R.: The Crime of Claudius Ptolemy. Johns Hopkins University Press, Baltimore, 1977.

Noordergraaf A.: Cardiovascular Concepts in Antiquity. Ch. 1 in: Analysis and Assessment of Cardiovascular Function. G.M. Drzewiecki and J.K-J. Li (eds.), Springer, New York NY, 1998.

Oppenheim A.L.: On the observation of the pulse in Mesopotamian medicine. Orientalia 3:27–33, 1962.

Ozanam Ch.: De la circulation veineuse par influence. Comptes Rendus hebd. des Séances de l'Académie des Sciences 93: 92–94, 1881.

Ozanam Ch.: La Circulation et le Pouls. Quatrième partie, Chapitre IV, J.B. Ballière et Fils, Paris, 1886.

Patel A.S.: Elimination of the discontinuity in the first interpretation of valveless flow. Project report in a course taught by A. Noordergraaf, Univ. of Pennsylvania, 2004.

Pirenne J.: Histoire de la Civilization de l'Egypte Ancienne. À la Baconnière, Neuchatel; Albin Michel, Paris, 1963.

Servetus M.: Christianismi Restitutio. Published anonymously in 1553.

Siegel R.E.: Galen's System of Physiology and Medicine. An Analysis of his Doctrines and Observations on Bloodflow, Respiration, Tumors and Internal Diseases. Karger, Basel, 1968.

Steuer R.O., Saunders J.B. de C.M.: Ancient Egyptian and Cnidian Medicine. University of California Press, Berkeley, 1959.

Weber E.H.: De Pulsu, Resorptione, Auditu et Tactu. Annotationes Anatomicae et Physiologicae, Lipsiae, 1834.

Wells R.A.: Astronomy in Egypt. In: Astronomy before the Telescope, C. Walker (ed.), British Museum Press, London, 1996.

Appendix

Questions

2.1 Compare Galenic to Harveyan concepts of the circulation. (List at least five concepts on which their theories differ.)

2.2 Which of Harvey's criticisms of Galenus' theory must be deemed to be incorrect?

2.3 Since Harvey rejected the existence of pores between the ventricles, could he sensibly be criticized for peripheral pores in his own theory?

2.4 Integration of Eq. 2.2

$$\int_0^T p_0 dt - \int_0^T p_1 dt = R_1 \int_0^T Q_1 dt = R_1 T \left[\frac{1}{T} \int_0^T Q_1 dt \right] = R_1 T \overline{Q}_1 = 0,$$

because the two integrals on the far left are each over one period and therefore vanish. With Eq. 2.9, $Q_2 = 0$, hence there is no steady flow around the circuit. This result does not square with the direct solution of Eqs. 2.1–2.8 and the resulting curve marked with dots in the top panel of Fig. 1.11c. Identify the cause of the contradiction.

2.5 Average flow in a closed loop, free of valves as in Fig. 2.10b, depends on the speed of release at the end of the compression phase. The faster the release, the smaller the steady flow around the loop. Explain this result.

2.6 Can shaking the two elastic tube model in its own plane along a straight line generate flow around the loop, if (a) the line is parallel to the line through the points where the elastic tubes connect, (b) if the line is perpendicular to the line under (a)?

2.7 In a normal cardiovascular loop with a beating heart, are all four cardiac valves ever open at the same instant of time?

Answers

2.1 Galenus: New blood is manufactured continuously in the liver; Harvey: The same blood flows around the closed system continuously.
Galenus: Blood contains spirits; Harvey: It does not.
Galenus: Blood flows from the liver to the organs through the veins; Harvey: Blood flows from the organs to the heart through the veins.
Galenus: Blood flows from the right ventricle to the left ventricle through the interventricular pores; Harvey: Those pores do not exist.
Galenus: The pulmonary vein carries two-way flow; Harvey: One-way, toward the left atrium.
Galenus: There is blood flow through the hollow nerves carrying animal spirit; Harvey: There is no such flow.
Galenus: The heart sucks in blood; Harvey: The heart does not exert suction.
Galenus: Contraction of the thorax forces blood into the pulmonary artery; Harvey: Right ventricular contraction is responsible for this.
Galenus: Blood is drawn from the left ventricle by the pulsatile properties of the arteries; Harvey: The other way around. The contractile properties of the heart make the arteries pulsate.

2.2 Actually, the heart does exert suction (Sect. 4.3 Chap. 8).

2.3 Pores provided the continuous pathway between the smallest arteries to the smallest veins in Harvey's thinking. The capillaries had not been seen yet (Sect. 5.1).

2.4 The function $p_0(t)$ contains a discontinuity that disallows integration.

2.5 Faster release, like faster compression promotes flow preference for the resistive channel, but in opposite directions.

2.6 (a) yes; (b) no.

2.7 No, not in the normal system.

Part II
Circulatory Sub-Systems

Chapter 3
The Venous Systems

Vis a fronte (Aristoteles, 384–322, B.C.E.)
Vis a tergo (Harvey, 1578–1657, C.E.)
Respiration (Valsalva, 1666–1723, C.E.)

Digest: The venous systems as the largest reservoirs of blood. Vis a fronte, vis a tergo, and Donders' claim that the respiratory system aids the return of blood to the central veins. Throat formation in steady flow. Picturesque terminology for flow in collapsible vessels explained via consideration of a three terminal port arrangement. Atrial and ventricular suction. The pulmonary venous bed equipped with two pulsatile sources, one at each end. Note: The nonlinear pressure-flow relations in collapsible vessels appear in Chap. 5 following the linear treatment of stiffer arteries. *The venous reservoirs facilitate moderate and strenuous exercise. Volume becomes the major attention getter.*

3.1 Prelude

In this book, it will be argued that the mammalian cardiovascular system is equipped with a large number of smaller pumps in addition to the cardiac pump. Furthermore, it will be emphasized that a variety of control mechanisms are able to modify the values of parameters defining the properties of these pumps. Such effects tend to become more pronounced during exercise.

A number of these phenomena sporadically appear in the literature, though without being conceptually organized or furnished with analytical underpinning. The introduction of impedance-defined flow will fill most of such gaps. This concept will, to some extent, also shift the emphasis away from discussions of blood pressure as a variable, to blood flow as the key variable in a transport system.

A. Noordergraaf, *Blood in Motion*, DOI 10.1007/978-1-4614-0005-9_3,
© Springer Science+Business Media, LLC 2011

In recognition of this, the organization of this book will deviate somewhat from the traditional pattern by starting out from the largest blood reservoir in the cardiovascular system, then follow the path of Harvey's circle.

3.2   Past Observations and Discussions

There is a general agreement that the systemic venous vessels contain somewhat more than 50% of the total blood volume in the mammal. This volume is maintained at low pressure. The veins, thin-walled soft vessels, thus serve as large low pressure reservoirs. Harvey called the venous vessels a "magazine" of blood (Harvey 1952).

Despite their thinness, most venous walls contain smooth muscle, which allows passive dilation when relaxed and contraction when stimulated. Morris and Swain (1978), e.g., reported a tenfold ratio between the diameters of a saphenous vein for the same blood pressure under conditions of maximal relaxation and maximal contraction of its smooth muscle, an early mammalian example of the generation of impedance-defined flow (Chaps. 2 and 8). As a consequence, the venous systems should be able to mobilize a large volume of blood for a restricted interval of time.

The central vessels, the venae cavae superior and inferior, feature at their junction a permanently wide open connection with the right atrium. Hence, central venous and right atrial pressures are close. Therefore, the path taken by the exit flow is clearly defined, while the blood enters the reservoir from the peripheral veins. The mechanism(s) that make(s) the blood enter the veins have(s) been debated for a long period, however.

There are several candidates for descriptions of the mechanism causing blood to flow, the oldest being attributed to Aristoteles. The valvular plane in the heart was observed to descend during ventricular ejection, thereby causing suction on the venous blood (vis a fronte). Harvey, who did not believe in suction, thought the driving pressure was the remnant of aortic pressure, providing a vis a tergo large enough to cause adequate filling flow despite the high peripheral resistance in between. Donders (1856) introduced the idea of the respiratory pump, which, he wrote, draws blood toward the thoracic cavity. Abel and Waldhausen (1969) as well as others, elaborated on this theme. Brecher (1956) summarized additional theories, now mostly defunct. The three theories listed here are considered operational, though at different levels. The respiratory pump will reappear in Sect. 11.2, as a significant contributor to venous return (filling).

Researchers have been sufficiently impressed by the venous systems to attribute to them a crucial role in the circulatory circuit by the oft repeated statement that they possess the unique property of delivering to the atria just as much blood as the ventricles pump into the arteries during the same time interval. This statement should be evaluated beyond its literal interpretation. Since all parts of the cardiovascular loop are capable of storing variable volumes of blood just like the venous systems, average inflow and outflow over one cycle do not have to be equal. But in conjunction with the

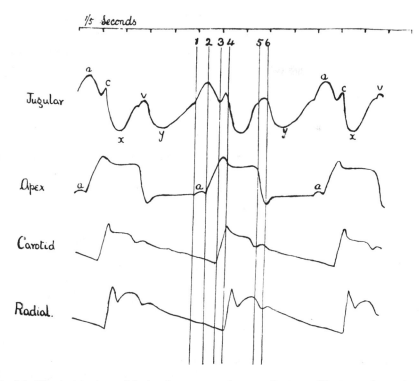

Fig. 3.1 Classical tracings of the jugular venous pulse, apex beat, carotid artery pulse, and radial artery pulse. The vertical lines indicate: (**1**) the onset of atrial systole, (**2**) the onset of ventricular systole, (**3**) the arrival of the pulse in the carotid artery, (**4**) same in the radial artery, (**5**) closure of the aortic and pulmonary valves, (**6**) opening of the atrioventricular valves. (From Mackenzie (1908)) For a description of the central venous waves see text

observation of modulation in aortic pressure at the respiratory frequency by Brecher (1956), as well as other considerations (vide infra), a number of investigators became convinced that the venous system exercises a powerful governing influence on average blood flow around the circuit. In essence, this is an alternative formulation of the first part of Starling's observations (Sect. 4.3) applied to respiratory-induced alteration of venous return. Guyton and Jones (1973) pointed out that a change in central venous pressure of a few millimeters of Hg may half or double cardiac output under some circumstances, as observed by Patterson and Starling (1914; Fig. 9.1).

The external jugular vein is so close to the right atrium and often sufficiently superficial that pulsations in it are easily observable in the reclining human subject. Largely due to the meticulous work of Sir James Mackenzie in the early part of the twentieth century, the time relationships between central venous pulsations on the one hand and cardiac phases and arterial pulsations on the other could be established (Fig. 3.1). The central venous pulse reflects atrial contraction (the a wave), followed by the X valley ascribed to atrial relaxation and the descent

Fig. 3.2 Abnormal jugular venous pulse, recorded on a patient suffering from congestive heart failure and tricuspid regurgitation. JVP stands for Jugular Venous Pressure and PCG stands for Phono Cardiogram. Line 1 and 2 indicate the time relation between the electrocardiogram and JVP. (Adapted from Massumi et al. (1974))

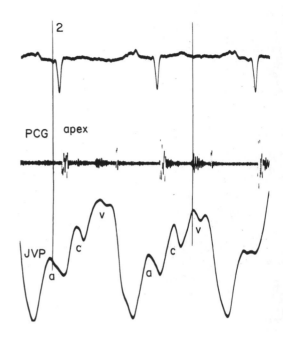

of the valvular plane during ventricular ejection. The downslope is interrupted by the c wave, ascribed either to crosstalk from the carotid artery (hence the c), and/or to bulging of the tricuspid valve when ventricular systole begins (Constant 1974). The v wave occurs when ventricular relaxation sets in, while the rapid ventricular filling phase causes the Y valley. In a wide variety of clinical situations, the jugular venous pulse exhibits drastic changes in shape (Fig. 3.2).

Furthermore, by observing the height to which the jugular vein refills when it is proximally occluded and when measured with respect to the level of the heart, a crude measure of the cardiac filling pressure is obtained in a noninvasive fashion. The jugular vein thus came to serve as a built-in manometer on the heart and was used extensively to diagnose abnormalities in cardiac performance (Lewis 1930; Borst and Molhuysen 1952; Massumi et al. 1974). Owing to the uncertainties involved – the debate about whether the venous pulse represents a pressure or a volume recording continued for decades – the electrocardiogram (Einthoven 1895) has largely replaced the venous pulse in diagnosis. Originally, this more conveniently obtained record was erroneously taken to contain the same mechanical information. Invasive measurements rely on an indwelling catheter tip micropressure transducer.

Although in earlier days of cardiovascular research a great deal much more accurate knowledge existed about the veins than about the arteries and the heart, the accumulation of new experimental data has failed to match the pace developed in other areas. Brecher (1969) blamed this on the invention of the mercury manometer by Poiseuille (1799–1869), which obviated the need for climbing benches to read the value of arterial pressure in the style of Hales (1733), but also made the accurate reading of such low pressures as commonly occur in veins more difficult. In addition, the evasiveness of veins to analytical treatment of the relationship between pressure and flow, and the need for high fidelity instrumentation to measure pressure and flow were, for a time, detracting from the venous system as a choice topic of study, despite the crucial role attributed to the venous system, above.

In many tissue locations, an artery and a vein are arranged as companions, carrying blood flow in opposite directions, the pair not infrequently being wrapped in a sheath. Of the companion artery and vein, the latter usually has the larger diameter and is the more distensible member, which provided the ancient characteristic to distinguish between arteries and veins (Chaps. 2 and 8).

These observations should be contrasted with several expressions of concern assembled in Sect. 3.3, the common denominator of which was that the heart is not sufficiently powerful to drive venous return.

3.3 Collapse Phenomena

3.3.1 Uniform Collapse

Choosing an unbranched, straight, uniform vessel of infinite length, Kresch and Noordergraaf (1972) studied the size and shape of such a vessel's cross section as a function of transmural pressure. This work was of a theoretical nature and focused on the negative transmural pressure range (external exceeding internal). Accordingly, in this study, it was assumed that the vessel's perimeter is constant, as was done by Tadjbakhsh and Odeh (1967), who solved part of this problem earlier. This assumption, which separates bending and stretch, was later validated for veins but found not to apply to arteries (Kresch 1977).

Taking into account the bending stiffness of the wall material, equilibrium conditions were written for the forces and moments that operate on the wall. These static equations were then solved numerically for a series of initial elliptical cross-sectional shapes. Samples of the results are shown in Figs. 3.3–3.6, and, in dynamic form, play a critical role in cardiopulmonary resuscitation (Chap. 11). Essentially, the results are similar to those obtained independently by Flaherty et al. (1972). Experimental confirmation was obtained by Moreno (1978) and Moreno et al. (1969, 1970). Both predicted and measured compliance, as a function of transmural pressure, show a pronounced maximum very close to zero transmural pressure. Since this maximum in compliance appears to fall close to the normal pressure range for central veins, it may have significant implications for venous return and filling of the heart. Kuhn and Drzewiecki (2003) demonstrated in model studies that arteries display a similar maximum, though deeper into the negative range of transmural pressures; with a sclerotic type of flow obstruction, the single peak may convert to a double one.

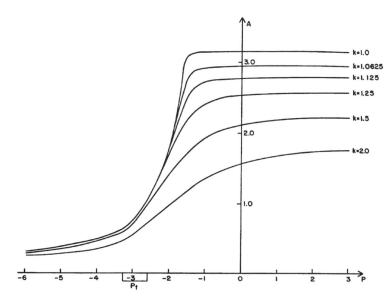

Fig. 3.3 Family of graphs of the normalized cross section A as a function of the normalized transmural pressure P for six values of initial venous eccentricity k. The cross-sectional area S of an actual vein is given by $S = r_0^2 A$, with r_0 its radius for zero transmural pressure. The actual transmural pressure, p_{tr}, in Figs. 3.3–3.5 is obtained from $p_{tr} = E_t h^3 P/6$ (Courtesy of Kresch and Noordergraaf 1972). P_t is the pressure range where opposite sides of a collapsing vein make contact

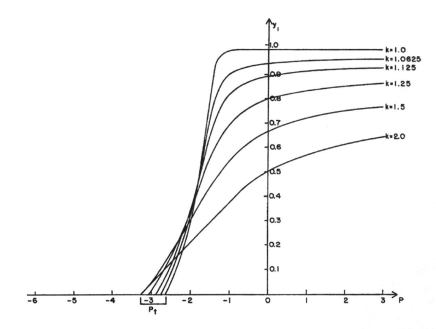

Fig. 3.4 Family of graphs of the y-axis intercept y_f as a function of normalized transmural pressure P. The conversion for the vertical axis reads $y_r = r_0 y_i$ (Courtesy of Kresch and Noordergraaf 1972)

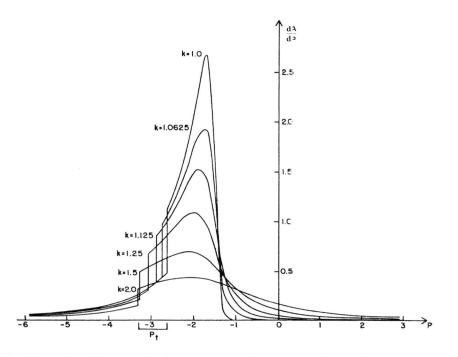

Fig. 3.5 As Fig. 3.3 for normalized compliance dA/dP. Actual compliance dS/dp_{tr} follows from $\dfrac{\mathrm{d}S}{\mathrm{d}p_{tr}} = \dfrac{6r_0^2}{E_t h^3}\dfrac{\mathrm{d}A}{\mathrm{d}P}$ The interval marked P_t displays a discontinuity, caused by opposite sides of the vessel beginning to touch (Courtesy of Kresch and Noordergraaf (1972))

3.3.2 Throat Formation in Steady Flow

The observation that veins may collapse in the in vivo situation is an old one, and has been traditionally attributed to the fact that their soft thin walls are unable to withstand even small negative transmural pressure.

Starling, in 1915, made use of the collapse phenomenon in his heart-lung preparation (Starling 1918), but the real ground-breaking work concerning the behavior of nonuniformly collapsing tubes was performed much later by Holt (1941). His experimental apparatus has since become the prototype for researchers who followed in his footsteps. Holt measured flow Q through a segment of collapsible tube as a function of the (steady) pressure just proximal to the collapsible segment (p_1), the pressure just distal to it (p_2), as well as of the pressure external to the collapsible tube, p_e. A typical result, measured on a section of Penrose tubing, which is a thin-walled rubber tubing once used as a surgical drain is displayed as Fig. 3.7. For downstream pressures exceeding external pressure ($p_2 > p_e$), the vessel is simply open over its entire length (p_1 is larger than p_2), and the slope of the $p_1 - p_2$ versus Q is determined by the flow resistance of a cylindrical vessel. The more intriguing result is the pressure flow relationship for $p_2 < p_e$, i.e., for conditions in which the tube is no longer circular in cross section, but partially collapsed. From inspection of Fig. 3.7, it will be clear that Holt observed flow to be

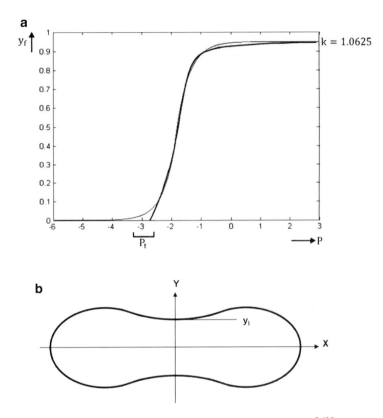

Fig. 3.6 (a) Mathematical approximation (*thin blue plot*) by $y_f = 38.5 \times e^{2.42P}$ for $P < -1.9$ and $0.95 - 0.0065 \times e^{-2.34P}$ for $P \geq -1.9$ (b) Illustration of the definition of y_i, which appears in Eq. 5.33 and in normalized form in Fig. 3.6b (Unpublished work, developed by Susanto (2009))

constant in that range. Holt described this as autoregulation, i.e., flow is no longer determined by $p_1 - p_2$, but by $p_1 - p_e$.

With almost cyclical intervening periods of several years, investigators returned to the study of the behavior of flow through collapsible tubes. Virtually all of the work since Holt's was experimental for more than two decades, when a wide variety of empirical relationships was determined, one example of which is reproduced as Fig. 3.8. This family of curves displays a downslope, which suggest the presence of a negative impedance. This led to the conclusion that the venous system, not the heart, should be viewed as the energy source driving the circulatory system (Conrad 1969).

The already confused situation was further compounded by the tendency of some investigators to attribute properties to collapsed tubes in picturesque terminology, such as "flow regulator" (Holt 1941, Fig. 3.7; Rodbard 1963), "vascular waterfall," as flow may be independent of the pressure downstream (Duomarco and Rimini 1954; Permutt and Riley 1963), and "negative impedance conduit" (Conrad 1969; Fig. 3.8).

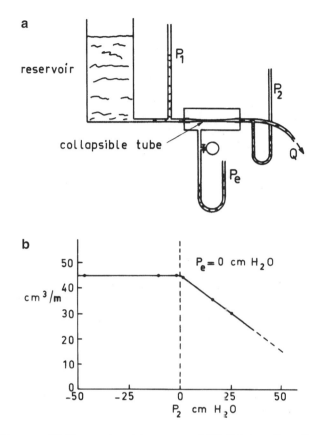

Fig. 3.7 (a) Diagram of Holt's experimental arrangement (1941) to investigate flow in collapsible tubes; p_1 denotes the pressure just upstream, p_2 just downstream of the collapsible tube, p_e the external pressure. Q denotes flow. (**b**) Flow measured in (**a**) as a function of downstream pressure with p_e and fluid level in the reservoir both constant (Adapted from Holt (1941, 1969))

Brower eliminated much of the confusion in 1970. He considered the phenomena in a broader sense and pointed out that since a collapsible tube constitutes a three-terminal device, only two independent pressure differences can be defined among the three available ones: $p_1 - p_2$, $p_e - p_2$, and $p_e - p_1$. The various other quantities, such as the pressure in an upstream reservoir that provides a pressure head, and the upstream and downstream resistances, while perhaps required in an experimental arrangement, are extraneous to the three-terminal device and, hence, should not enter into the formulation of its properties. Brower (1970) wrote for steady flow $p_1 - p_2 = f(Q, p_e - p_2)$ and determined the function f, which contains various critical parameters, such as the elastic properties of the tube or vessel, its dimensions, as well as the properties of the fluid (Seymour et al. 1993). The function turned out to be a surprisingly straightforward one for a given tube and is reproduced as Fig. 3.9 in the form of the dependence of

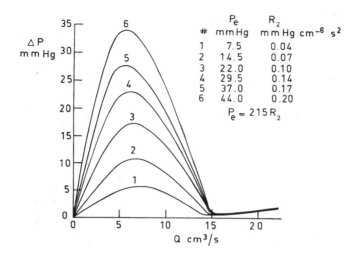

Fig. 3.8 Results of a series of experiments in which the difference between upstream and downstream pressures Δp was measured as a function of flow, Q, for each of the stated combinations of external pressure, p_e, and downstream resistance R_2. The range of apparent negative impedance may be noted. In this range, rapid fluctuations in outflow tend to occur (Courtesy of Conrad (1969))

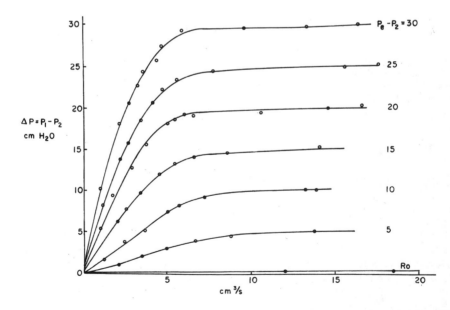

Fig. 3.9 Experimentally determined characteristic pressure-flow curves for a segment of axially stretched Penrose tube. The *bottom* curve defines the resistance R_0 for the completely open tube (From Brower and Noordergraaf (1973), by permission)

$p_1 - p_2$ on Q, with $p_e - p_2$ serving as the parameter. Three features may be noted here: (a) the simplicity of the function; (b) the disappearance of the negative impedance; (c) the closeness of the values for $p_1 - p_2$ and $p_e - p_2$, and thus for p_1 and p_e, in the nearly horizontal sections of the curves.

The question then arose whether the relationships depicted in Fig. 3.9 permit the interpretation of all previously reported relationships, if the individual experimental arrangements are taken into consideration. To this end, the relations of Fig. 3.9 were recast into a formula, which is empirical in nature.

$$p_1 - p_2 = (Q/Q_c)(p_e - p_2)[1 + (Q/Q_c)^6]^{-1/6} \qquad (3.1a)$$

provided

$$p_1 - p_2 > R_0 Q,$$

otherwise

$$p_1 - p_2 = R_0 Q \qquad (3.1b)$$

Equation 3.1b applies for the completely open (circular) tube; its flow resistance is R_0.

Q_c is an empirical quantity, which for the tube under consideration could be described by

$$Q_c = 4.7 + 8.1 e^{-(p_e - p_2)/7.5} \qquad (3.1c)$$

and represents the value for flow at which the tangents to curves, drawn at both ends, intersect.

Brower and Noordergraaf (1973) were able to show that the characteristic curves of Fig. 3.9, in conjunction with the different experimental arrangements employed by various authors, indeed covered the broad variety of relationships reported by these authors in at least a qualitative sense (incomplete definition of the original experimental arrangements often precluded rigorous quantitative tests). Stated in other words, a collapsible tube tends to interact strongly with the circuit in which it is embedded. The conclusion seems warranted that all steady state relationships so far reported have as their single common denominator the characteristic pressure-flow curves.

Brower and Noordergraaf (1978) demonstrated that the characteristic curves can be predicted on the basis of the Navier-Stokes equations coupled to the elastic properties of the wall material by considering a nonuniformly collapsing vessel as conceptualized in Fig. 3.10. Throat formation (partial or total collapse at the downstream end), as a special case, could be predicted as well. Figure 3.11 displays a computed example of an expanding throat. Measured and computed phase velocities are depicted in Fig. 3.12.

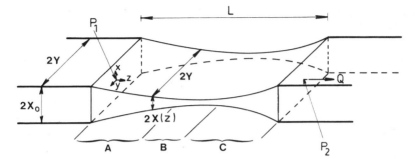

Fig. 3.10 Conceptualization employed to analyze flow in a collapsible tube. The side walls are rigid, while the *top* and *bottom* walls deflect. In region A the tube is convergent, in region B it is almost uniform, while in region C the tube is divergent (From Brower and Noordergraaf (1978))

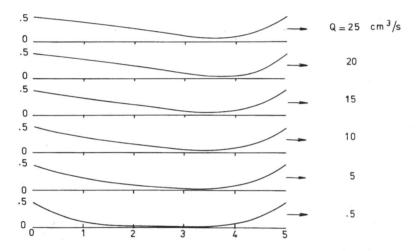

Fig. 3.11 Computed shape of the upper membrane in Fig. 3.10 for several values of flow, Q, and a constant value of $p_e - p_2$ as in Fig. 3.10 (Courtesy of Brower and Noordergraaf (1978))

3.4 Venous Pulses

3.4.1 Arterial and Cardiac Determinants of Venous Pressure and Flow Pulses

3.4.1.1 Systemic and Pulmonary

Brecher (1956) performed extensive investigations for the purpose of establishing whether or not the heart significantly influences venous return. Galenus had referred to this as suction generated by the heart. Harvey subsequently rejected it. Brecher concluded from his pioneering measurements of flow that the descent of the

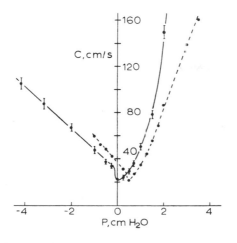

Fig. 3.12 Phase velocity as a function of transmural pressure for a Penrose tube with an unstressed diameter of 12.7 mm. *Fully drawn line* depicts measured results, *broken line* computed using the approximation by the Moens-Korteweg formula (Eq. 5.8c) (From Brower and Scholten (1975))

atrioventricular junction during ventricular ejection actively promotes venous return. When the ultrasonic flow probe became available, Brecher's idea was confirmed and could be expanded, e.g., by Morgan et al. (1966) in dogs, and by Kalmanson et al. (1971) in patients with arrhythmias. Flow into the right atrium generally reverses during right atrial contraction. The two forward surges in flow were attributed to the descent of the atrioventricular plane during ventricular ejection, confirming Brecher's idea, and to the filling phase during ventricular diastole (Fig. 3.13). The presence of suction appears well established, though the negative transmural pressure that the atrial wall can sustain amounts to only a few mmHg. It may be interesting to compare "a few" to the numbers quoted in Sect. 4.3.

Moreno (1978) studied the influence of respiratory dynamics on the events in central veins. His conclusions support only in part the classical concept of abdominal compression during inspiration. Simultaneous measurements of intra-thoracic and intra-abdominal pressures in a lightly anesthetized dog during a respiratory cycle show a decrease in both pressures rather than a decrease in intrathoracic pressure combined with an increase in intra-abdominal pressure during inspiration, though this effect could be reversed by selective cooling of the upper segments of the spinal cord. The effect of ambient pressure changes on blood flow is illustrated in Fig. 3.14 and dramatizes the softness of the venous walls.

Further studies were focused on the effect of the interposition of the liver's capillary bed between the blood returned from the splanchnic system and the inferior caval system. Moreno observed that the respiratory cycle affects flow through the portal veins and through the inferior vena cava in opposite fashion (Fig. 3.14), with the sum total, however, increasing during respiratory activity, thus

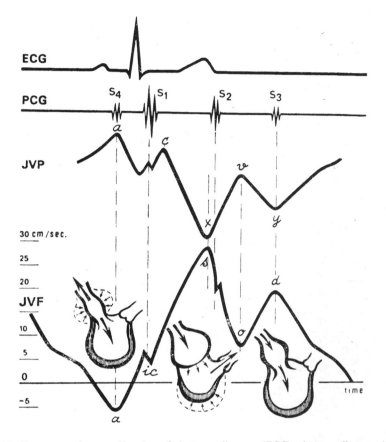

Fig. 3.13 From *top* to *bottom*: Sketches of electrocardiogram (*ECG*), phonocardiogram (*PCG*), jugular venous pressure (*JVP*), and jugular venous flow (*JVF*) velocities in opposite directions with their time relations for a normal subject (Courtesy of Kalmanson and Veyrat (1978)). S_1 = Closure of AV valves. S_2 = Closure of aortic + pulmonary valves. S_3 = Vibration of blood between walls of ventr. S_4 = Atrial contraction

indicating that venous return phenomena are much more finely tuned than supposed by Donders. The decrease in portal flow during inspiration had been observed before (e.g., Selkurt and Brecher (1956)).

Investigators have occasionally probed systemic veins for the purpose of measuring pulse wave velocity (Chap. 5), the idea being that right atrial contraction generates a (modest) pressure disturbance, which one would expect to travel upstream through the larger veins. This is in partial analogy to the left ventricle's contraction generating a wave that propagates downstream through the systemic arteries. It was found, e.g., by Duomarco and Rimini (1954) and later by Kresch and Noordergraaf (1978), that the expected pulsation could be detected in the vena cava immediately outside the heart, but not at some distance from the heart, the pulse never leaving the thoracic cavity, according to the observations by the former team.

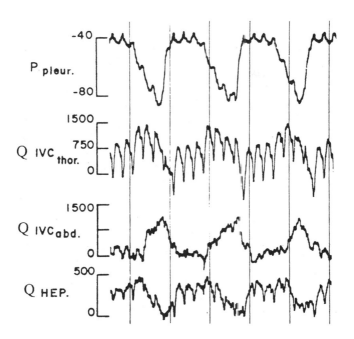

Fig. 3.14 Moreno's records, taken on a dog, of intrapleural pressure (*top*) and three flow curves, marked Q. Splanchnic flow Q_{HEP} is shown to decrease during inspiration, attributed to compression of the liver by the diaphragm. Systemic inferior vena caval flow increases nonetheless, as does thoracic inferior caval flow (Modified from Moreno (1978))

However, Moreno (1978) observed that the cardiac pulse travels all the way to the feet when the veins are distended. A possible interpretation of these differences could be that at low transmural pressures partial collapse occurs where veins enter the thoracic cavity, effects that may be reduced or absent under high distending pressure. Partial collapse would introduce wave reflection for waves generated by cardiac activity. As described above, abdominal venous return is complex during superficial respiration.

A direct result of the fact that the right ventricle pumps blood into the pulmonary artery in an intermittent fashion is that pulmonary arterial pressure and flow possess pulsatile components. But unlike in the systemic circulation, the peripheral vasculature in the pulmonary circuit does not isolate pulsatile events in the arteries from those in the veins.

There is both theoretical and experimental evidence supporting this conclusion. The theoretical evidence is based on the distribution of impedance between right ventricle and left atrium. Experimental evidence comes from the fact that pulmonary capillary flow may be measured directly by means of the detection of gas absorption. Such measurements show convincingly that capillary blood flow pulsates with a frequency equal to that of the right ventricle. Also, this pulsation follows ventricular contraction with a time delay aptly attributed to the transmission time through the arteries. The movement of radioopaque material injected into a small pulmonary artery through a wedged catheter has been observed to be affected by the arterial pulse by means of cineradiography (Morkin et al. 1964, 1965).

Hence, the pulmonary venous vasculature is equipped with two pulsatile sources, one at each end: at the peripheral input, transmitted effects generated by the right ventricle; at the cardiac end, by the alternating contraction and relaxation of the left atrium. As a result, it would be expected that flow and pressure in the pulmonary veins are pulsatile in nature. That this is indeed the case has been documented. The wave patterns have been reported as highly variable, both in time and among subjects or animals, including shapes very similar to those observed in the vena cava. Although it is agreed that the pulmonary venous pressure and flow pulses are formed by two generators, there remains a wide variety of opinions as to the relative magnitude of their contributions, ranging all the way from one dominating the other such that the latter is vanishingly small, to the converse. For a critical comparative study, reference is made to Guntheroth et al. (1974).

Additional material on veins with positive and negative transmural pressures may be found in Chap. 5, for negative transmural pressure in Chap. 10, and in Chap. 4, for the coronary veins.

3.5 Conclusions

Only recently have the veins, the most disadvantaged part of the circulatory system, reached maturity in understanding and modeling. These collapsible vessels constitute three-terminal networks with only two independent pressure differences defining characteristic curves with pressure-flow curves as their common denominator.

Early suggestions that they be granted major pump status within the circulatory system, perhaps compensating for their early neglected status, now seem exaggerated. Once reconciled with their role within the system, their function as reservoirs, actively participating in the circulation, cannot be understated or ignored.

3.6 Summary

Chapter 3 analyzes the venous systems. By coupling a simplified form of the Navier–Stokes equation with the elastic properties of a collapsible vessel, the reasons could be pinpointed underlying the wide variety of pressure-flow relations observed in different experimental arrangements by different investigators employing fluid dynamic models. This embodies variable throat formation in steady flow, and resulted in normalized collapse relations for cross-sectional area and compliance, suitable for vital practical studies such as resuscitation (in Part III), while eliminating the need for colorful designations.

The nineteenth century produced a series of views essentially doubting that the heart is powerful enough to take proper care of venous return. These rather undifferentiated claims proved to be in the need of refinement: in the resting state, the heart itself is able to pump a small amount of blood around the closed loop. This flow, amounting to around 60% of the widely accepted normal cardiac output under resting conditions, might be adequate to sustain the bodily functions. Thus, the heart appears to be capable of handling baseline requirements.

But even under such conditions, the heart receives some small support from the respiratory system. During inspiration, the intrathoracic pressure decreases, thereby promoting venous return to the right heart, in turn augmenting cardiac output of both right and left heart, though respiration is shallow and occurs at a low frequency.

References

Abel F.L. and Waldhausen J.A.: Respiratory and cardiac effects on venous return. Am. Heart J. 78: 266–275, 1969.

Borst J.G.G. and Molhuysen J.A.: Exact determination of the central venous pressure by a simple clinical method. Lancet 2: 304–309, 1952.

Brecher G.A.: Venous Return. Grune and Stratton, New York, NY, 1956.

Brecher G.A.: History of venous research. IEEE Trans. Biomed. Eng. 16: 233–247, 1969.

Brower R.W.: Pressure-Flow Characteristics of Collapsible Tubes. Ph.D. Dissertation, Univ. of Pennsylvania, Philadelphia PA, 1970.

Brower R.W. and Noordergraaf A.: Pressure-flow characteristics of collapsible tubes: a reconciliation of asumingly contradictory results. Ann. Biomed. Engs. 1: 333–355, 1973.

Brower R.W. and Noordergraaf A.: Theory of Steady Flow in Collapsible Tubes and Veins. Ch. 27 in Cardiovascular System Dynamics, J. Baan et al. (eds.), MIT Press, Cambridge, 1978.

Conrad W.A.: Pressure-flow relationships in collapsible tubes. IEEE Trans. Bio-Med. Eng. BME-16: 284–295, 1969.

Constant J.: The X prime descent in jugular contour nomenclature and recognition. Am. Heart J. 88: 372–379, 1974.

Donders F.C.: Physiologie des Menschen, Hirzel, Leipzig, 1856.

Duomarco J.L. and Rimini R.: Energy and hydraulic gradients along systemic veins. Am. J. Physiol. 178: 215–220, 1954.

Einthoven W.: Über die Form des menschlichen Electrocardiogramms. Pflügers Arch. 60: 101–123, 1895.

Flaherty J.E., Keller J.B. and Rubinow S.I.: Post buckling behavior of elastic tubes and rings with opposite sides in contact. SIAM J. Appl. Math. 23: 446–455, 1972.

Guntheroth W.G., Gould R., Butler J. and Kinnen E.: Pulsatile flow in pulmonary artery. capillary, and vein in the dog. Cardiovasc. Res. 8: 330–337, 1974.

Guyton A.C., Jones C.E.: Central venous pressure: Physiological significance and clinical implications. Am. Heart J. 86: 431–437, 1973.

Hales S.: Statical Essays: Containing Haemostaticks, or an Account of some Hydraulick and Hydrostatical Experiments made on the Blood and Blood-Vessels of Animals; etc., Vol. 2. Innys and Manby, London, 1733.

Harvey W.: On the Motion of the Heart and Blood in Animals (Translated by R. Willis). On the Circulation of the Blood. On the Generation of Animals. Encycl. Britannica, pp. 263–496, 1952.

Holt J.P.: The collapse factor in the measurement of venous pressure: The flow of fluid through collapsible tubes. Am. J. Physiol. 134: 292–299. 1941.

Holt J.P.: Flow through collapsible tubes and through in situ veins. IEEE Trans. Bio-Med. Eng., BME-16: 274–283, 1969.

Kalmanson D. and Veyrat C.: Clinical Aspects of Venous Return: A Velocimetric Approach to a New System Dynamics Concept. Ch. 31 in: Cardiovascular System Dynamics, J. Baan et al. (eds.), MIT Press, Cambridge, 1978.

Kalmanson D., Veyrat C. and Chiche P.: Atrial versus ventricular contribution in determining systolic venous return. Cardiovasc. Res. 5: 293–302, 1971.

Kresch E.: Cross-sectional shape of flexible tubes. Bull. Math. Biol. 39: 679–691, 1977.

Kresch E. and Noordergraaf A.: Cross-sectional shape of collapsible tubes. Biophys. J. 12: 274–294, 1972.

Kresch E., Granelli M. and Melbin J.: Wave Experiments in Collapsible Tubes. Ch. 26 in: Cardiovascular System Dynamics, J. Baan et al. (eds.), MIT Press, Cambridge, 1978.

Kuhn I. and Drzewiecki G.: Model investigation of the changes in mechanical properties of a blood vessel with a blood flow obstruction. Abstract, Second Int. Conf. on Cardiovasc. Med. and Science, J. Vossoughi (ed.), Bethesda MD, 2003.

Lambert R.K. and Wilson T.A.: Flow limitation in a collapsible tube. J. Appl. Physiol. 33: 150–153, 1972.

Lewis T.: Early signs of cardiac failure of the congestive type. Br. Med. J. 1: 849–852, 1930.

Mackenzie J.: Diseases of the Heart. Oxford University Press, London, 1908.

Massumi R.A., Zelis R., Ali N. and Mason D.T.: External Venous and Arterial Pulses. In: Noninvasive Cardiology, A.M. Weissler (ed.), Grune & Stratton, New York, 1974.

Moreno A.H.: Dynamics of Pressure in the Central Veins. Ch. 28 in: Cardiovascular System Dynamics, J. Baan et al. (eds.), MIT Press, Cambridge, 1978.

Moreno A.H., Katz A.I. and Gold L.D.: An integrated approach to the study of the venous system with steps toward a detailed model of the dynamics of venous return to the right heart. IEEE Trans. Biomed. Eng. 16: 308–324, 1969.

Moreno A.H., Katz A.I., Gold L.D. and Reddy R.V.: Mechanics of distension of dog veins and other very thin-walled tubular structures. Circ. Res. 27: 1069–1080, 1970.

Morgan B.C., Abel F.L., Mullins G.L. and Guntheroth W.G.: Flow patterns in the cavae, pulmonary artery, pulmonary vein, and aorta in intact dogs. Am. J. Physiol. 210: 903–909, 1966.

Morkin E., Levine O.R. and Fishman A.P.: Pulmonary capillary flow pulse and the site of pulmonary vasoconstriction in the dog. Circ. Res. 15: 146–160, 1964.

Morkin E., Collins J.A., Goldman H.S. and Fishman A.P.: Patterns of blood flow in the pulmonary vein of the dog. J. Appl. Physiol. 20: 1118–1128, 1965

Morris T.W. and Swain M.L.: Peripheral Vein: Diameter-Pressure Relationship, Structure and Control. Ch. 29 in: Cardiovascular System Dynamics, J. Baan et al. (eds.), MIT Press, Cambridge, 1978.

Noordergraaf A.: Circulatory System Dynamics. Academic Press, New York NY, 1978.

Patterson S.W. and Starling E.H.: On the mechanical factors which determine the output of the ventricles. J. Physiol. 48: 357–379, 1914.

Permutt S. and Riley R.L.: Hemodynamics of collapsible vessels with tone: the vascular waterfall. J. Appl. Physiol. 18: 924–932, 1963.

Poiseuille J.L.M.: Récherches expérimentales sur le mouvement des liquides dans les tubes de très-petits diamètres. Comptes Rendues de l' Académie de Science, Paris 11: 1041–1048, 1840.

Rodbard S.: Autoregulation in encapsulated, passive, soft-walled vessels. Am. Heart J. 65: 648–655, 1963.

Selkurt E.E. and Brecher G.A.: Splanchnic hemodynamics and oxygen utilization during hemorrhagic shock. Circ. Res. 4: 693–704, 1956.

Seymour R.S., Hargens A.R. and Pedley T.J.: The heart works against gravity. Am. J. Physiol. 265: R715-R720, 1993.

Starling E.H.: The Linacre Lecture on the Law of the Heart, Delivered at St. John's College, Cambridge, 1915. Longmans, Green, London, 1918.

Susanto: Personal information (2009)

Tadjbakhsh I. and Odeh F.: Equilibrium state of elastic rings. J. Math. Anal. Appl. 18: 59–74, 1967.

Appendix

Questions

3.1 Is the "unique" property referred to in Sect. 3.2 actually unique to the venous system?

3.2 What should be the response to the long debated issue whether the venous pulse is a pressure or a volume pulse?

3.3 Lambert and Wilson (1972) stated that flow limitation in nonuniformly collapsing tubes can be predicted on the simple basis of combining Bernoulli's equation with vessel deformation caused by a transmural pressure difference. Show this by a reasoned argument.

3.4 Compare the resistances to steady flow for two vessels of length l, one with a circular cross section, the other with an ellipsoidal cross section and the same circumference.

3.5 Explain the origin of "negative impedance" (Fig. 3.8) in words.

3.6 Verify the applicability of Eq. 3.1a for the nearly horizontal parts of the characteristic curves in Fig. 3.9.

3.7 Borst and Molhuysen (1952) use the adjective "exact" in the title of their paper about noninvasive measurement of central venous pressure. What would be the estimated error of measurement?

3.8 Show that for $P = -1$ in Fig. 3.5, the denormalized pressure is, from a practical point of view, indistinguishable from zero.

3.9 The external pressure $p_e(t)$ exhibits a negative mean value during resting respiration (Fig. 10.4). This value becomes more negative during exercise. One would expect this to enlarge the vessel's diameter and facilitate flow. Does Eq. 5.32 reflect this?

Answers

3.1 No; one can make similar statements with respect to any organ.

3.2 For a compliant vessel, the relation is determined by the compliance $C' = dS/dp$, in which C' may well be a function of pressure.

3.3 For a vessel mounted as in Fig. 2.12, collapse will start close to the downstream end as pressure decreases from p_1 to p_2 along the tube (due to fluid viscosity). Neglecting viscous effects from here on, Bernoulli's law states

$$p_1 + \frac{1}{2}\rho v_1{}^2 = p_2 + \frac{1}{2}\rho v_2{}^2 \tag{3.2}$$

where index 1 refers to the inlet and index 2 to the narrowest point of the collapsible vessel. If p_2 were lowered, the cross-sectional area S_2 would tend to diminish and v_2 would increase, even with v_1 and p_1 unchanged. Hence, the right-hand member of the Bernoulli expression tends to be unchanged. Formulated in terms of flow Q

$$Q = v_1 S_1 = v_2 S_2 \tag{3.3}$$

Elimination of v_2 yields, by approximation,

$$Q = S_2 \left[\left(\frac{2}{\rho} \right) (p_1 - p_2) \right]^{\frac{1}{2}} \tag{3.4}$$

which is about constant under these conditions.

3.4 Flow resistance for a circular cross section R_c equals $R_c = 8\eta l / \pi r_0^4$. For an elliptic cross section, $R_e = (4\eta l / \pi)(a^2 + b^2)/a^3 b^3$, where a and b are the major and minor semiaxes. Since the perimeters are equal, $2\pi r_0 = 2\pi [(a^2 + b^2)/2]^{1/2}$. Thus, $R_e/R_s = 8a^3 b^3/(a^2 + b^2)^3$.

3.5 With increasing flow $(\Delta Q > 0)$, downstream pressure increases in accordance with $p_2 = R_2 Q^2$. As a consequence, p_2 must eventually approach p_e. In the process, the degree of collapse diminishes. As the vessel rounds out, $\Delta p < 0$, and the ratio is negative.

3.6 For $Q > Q_c$, Eq. 3.1a reduces to $p_1 - p_2 = p_e - p_2$, which is the parameter in these experiments.

3.7 A few mmHg. The percentage error depends strongly on the level of the central venous pressure.

3.8 For $P = -1$ with $10^{\pm n}$ written as $(e \pm n)$

$$p_{tr} = \frac{E_t h^3}{6} P = \frac{4.5(e+5)[2(e-2)]^3}{6} [-1] = -0.45(e-3) \text{mmHg} \tag{3.5}$$

which means, in practical terms, that the maximal compliance occurs very near to zero transmural pressure, in agreement with the experiment (Fig. 5.9 in Noordergraaf A 1978).

3.9 Yes, the second term on the right takes care of this.

Chapter 4
The Heart

Cordis meatus ita à natura paratos esse, vt ex vena caua
intromissio fiat in Cordis ventriculum dextrum, vnde patet
exitus in pulmonem: Ex pulmone praeterea aliu ingressum
esse in cordis ventriculum s nistrum, ex quo tandem patet
exitus in arteriam Aortam, membranis quibusdam ad ostia
vasorum appositis, vt impediant retrocessum: sic enim
perpetuus quidam motus est ex vena caua per cor &
pulmones in arteriam Aortam: vt in questionibus
peripateticis explicauimus.

— Andreas Caesalpinus (1593)

Digest: Unscrambling the morphology of the four chambered mammalian heart requires long term devotion, but reaches a new level of success when the band structure is found. The electrical stimulation pathways do not appear to adhere to the band's filaments. The lack of critical experimental techniques allowing particular observations during the dynamic process hampers discovery of the contractile force production mechanism and continues to invite speculation, leaving the crossbridge theory of the Huxleys in the most favored position. A recent distributed model founded on this theory suggests why no trigger for muscle relaxation was unearthed until recently. Starling's law proves to be a generalization of the Frank mechanism. The ejection effect is quantified and shows that the ventricle is not a pure pressure source, which triggered the development of a unifying theory for all ventricular properties. Ventricular elastance can be determined for the entire cardiac cycle. A noninvasive method to evaluate contractile properties based on changes in ventricular shape is summarized.

The heart qualifies as our most powerful source of impedance-defined flow.

4.1 Morphology and Stimulation

Harvey placed the responsibility for keeping the blood in motion squarely on the heart, which created a new interest in the organization and contractile behavior of its muscular walls. Lower, in his book published in slightly different versions in

A. Noordergraaf, *Blood in Motion*, DOI 10.1007/978-1-4614-0005-9_4,
© Springer Science+Business Media, LLC 2011

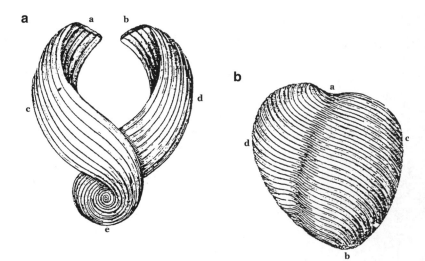

Fig. 4.1 (**a**) Lower's Fig. 7 in his Tabularium 2 (1669) showing how the fibers of the inner LV wall (*d*) and outer LV wall (*c*) together form the whorl near the apex. (**b**) Lower's Fig. 3 in his Tabularium 2 showing superficial fibers running across the sulcus at the boundary between the two ventricles (the RV is marked *d*). In the sulcus, below the superficial fibers the descending branch of the left coronary artery is found. The lines of the inner parts, a, b, c etc (small) indicate fiber orientation

both London and Amsterdam in 1669, exposed the complex architecture of the ventricular walls. He described muscle fascicular orientation using phrases such as up and down, left to right, oblique, inside to outside, etc. and provided engravings to illustrate some of his astute observations (Fig. 4.1a).

This led to the question of whether muscular layers can be identified. Over time, this question has been answered affirmatively as well as negatively. Pettigrew (1864) concluded that there are seven layers in the ventricles, together forming an imperfect figure eight. Lev and Simkins (1956) demonstrated that despite the presence of intercommunicating fasciculi, multiple cleavage planes can be found and layers can be partially unrolled. Other investigators pursued more detailed studies of bundle orientation through the thickness at particular sites of the free wall and found large differences at various depths (e.g., Streeter et al. 1978). Eventually, such anatomical studies guided Torrent-Guasp to his discovery of an overall structure which, in view of its appearance, was called the ventricular band (1980). Since that time, a ventricular band has been recognized in a variety of species.

The main phases to achieve this result can be described succinctly. The specimen, depending on size, is boiled in water for a few minutes to several hours to soften the collagenous connecting tissue. The atria are removed. In the dissection of the ventricles, three anatomically defined cleavage planes are utilized. Much of the dissection can be achieved using a blunt instrument.

The first cleavage plane is located at the anterior ventricular sulcus (along which runs the descending branch of the left coronary artery). The sulcus is covered by a thin layer of fasciculi as shown in Fig. 4.1b. These must be cut. Cleavage along this

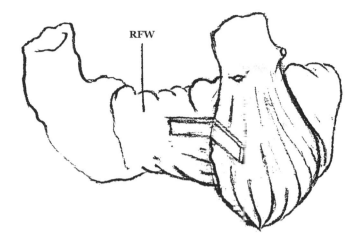

Fig. 4.2 Cleavage along the anterior ventricular sulcus exposes the first part of the band, containing primarily the right ventricular free wall (*RFW*) (Adapted from Torrent-Guasp (1980))

sulcus exposes the first part of the band, its main component being the right ventricular free wall, with the root of the pulmonary trunk at its outer end. The drawing in Fig. 4.2 shows this, up to the level of the beginning of the second cleavage plane.

The second anatomical cleavage plane starts at the linear posterior limit of the right ventricular cavity, which coincides with the posterior interventricular sulcus (along which runs the right coronary artery). This posterior limit is given by the dihedral angle formed between the right free wall and the septum. The angle is marked in Fig. 4.2. Following this cleavage plane, the myocardial band can be separated until it turns toward the apex to form the inner layer of the left ventricular free wall (Fig. 4.3).

The third anatomical cleavage plane is found at the septum where two layers of fibers cross at about 90°, which can also be seen in Fig. 4.3. Separation along this cleavage plane is then performed, with the result drawn in Fig. 4.4. This completes the dissection of the muscular band. The root of the aorta appears at the opposite end compared to the root of the pulmonary trunk.

Rewinding of the band reconstitutes the two chambers with their septum, sans intercommunicating fasciculi and connective tissue fibers cut or torn during the dissection procedure. The atria show a similar architecture. Against the background of the band structure, much of the complexity of the fascicular organization, referred to above, can be easily understood. In the design of ventricular wall anatomical models, the band structure has been, thus far, largely ignored (e.g., Nielsen et al. 1991; Arts et al. 1982; Hunter and Smaill 1988).

Proceeding to the microscopic level, Fig. 4.5a displays myocardium with its conspicuous architecture of branching fibers as seen under the light microscope. Figure 4.5b shows part of one fiber (myocyte) at a higher enlargement as reconstructed from electron micrographs. Fibrils are seen, arranged in parallel,

Fig. 4.3 Following the
second cleavage plane, the
band can be separated until it
turns toward the apex to form
the inner layer of the *left*
ventricular free wall (Adapted
from Torrent-Guasp (1980)
and Torrent-Guasp et al.
(1997). (The sketches in
Figs. 4.2–4.4 were drawn for
the author by Dr. Torrent-
Guasp))

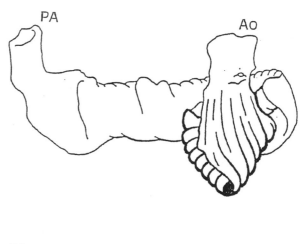

Fig. 4.4 Separation along the
third cleavage plane exposes
the LV's outer layer ending in
the aortic root (*Ao*) (Adapted
from Torrent-Guasp (1980)
and Torrent-Guasp et al.
(1997))

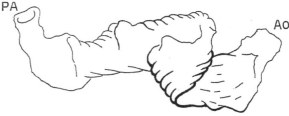

with each fibril consisting of a series arrangement of sarcomeres. A single sarcomere with a representation of overlapping myofilaments is provided in Fig. 4.5c.

In addition to the branching structure of the myocytes, an extracellular matrix of
collagen fibers lends structural integrity to the cardiac walls. Scanning electron
microscopy made it possible to demonstrate a skeleton of such fibers connecting
myocyte to contiguous myocyte and myocyte to contiguous capillary at many sites
and often in directions roughly perpendicular to the cell's or vessel's longitudinal
axis (Caulfield and Borg 1979).

Just as the heart is hemodynamically divided into two pairs of chambers
(Chap. 2), there is a division into two pairs for the electrical system that provides
the trigger for myocardial (heart muscle) contraction. The arrangement of pairs is
quite different for the two cases. For the fluid system, the division is between the
right and left side of the heart and is provided by the septum (Figs. 2.4 and 2.7); for
the electrical system, the division is between the atria and the ventricles, i.e., by the
plane in which the four valves lie. The organization of the electrical system is
intimately related to the efficiency of the fluid pump.

The heart's electrical system is basically self-contained (Fig. 4.6). Under
normal circumstances, a small fraction of the cardiac cells is capable of periodic
impulse generation. These cells belong to the so-called specialized tissue that
includes the sino-auricular (SA) node, a small section of the wall of the right
atrium near the point of entry of the superior vena cava, the atrioventricular (AV)

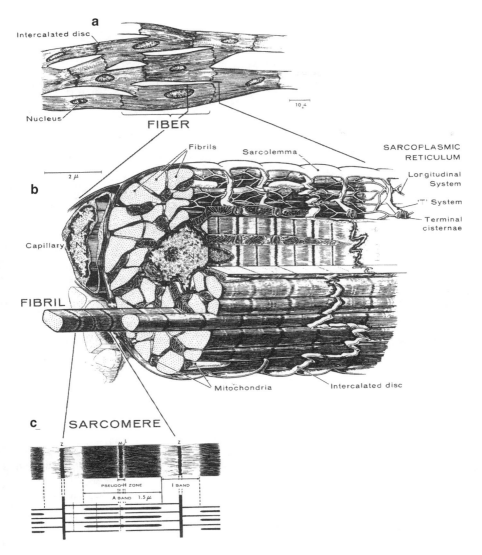

Fig. 4.5 (**a**) Myocardium as seen under the light microscope. Branching fibers, each with a centrally located nucleus, can be distinguished clearly; (**b a**) myocardial fiber, reconstructed from electron micrographs, showing parallel arrangement of fibers and series arrangement of sarcomeres that make up the fibril; (**c**), An individual sarcomere, with diagrammatic representation of overlapping myofilaments (Adapted from Braunwald et al. 1968)

node, located at the base of the interatrial septum, the His bundle, and finally, the perforating transmissional endings, the Purkinje fibers in the atria and the ventricles.

During rest, regular tissue cells exhibit a constant potential difference across their membranes, with the outside positive with respect to the inside. This is called

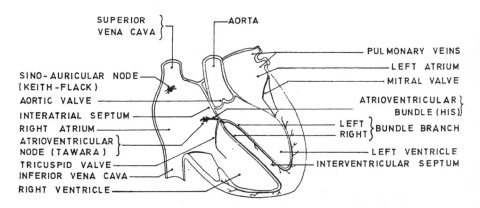

Fig. 4.6 Sketch to show the heart's main locations of the electrical system relative to its anatomy (Modified from Burger 1968)

the resting potential. For the specialized tissue cells, this membrane potential decreases in time with different characteristic times for different tissues. The fastest rate, under normal conditions, is found in the SA node cells. As soon as the membrane potential has diminished to the threshold value, a so-called action potential will occur, i.e., a current will flow: the membrane potential goes to zero (the cell depolarizes), changes sign briefly, then returns more slowly to reestablish the resting potential (the cell repolarizes, Fig. 4.7). The cell that initiates the impulse, i.e., depolarizes first, is referred to as the pacemaker cell. Normally, the tissue that makes up the SA node fills this role. Accordingly, the SA node is called the pacemaker. All other potential pacemakers are denoted subsidiary pacemakers.

The action potential of a pacemaker cell depolarizes neighboring cells to their thresholds, which, in turn, initiate action potentials, etc. This process of propagation of the action potential continues as long as there is excitable tissue available (Glitsch 1982). Excitation phenomena propagate over the atrial musculature with a speed of about 40 cm/s. In view of the distance to be covered, it requires about 80 ms to reach the most distant points, although specialized pathways permit varying rates of pulse propagation to occur. The spread of the excitation wave is followed by shortening of the atrial musculature, i.e., by contraction and pumping of both atria.

The atrial excitation wave also reaches a volume of specialized tissue located on the right side of the atrial septum in the proximity of the valve plane. This volume is designated the AV node (Fig. 4.6). Subsequent to the arrival of the electrical signal, the AV node issues an impulse after a delay in the order of 100 ms. The impulse is conducted through a cable, the His bundle, which penetrates the valve plane. Inside the ventricles, the cable branches, forming the two left and the right bundles, which are embedded on opposite sides of the interventricular septum. The bundle branches eventually differentiate to a large number of fibers, the Purkinje (Purkynv) fibers,

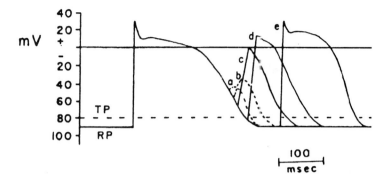

Fig. 4.7 Spontaneous transmembrane action potential followed by responses to a series of stimuli (*a–e*) applied during and after the end of repolarization. Response *c* is the earliest propagated response and marks the end of the refractory period. Response *d* is elicited at the time when the potential difference across the membrane is close to the level of the threshold potential (*TP*). *RP* denotes the level of the resting potential (Modified from Hoffman 1969)

which in the human are distributed over a part of the inner surface of the ventricles and terminate within the myocardium (Fig. 4.8).

The velocity of propagation along the specialized stimulus-conducting pathways is 2–4 m/s, thereby providing rapid signal transmission to many points of the ventricular muscle mass. Conduction over the muscle fibers themselves, again with a speed of about 40 cm/s, completes the excitation phase. From the time of AV node firing, it requires about 75 ms to fully excite the ventricles (Durrer et al. 1970). Electrical stimulation is followed by shortening of the muscle fibers and ventricular pumping (excitation-contraction coupling). Elaborate collection of experimental data, employing multiple electrodes embedded throughout the myocardium (Scher 1965; Durrer et al. 1970) show that the depolarization sequence does not follow the band structure (Figs. 4.4 and 4.9).

Although the heart's firing system is basically self-contained, it is connected to the central nervous system and hence reflects central control. Both sympathetic and parasympathetic nerves reach the heart and are distributed profusely in the areas near the SA and AV nodes and variably in the muscular walls of atria and ventricles. The two nerve types exercise antagonistic influences on the heart, with respect to both rate and strength of contraction.

It has been found that the excitation front traveling through the myocardium has a thickness of only 1 mm. This is relatively thin with respect to the thickness of the myocardium (1 mm atrial to 10 mm ventricular) so that the excitation front is often conveniently viewed as a propagating dipole shell. This electrical dipole layer generates a transient electrical field in the body. Hence, potential differences can be recorded between various points inside the body, as well as on its surface.

Examples of potential differences recorded between pairs of points on the body surface (electrocardiograms, ECG's) are reproduced in Fig. 4.10. A number of

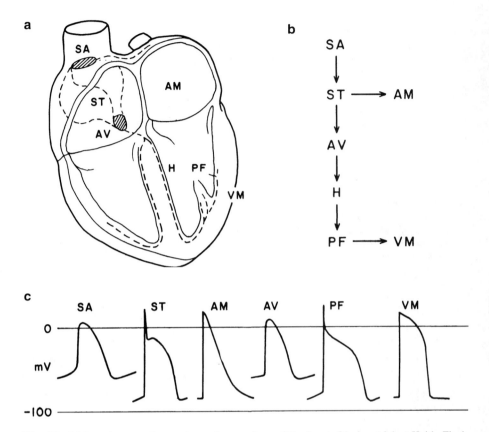

Fig. 4.8 (a) Impulse spread over the various regions of the heart. *SA* sinoatrial or Keith–Flack node, named after the first investigators who suggested its significance in 1907, *ST* specialized tracts, *AM* atrial musculature, *AV* atrioventricular node, *H* bundle of His, *PF* Purkinje fibers, *VM* ventricular musculature. (Modified from Tsien and Hess 1986). (**b**) The same as 4.8a, schematically. (**c**) The same as 4.8a, experimentally

wave components can be easily recognized (Fig. 4.10a). The P wave reflects stimulus conduction through the atrial muscle mass, and the QRS complex through the ventricular myocardium. The pause between the termination of the P wave and the onset of the QRS complex arises from the slow impulse propagation through the AV node, as well as, to a small extent, from conduction through the His bundle and its branches. The electrical fields accompanying nodal activity and conduction through the pathways are too weak to be recorded on the body's surface, although they can be discerned by electrodes placed in their immediate vicinity. A small wave hidden in the QRS complex and the T wave are related to the recovery process of the atrial and ventricular myocardium, respectively.

Einthoven (1913) introduced the concept that the electrocardiograms which can be recorded between any pair of points (so-called leads I, II, III) are actually

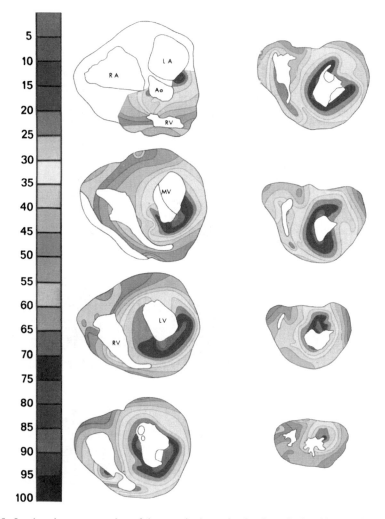

Fig. 4.9 Isochronic representation of the ventricular activation in an isolated human heart, based on measurements at 870 intramural electrode terminals. The horizontal planes into which the multielectrodes were inserted, and into which the heart was sectioned, are depicted. Zero time is the beginning of the left ventricular cavity potential. Color coded bar in milliseconds. *RA* right atrial cavity, *LA* left atrial cavity, *Ao* aorta, *LV* left ventricular cavity, *RV* right ventricular cavity, *MV* mitral valve (Durrer et al. 1970. Reproduced by permission)

projections of a vector quantity, the magnitude and direction of which is defined by the propagating dipole shell. For example, lead I is $RA^- - LA^+$ He designated this quantity the "manifest value," but it has since become known as the "heart vector." Appropriate combinations of three leads recorded in the three spatial dimensions make it possible to derive the heart vector in good approximation and to display its variation in magnitude and direction during the heart cycle. An example is shown in Fig. 4.11. Despite the expenditure of considerable efforts, researchers have not yet

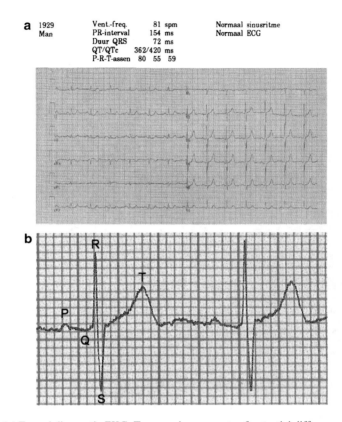

Fig. 4.10 (**a**) Formal diagnostic EKG. Two synchronous sets of potential differences, electrocardiograms, between pairs of points on the body surface. (*left*) *Top*, between both arms (*lead I*); *center*, between *right* arm and *left* leg (*II*); *bottom*, between *left* arm and *left* leg (*III*) aVR, aVL, aVF. (*right*) From *top down*, V_1,–V_6, between selected points on the chest close to the heart and a weighted combination of the limb potentials. Subject A.N. One millivolt vertical calibration. Horizontal calibration: 5 large divisions per second. (**b**) Enlarged segment of lead *I* to show traditional names of ECG waves

been able to derive the detailed propagation phenomena from surface leads. This inverse problem may, in fact, be irresolvable for practical reasons (Quick et al. 2006, in a related issue).

Exposure of the intact heart to a sufficiently intense pulse of ultrasound offers a (mechanical) alternative to initiate the excitatory process (electrical, either natural or artificial) followed by contraction (below and Sect. 9.2).

4.2   Contraction and Relaxation

Cardiac muscle has the long established ability alternately to contract, i.e., generate a force, and relax, i.e., become passive, in a quasiperiodic fashion. Where conditions permit, muscle contraction is accompanied by muscle shortening.

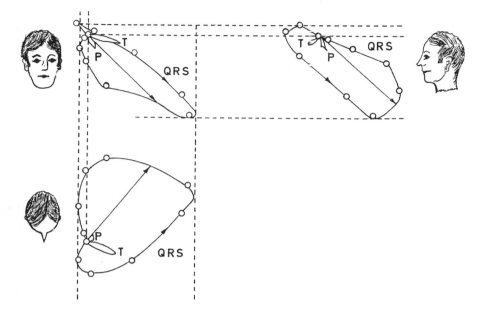

Fig. 4.11   A normal vectorcardiogram in three projections. Lettering as in Fig. 4.10b. Time marks 10 ms apart. The projections of the heart vector itself are shown for one given instant in time (Modified from Burger 1968)

Within physiological limits, shortening muscle can partially sustain its contractile force. Contraction is followed by relaxation through an automatic mechanism. In the human, the contractile state has a duration of one fourth to one third of the duration of one heart cycle. The signal that normally induces contraction has been known for about a century (above). Notwithstanding diligent searches, a similar signal to induce the onset of relaxation has never been discovered. Possibly as a consequence, muscle contraction has often been judged more intriguing than its relaxation. Particularly in the early phases, most of muscle research dealt with skeletal muscle, primarily owing to its ease of accessibility.

In skeletal muscle, Galenus attributed the facility to contract to the flow of animal spirit. In spite of Harvey's effort at abolition, this type of idea proved to be persistent: Croone in 1664 viewed contraction as the result of a change in volume, induced by the flow of spirituous liquor into the muscle (Wilson 1961), though Swammerdam[1] (1663, 1737) demonstrated experimentally that muscle contraction is either an isovolumic event or the volume diminishes slightly.

---

[1]Jan Swammerdam (1637–1680) did not publish his extensive notes written in Dutch, but Herman Boerhaave later purchased them, had a Latin translation made and published the entire collection as three large volumes in two languages, printed side by side. Volume three contains Swammerdam's drawings, with captions.

Mayow (1674) was instrumental in providing a primitive transition to the inclusion of metabolic activity. Thus, Weber (1846) could state as his view that muscle is an elastic material which changes state as a consequence of activation due to conversion of chemical energy. Helmholtz (1845) demonstrated this experimentally and confirmed production of heat (1848). For a long period, this view was simplified by considering muscle as an elastic material only: muscle behaves like a stretched spring. Upon activation, the stretched state stores potential energy which can be used to do work via shortening. The generalization from an elastic to a viscoelastic material to explain heat production during contraction was rejected by Heidenhain as early as 1864, primarily because heat production was found to be maximal when muscle length was kept constant (isometric contraction). Yet, the viscoelastic feature reappeared time and again. Hill, e.g., tried to popularize it in 1922. In support of this, Gasser and Hill (1924) even described a viscoelastic fluid-mechanical model claimed to reproduce the phenomena observed on active skeletal muscle.

The concept of the stretched spring seemed to be supported by Fick's observation (1882), confirmed innumerable times since that isometric force increases with length within physiological limits. First suspected by Laulanié in 1890, Hill (1939) complimented this with his force–velocity relation, suggesting that the rate of energy conversion in shortening muscle is subject to an upper bound. Marriage between the two observations was proposed by the idea of conformational change in long macromolecules, a popular theory for some time. Coiling of long molecules from an extended state would manifests itself as muscle shortening, occurring more slowly at higher muscle loads. This idea was presented in several variations (Meyer 1929; Polissar 1952).

Viscoelastic models of muscular tissue, such as the once popular three-element model consisting of a configuration of two springs and a dashpot, failed to match tissue behavior for reasons clarified much later (Quick et al. 1994). Incorporation of Hill's contractile element into the three-element model, which featured both active as well as passive force–length (spring) relations and a force–velocity relation, allowed for internalized energy conversion. But this, even with augmentation by a number of holdover passive elements (Parmley et al. 1969), did not remedy the basic deficiency. Such models share the absence of any correlation between tissue and model structures. Nonetheless, the elastic and viscoelastic features themselves survived.

Some of the older theories yielded their position to the idea of the sliding filament mechanism, at least for striated muscle, which was proposed in 1954 simultaneously by A.F. Huxley and Niedergerke and by H.E. Huxley and Hanson. This concept describes shortening and lengthening of muscle by a change in the relative position of molecules instead of by changes in shape. It leaves unanswered the question of the generation of the forces that cause the sliding. Subsequently, a variety of theories has been advanced for the purpose of identifying the force generating mechanism itself.

A claim by a veteran contributor, and avid collector of theories, to have in his possession more than a hundred published theories about muscle activity, demonstrates the level of interest in devising mechanisms of muscle contraction. In these theories different physical principles are invoked to account for force generation. In addition, there are many variations in the details of the biochemistry at the molecular level.

The assumption of the same or opposite polarity of distributed electrical charges is often found to be favored. For example, it has been argued that the repulsive force between the filaments arising from electrical charges of the same sign leads to radial extension of the muscle and thus, in view of constant muscle volume, to axial shortening (Shear 1970; Elliott et al. 1970). This is reminiscent of Croone's view, with electrical charges replacing fluid infusion. Other theories assume electrical charges of equal sign on the filaments, the sign of one of which is reversed upon activation of the muscle (Spencer and Worthington 1960), or charges of opposite sign on the filaments (Ingels and Thompson 1966) as the origin of the contracting force.

In Iwazumi's theory (1970, 1978), the myosin filaments are argued to form a stable superstructure through their protrusions. In other words, the protrusions are considered to form steady bridges between the thick filaments. Each protrusion is regarded as charged positively at its outer end and negatively at its base on the thick filament. Such a charge distribution gives rise to strong, local, electrical fields in the myosin space. The actin filaments thus find themselves in a nonuniform electrical field. Provided that the actin filaments have electrical properties (dielectric constant, conductivity) different from their fluid environment, they will experience a force directed along their longitudinal axis.

In Pollack's theory (1990), the myosine superstructure is retained, though in a slightly modified form. During contraction, the actin filaments are presumed to attach themselves to the superstructure's bridges, thereby creating a path for force transduction to the outside, while the forces are proposed to be generated by shortening of particular sections of the thick filaments. This shortening is called melting and is visualized as a helix to coil transition. Relaxation comes about by the inverse transition. Both are reminiscent of conformational changes in long macromolecules proposed earlier.

By far, the most popular theory of muscle contraction is the crossbridge theory (Huxley 1964, 1969; Huxley and Simmons 1971). Its essential feature is the assumption that the protrusions on the thick filaments form mechanical bridges between the two types of filaments. This theory has been scrutinized in great detail and strong support has been marshaled. This does not mean that this theory is free of problems (Noble and Pollack 1977). Specifically, limitations in resolution have so far prevented direct observation of the bridges themselves during the dynamic process.

The mechanism of force production is often visualized as sketched in Fig. 4.12. Rotation of the myosin head generates an almost longitudinal force, but can only execute a small stroke. Therefore, for the sarcomere to achieve significant shortening, the bridges are supposed to perform a cyclic motion with the net effect of a more widely ranging axial contractile force. Biochemical studies have indicated that the necessary energy for contraction is derived from ATP. In the biochemical machinery, Ca^{2+} ions play the role of trigger.

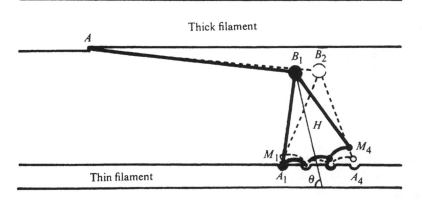

Fig. 4.12 Concept of crossbridge operation as visualized by Huxley and Simmons (1971). Rotation of the myosin head H, from the position marked by fully drawn lines to that marked by broken lines, causes shortening (Reproduced by permission of the senior author)

The majority of muscle models has never been subjected to quantitative evaluation, which allows for much room to speculate about possible mechanisms of contraction. The crossbridge theory is one of the few that has been modeled in some detail, allowing for quantitative comparison with experimental data and prediction of features not appreciated before.

Classically, papillary muscle has been found to offer ideal material for the performance of experiments on living heart muscle (strip experiments). Such studies permit scrutiny of muscle under a variety of conditions, including isometric contraction, shortening against a constant load, isometric contraction with a quick release, or a quick stretch, or a quick alteration in load superimposed. At the other end of the spectrum, experiments were designed and executed where through the application of feedback, sarcomere length was kept constant better than in a standard isometric contraction in which the ends of the strip tend to stretch.

As illustrated in Fig. 4.13, stimulated cardiac muscle, held isometric, first builds up a force, which reaches a maximum; it is followed by a gradual reduction in force, eventually resulting in complete relaxation when the available energy has been expended. The time course of this expenditure can be modified by external conditions as demonstrated in Fig. 4.14. The velocity of shortening appears to play a critical role: superimposition of a sudden small shortening (quick release) on an otherwise isometric contraction causes a sudden drop in generated force, which is generally followed by partial restoration of the contractile force terminating earlier than in the undisturbed case (Fig. 4.15). In contrast, when an effort is made to keep sarcomeres at constant length, relaxation proceeds at a slower pace than in an ordinary isometric twitch (Huxley and Simmons 1973). In an effort to clarify these experimental observations, a distributed model of the cross bridge theory proved to furnish a powerful tool.

Palladino's model (1990) incorporates the main features of the crossbridge theory. It avoids gross lumping by preserving the individuality of participating

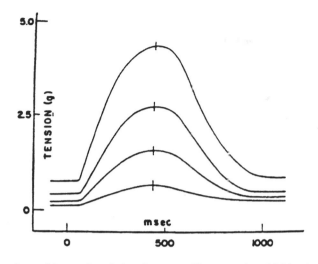

Fig. 4.13 Experimental isometric twitches for cat papillary muscle exhibiting larger forces for increased initial lengths. Original muscle length 8.5 mm with increments of 0.5 mm (Adapted from Sonnenblick 1962)

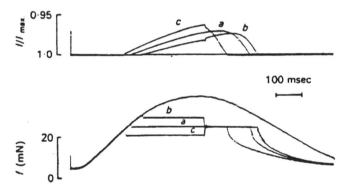

Fig. 4.14 Variable load clamps for cat papillary muscle. *Bottom*: Force-time curves. Curve *a* illustrates constant load, *b* shows a reduction, and *c* an increase in load imposed during the shortening process. *Top*: Shortening versus time for the same conditions. Energy expenditure is clearly modified by load manipulation (Adapted from Brutsaert et al. 1978)

elements. The model represents that the sarcomere consists of overlapping thin and thick filaments. In passive muscle, thick filaments are in stable suspension at the center of the sarcomere, which contributes to the muscle's passive elastic properties (Winegrad 1974). Calcium ions serve as the trigger that allows bond formation. Bonds are stretched at the expense of biochemical energy, thereby developing force. This stretching results from myosine heads flipping from one position to another (Huxley and Simmons 1973). The number of bonds formed depends on the degree of overlap between thick and thin filaments (Gordon et al. 1966). Asynchrony in bond formation and unequal numbers of bonds formed in each half

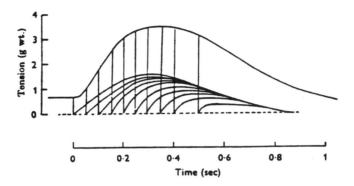

Fig. 4.15 Compilation of quick releases in cat papillary muscle to zero force. The release was only 2% of initial muscle length with a velocity of 75 mm/s (Adapted from Brady 1966)

sarcomere, as well as disturbances such as sarcomere shortening and imposed length transients, cause movement of thick filaments with respect to thin filaments. Taking into account myofilament masses make these movements take the form of damped vibrations with a spectrum of frequencies due to the distributed system properties. When the stress in a bond falls to, or below, a threshold value (set at zero here) the bond detaches (Huxley and Simmons 1973). Myofilament motion and stress relaxation in bonds lead to bond detachment and therefore cause relaxation.

In this model the crossbridge is formulated as follows. Since biomaterials consistently appear to manifest viscoelastic properties, bonds between thin and thick filaments are described as viscoelastic material and can exhibit stress relaxation and creep. The relation between change in bond length Δl and stress σ, the force F per bond cross-sectional area A, can, in its simplest form, be written as a first-order linear differential equation in the time domain (Fig. 4.16):

$$\sigma(t) + \frac{\beta l_1}{AE_2}\frac{d\sigma}{dt} = \frac{E_1}{l_0}\Delta 1(t) + \left[\frac{\beta}{A} + \frac{\beta l_1 E_1}{Al_0 E_2}\right]\frac{dl}{dt} \tag{4.1}$$

The pattern for the arrangement of some 5,000 bonds is indicated in Fig. 4.17. A few results are reproduced in Figs. 4.18 and 4.19.

The results obtained from the model suggest why no relaxation initiating signal was ever found: Contracting striated muscle is unstable. Left to itself, it will relax owing to the vibrations of the thick filaments and the consequential detachment of bonds. Mechanical disturbances, such as muscle shortening, quick release, or quick load alteration would be expected, and are predicted by the model to enhance the rate of relaxation and this was indeed observed in muscle experiments (e.g., in Fig. 4.14). Such disturbances are deemed to enhance heat production.

The model also suggested two new experiments. The simpler of the two was the consideration that since the thick filaments are computed to vibrate with a frequency in the megahertz range, exposure of a contracting ventricle to a very short intensive burst of ultrasound should accelerate the onset of ventricular diastole.

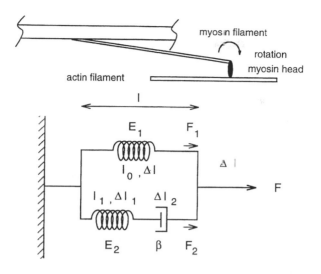

Fig. 4.16 *Top*: Sketch of a crossbridge bond between myosin and actin filaments. The bond is stretched by rotation of the myosin head (cf. Fig. 4.12). *Bottom*: Mechanical representation of a viscoelastic crossbridge of length l. E_1 and E_2 are elastic moduli, β is viscous damping, and l_0, l_1 are initial lengths. The lower branch converts energy into heat. A change in bond length Δl generated by force F produces forces F_1, F_2 with changes in length Δl_1, Δl_2 as shown (From Palladino and Noordergraaf 1998)

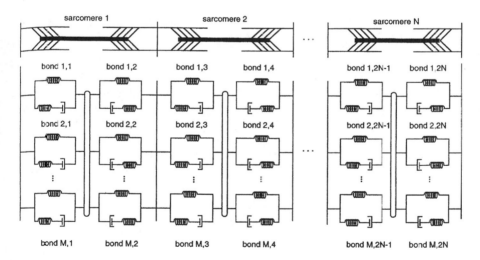

Fig. 4.17 Schematic representation of a muscle fiber composed of N series sarcomeres, each with M parallel pairs of active viscoelastic bonds. Each bond is modeled as in Fig. 4.16 and Eq. 4.1 (Reproduced from Palladino et al. 2000a)

Experiments on frog hearts confirmed this (Dalecki et al. 1997). The other experiment suggested by the model is that contracting muscle in a strong magnetic field environment should display a tiny, rapidly varying induced voltage on the basis of Maxwell's law.

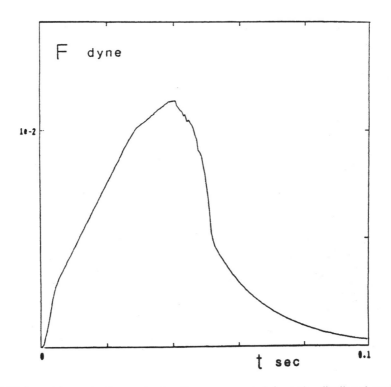

Fig. 4.18 Isometric contraction and relaxation as computed from the distributed model in Fig. 4.17 (From Palladino 1990)

Two other aspects deserve attention. The first is that a burst of ultrasound, administered during ventricular diastole proved capable, experimentally, of initiating contraction (i.e., serve as a mechanical pacemaker, Dalecki et al. 1991). The second is that as long as the energy supply in muscle is not exhausted, muscle can fight the instability feature by reattaching crossbridges that became detached, thereby extending the duration of the contraction period (Sect. 4.3).

4.3   Cardiac Discharge and Filling

Otto Frank discerned that the mechanical activity of skeletal muscle had been widely studied under the most varied conditions, while relatively little had been done with cardiac muscle. He set out to rectify the situation. In view of the experimental difficulties that had to be overcome, Frank restricted himself to studies of the isolated frog heart, as had Roy before him. The experiments concerned the isovolumic pressure curves of the atrium and of the ventricle with the volume of blood contained by the chamber and time as independent variables.

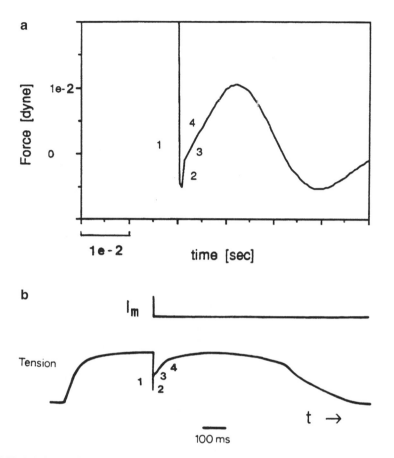

Fig. 4.19 Huxley and Simmons (1973) identified four phases in a quick release experiment (**b**), which are also seen in the model of Fig. 4.19 (**a**) (From Palladino 1990)

Although Frank did not measure atrial or ventricular volume directly, his results clearly show that maximum isovolumic pressure first rises and subsequently falls with increasing intracavitary volume (Fig. 4.20). He thus established the needed transition from skeletal to cardiac muscle by observing that for both "the maximum tension [. . .] at first increases with augmentation of the initial length" (Fig. 4.21).

The formulation of the mechanism that Starling termed "the law of the heart" may be viewed as a follow-up on Harvey's nomination of the heart as the central and only pump, comprising two sets of valves (Chap. 8), within the mammalian cardiovascular system. This newer work represented a crystallization of ideas about the heart, ejecting into high pressure reservoirs that evolved from earlier studies of cardiac phenomena by several scientists including Charles Roy, who published in 1879.

Starling studied the mechanism of adaptation for the warm-blooded animal in his heart-lung preparation. This preparation approximated, in several ways, actual conditions in life more closely than was achieved by Cyon (1866), Roy, or Frank. The heart and the lungs were removed from the body while preserving their interconnections. The left ventricle pumped into an air-cushioned reservoir

Fig. 4.20 The amplitude and
duration of contractions
increase with increasing
volume (*#1,2,3*). When the
stretch becomes extreme
(*ventricular graph 4*) the
effect is reversed (*#4*), all of
the ventricle (Frank 1985)

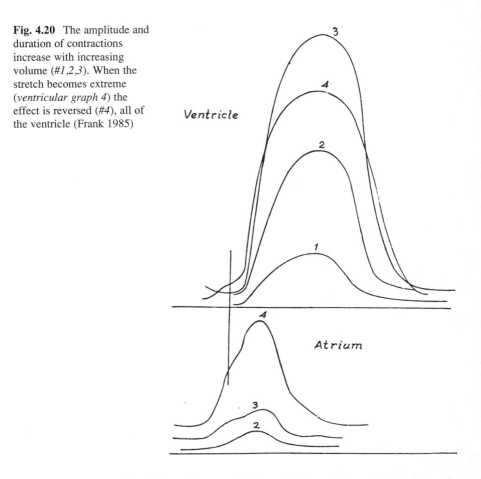

supplied with an adjustable outflow resistance. Filling of the right atrium was
provided from a low pressure reservoir, while the lungs were subjected to artificial
respiration. In these experiments, systemic arterial pressure was controlled by
manipulating the air pressure surrounding the partially collapsed tube, which
determines the outflow resistance (cf. Chap. 3). The volumes of the ventricles
were measured by means of a cardiometer.

In 1915, Starling presented two observations pertinent to the dynamic behavior
of the ventricles (Starling 1918). First, cardiac output initially increased rapidly, but
declined eventually, when venous inflow was augmented, while systemic arterial
pressure was maintained at the same level (Starling curve, Fig. 4.22). Starling
observed that the heart, when operating on the ascending limb, is therefore induced
to perform more work when inflow increases. The work per beat, W, can be
calculated from

$$W = \int_0^T p_{ao}(t)Q_{ej}(t)dt \qquad (4.2a)$$

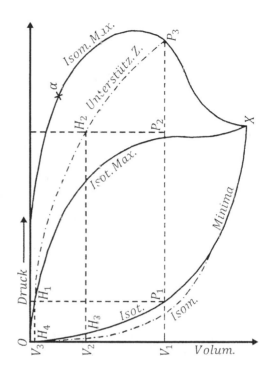

Fig. 4.21 Pressure
(*Druck*)–volume
(*Volum*)–time relations,
projected on the
pressure–volume plane, for
the excised frog heart beating
under a variety of conditions.
The top and bottom curves
relate maximum and
minimum pressures to
volume for isovolumic
(*Isom.*) contractions (Adapted
from Frank 1899)

or approximated by

$$W = \bar{p}_{ao} V_s \tag{4.2b}$$

where $p_{ao}(t)$ denotes instantaneous root aortic pressure, $\bar{p}_{ao}$, its mean value, $Q_{ej}(t)$ instantaneous ejection flow, V_s stroke volume, and T the duration of a heart cycle. Second, the experiment showed cardiac output to be nearly independent of aortic pressure (or total peripheral resistance) in the physiologic range, as long as inflow remained constant. In other words, cardiac output was found virtually insensitive to afterload, a term already used by Starling. Hence, it is the cardiac work which increases with increasing aortic pressure (Eqs. 4.2). Searching for the nature of the automatic arrangement that induces the heart to respond to such changing conditions, Starling concluded that "within physiological limits, the larger the volume of the heart, the greater are its energy of contraction and the amount of chemical change at each contraction."

The interpretation that left ventricular discharge is insensitive to conditions in the aorta is unwarranted in the breadth over which it has been applied. To illustrate, when end-diastolic volume is kept constant, rather than venous return, stroke volume drops with increasing peripheral resistance (Porter et al. 1982). With constant venous return, end-diastolic volume will find a new and stable steady state, compatible with cardiac output, equal to venous return, for a given arterial load as shown experimentally by Roy and Adami as early as 1888. Hence, if

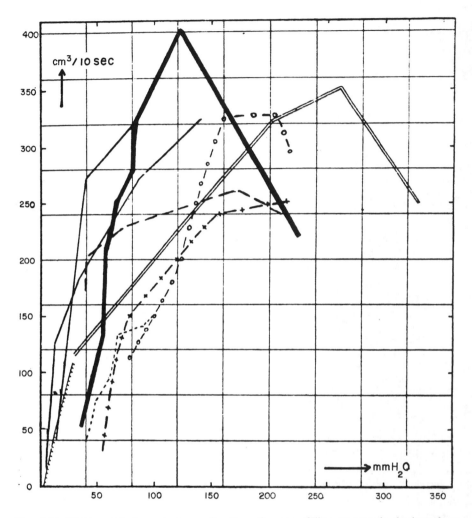

Fig. 4.22 Right ventricular output as a function of venous filling pressure in the heart-lung preparation of a dog (original axes interchanged. Modified from Patterson and Starling 1914)

end-diastolic volume is kept constant, discharge becomes a function of the arterial afterload in a futile effort to meet the compatibility requirement. Formulated differently, ventricular performance is sensitive to both upstream and downstream conditions, except under a few, very carefully selected, circumstances.

In the pumping ventricle, ventricular pressure, p_v, and ventricular volume, V_v, are both functions of time, t. By eliminating time, pressure can be plotted against volume (Fig. 4.23), resulting in the "work loop," so-called because the enclosed area equals the amount of work done by the ventricle while ejecting the stroke volume. In addition, the stroke volume can be read from the graph as well as maximum ventricular pressure reached, while the ejection fraction can be

Fig. 4.23 Idealized sketch of the (dynamic) ventricular work loop situated between the (static) maximally activated and relaxed states. At interval AB filling occurs. At interval CD emptying occurs

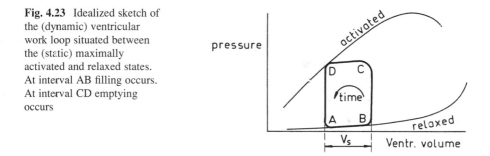

calculated. It has also been attempted to extract the contractile properties of the ventricle, but this effort was not altogether successful (Campbell et al. 1986).

To show why this was the case, it is instructive to look at the expressions employed. One possibility to describe global contractile properties is to define the ventricle's elastance, E_v, or its reciprocal, compliance C_v, as

$$E_v = \frac{1}{C_v} = \lim_{(\Delta V_v = 0)} \frac{\Delta p_v}{\Delta V_v} \qquad (4.3a)$$

where the limit denotes the ratio between an incremental change in pressure, Δp_v, and its accompanying incremental change in volume, ΔV_v. for ΔV_v going to zero. For the elastance, this may be rewritten as

$$dp_v = E_v dV_v \qquad (4.3b)$$

which may be integrated, provided that E_v is independent of volume, to yield

$$p_v = E_v V_v + k \qquad (4.3c)$$

with k serving as an integration constant equal to $-E_v V_c$ causing pressure to become zero for $V_v = V_c > 0$ instead of for $V_v = 0$. For elastance and compliance, it follows

$$E_v(t) = p_v(t)/(V_v(t) - V_c) \quad \text{and} \quad C_v(t) = (V_v(t) - V_c)/p_v(t) \qquad (4.3d, e)$$

two expressions that found extensive application for decades (Suga 1971; Sagawa et al. 1978).

Frank's work, however, clearly demonstrated that ventricular pressure is a strong function of both volume contained and of time, symbolically expressed as $p_v = p_v(V_v, t)$. This means that Eq. 4.3a needs accommodation to the fact that pressure is a function of at least two variables (Shoucri 1998). Hence,

$$\Delta p_v = \frac{\partial p_v}{\partial V_v} \Delta V_v + \frac{\partial p_v}{\partial t} \Delta t \qquad (4.4a)$$

which leads to

$$\frac{\Delta p_v}{\Delta V_v} = \frac{\partial p_v}{\partial V_v} + \frac{\partial p_v}{\partial t}\frac{\Delta t}{\Delta V_v} \qquad (4.4b)$$

Returning to the work loop, despite the considerations above, investigators attempted to extract C_v or E_v, basically applying Eq. 4.3a, though employing incremental differences for practical reasons. However, during ejection, $\frac{\Delta t}{\Delta V_v} = -\frac{1}{Q_{ej}}$, hence, the left-hand side of Eq. 4.4b is contaminated with arterial effects. This could be the reason why left ventricle–arterial system interaction manifests much complexity when Eq. 4.3d is invoked to analyze such interaction (Burkhoff et al. 1993). When all the valves are closed $\Delta V_v = 0$ and the left-hand side of Eq. 4.4b tends to $\pm$ infinity.

The original reasoning employed to describe quantitatively the pumping properties of the heart revolved around answering the question how much blood it pumped, or in other words, determining cardiac output (CO). Since CO $= f \times V_s$, where f denotes heart rate and V_s stroke volume, two avenues are open. One can either determine stroke volume and multiply by heart rate, which can be easily determined, or one can measure average flow over a period longer than the duration of one heart beat. Several methods have been worked out following both lines of thought and were adopted in practice (Noordergraaf A 1978). However crucial the amount of flow may be for the maintenance of the peripheral organs, it proved not to offer a useful measure of the quality of the pump itself. Other approaches were sought.

At first, investigators turned to the design and construction of fluid-mechanical models. This required overcoming a host of technical difficulties. When it was realized that the utilization of electrical or mathematical models should be more attractive, researchers turned toward such tools, immediately discovering a new problem of immense magnitude. When an electrical circuit is designed, or an equation is developed, the procedure requires specifications of precisely what elements make up the circuit, or which terms go into the equations. In other words, the designer or developer is forced to formulate his/her concept on how the biological object operates. Such requirements were far less stringent for fluid-mechanical models.

Buoncristiani et al.'s 1973 model of the left ventricle may serve as an illustration. Starting from the concept that the average ventricular pressure, $\bar{p}_v$ and source resistance R characterize the ventricle, their relationship with mean aortic pressure $\bar{p}_{ao}$ and average ejection flow $\bar{Q}$ was written as

$$\bar{p}_{ao} = \bar{p}_v - R\bar{Q} \qquad (4.5a)$$

If the pressure in the aorta is changed, this relationship modifies to

$$\bar{p}'_{ao} = \bar{p}_v - R\bar{Q}' \qquad (4.5b)$$

which yields two equations in the two surmised characteristics. They, $\bar{p}_v$ and R, proved, however, to be sensitive to the magnitude of the aortic pressure change. Of course, the implied statement of Eqs. 4.5 is that muscle is viewed as a viscoelastic material, which was rejected by Heidenheim in 1864 and repeatedly since, though it is an intuitively attractive way to automate the transition from the ventricular isovolumic pressure level to the pressure level normally observed during ejection.

As early as 1959, Warner reintroduced the concept that the ventricle should be considered as an elastic chamber of which the compliance, or its inverse, elastance, changed during the cycle. In a crude approximation, he assigned two values, one during systole and another during diastole and demonstrated the pumping property. After a number of suggestions by other investigators, this led to the proposal of a continuously time-varying elastance, $E_v(t)$, defined by Eq. 4.3d (Suga 1971; Suga and Sagawa 1974), which gained a high degree of popularity, particularly after the maximal value of the left-hand side was proposed as a measure of the contractile properties of the left ventricle. This maximal value was obtained from the slope of the tangent common to two or more work loops plotted for different end diastolic volumes. It took a few decades to realize that this seemingly straightforward definition of ventricular elastance, containing only ventricular quantities, was impure owing to its sensitivity to ejection flow, as discussed in the context of Eqs. 4.3 and 4.4 above.

When experimental difficulties arose in predicting ventricular pressure and volume from time-varying elastance (Eq. 4.4), recourse was once again taken to the addition of R, a viscous quantity. Campbell et al. (1985) compared the predictions of the best of 14 variations on Eqs. 4.3 with experiments and found all of them wanting, as demonstrated by their failure to predict flow accurately later in systole. In these studies, $E_v(t)$, once determined for a given heart, remained unchanged.

It will be recalled that the Frank mechanism deals with isovolumic contraction while Starling's observations focus on the ejecting ventricle. Both phenomena can be integrated into a single analytical expression describing ventricular pressure, p_v, as a function of ventricular volume, V_v, time, t, and ejection flow, Q_{ej}. This can then be formally written as $p_v(V_v,t,Q_{ej})$. In this equation, ventricular volume and ejection flow may be time dependent. Once the parameters of a given ventricle have been determined, ventricular elastance E_v (and compliance C_v), including their variation with time, can be computed for the entire heart cycle.

In a first step to determining whether this is in fact true, Mulier (1994), like several earlier workers, noted the nonlinear relation between canine diastolic ventricular pressure and volume. This was written as

$$p_v(V_v) = \pm a(V_v - b)^2 \tag{4.6a}$$

The parameter a relates to diastolic compliance, and b denotes the diastolic volume for which pressure equals zero. The negative sign applies only when $V_v < b$, thereby reintroducing suction (Ingels et al. 1996, and, by implication, by Little (1949) for the atria as well). Half a century earlier, Goltz and Gaule reported in dogs a left ventricular suction pressure of 52, in the right ventricle of 17 and in the right atrium of 11 mmHg.) Suction played a key role in Galenus' theory, but was rejected by Harvey (Chap. 2).

Fig. 4.24 Isovolumic
ventricular pressure, p_{iso},
ejecting ventricular pressure,
p_v, and root aortic pressure,
p_{ao}, computed from Eq. 4.6b
for a set of control parameter
values. The ventricle ejects
into a three-element arterial
model (Fig. 5.8). Note the
difference between the
amplitudes of the ventricular
pressures (From Danielsen
and Ottesen 2001)

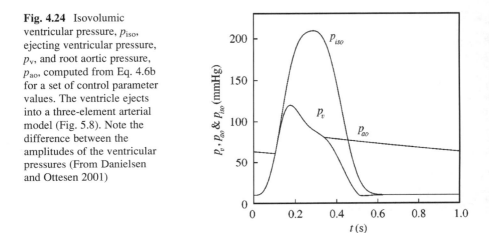

The next step, also executed by Mulier, considers isovolumic contraction in isolated dog hearts. Attachment and detachment of bonds is described by exponential functions, one for each, the steepness of which and their separation in time can be adjusted as mandated by the chamber under study. The experiments indicated that systolic ventricular pressure, known to be a strong function of the volume contained, V_v, and of time, t, could be described by a term to be added to the right-hand side of Eq. 4.6a, yielding

$$p_v(V_v, t) = \pm a(V_v - b)^2 + (cV_v - d)f(t) \qquad (4.6b)$$

in which the parameters c and d determine the volume associated and nonvolume associated components of developed pressure, while $f(t)$ is a normalized function describing transient crossbridge formation and detachment by exponential functions of the type $1 - \exp - (t/\tau_c)$, which are more completely formulated in Sect. 11.3. The time constants τ_c and τ_r characterize attachment and detachment processes, while α is a measure of their overall rates of development and τ_d the time delay (of about 0.3 s) between the onsets of attachment and detachment (Palladino 1990; Danielsen 1998; Palladino et al. 1997, 2000b; Eqs. 11.9a, b and 11.10).

When this description of the isovolumically contracting ventricle is furnished with a source of venous blood and a representation of the arterial system, it operates as a pump displaying Starling's law. Hence Starling's law may be considered an extension of the Frank mechanism, which, in a strict biophysical sense, disqualifies it as a "law." Their combination was, for a time, referred to as the Frank–Starling mechanism, or the generalized Frank mechanism. As is illustrated in Fig. 4.24, Eq. 4.6b embodies the major features of a normal pumping ventricle, excluding the effect of the respiration. Specifically, the large drop in pressure from the isovolumic level is accounted for by the decrease in volume contained by the cavity. But detailed scrutiny of the pressure and ejection flow curves during their downstrokes shows them to tend to concavity instead of to the convexity commonly observed in the experiment.

When a comparison is made between measured ventricular pressure and that predicted by Eq. 4.6b the so-called ejection effect is exposed: early into ejection, the predicted pressure is higher, later in ejection it is lower. The two differences are denoted "deactivation" and "hyperactivation," respectively. Together they constitute the ejection effect. This creates the possibility to differentiate between isovolumic contraction properties and those during (significant) muscle shortening.

To describe the ejection effect quantitatively, Eq. 4.6b requires modification of $f(t)$ by the introduction of ejection flow. It then becomes

$$p_v\left(V_v, t, Q_{ej}\right) = \pm a(V_v - b)^2 + (cV_v - d)F_1(t, Q_{ej}) \qquad (4.6c)$$

with

$$F_1 = f(t) - k_1 Q_{ej}(t) + k_2 Q_{ej}(t - \tau)$$

or

$$p_v\left(V_v, t, Q_{ej}\right) = \pm a(V_v - b)^2 + (cV_v - d)F_2\left(t, Q_{ej}\right) \qquad (4.6d)$$

where

$$F_2 = f(t) - k_1' Q_{ej}(t) + k_2' Q_{ej}^2(t - \tau)$$

Each generalization contains three additional parameters, which characterize the ejection effect, and move the ejecting ventricle further away from viewing it as a pressure source. Both generalized expressions reduce to Eq. 4.6b when ejection flow is zero. Figure 4.25 illustrates the effect of the introduction of ejection flow (Danielsen and Ottesen 2001; Rabbany et al. 2001; Palladino and Noordergraaf A 2002). The sensitivity of pressure to ejection flow testifies that the ventricles are not pressure sources, despite published assurances that they are. Sample computations indicated that inclusion or exclusion of both k'_1 and k'_2 modified external work of the left ventricle insignificantly, suggesting a shift of energy along the time axis. Equations 4.6a–d for ventricular pressure and its generalizations permit the computation of ventricular elastance during the entire heart cycle. Utilizing a classical definition,

$$E_v(t) = \frac{\partial p_v}{\partial V_v} \qquad (4.7)$$

It may be noted that the first term on the right of Eqs. 4.6 remains unchanged. Differentiation yields
for Eq. 4.6b:

$$E_v(t) = 2a|V_v - b| + cf(t)$$

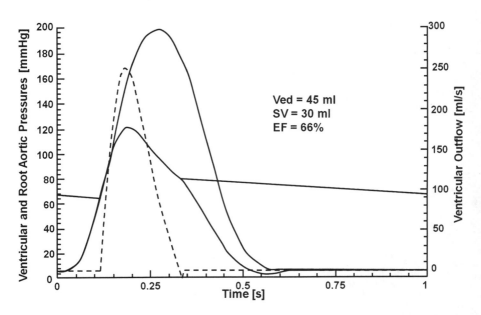

Fig. 4.25 Computed ventricular and root aortic pressures with inclusion of the ejection effect as described by Eq. 4.7c. Note the change from concave downstroke in pressure and flow (the latter not shown here) to the familiar convex patterns for both pressure and flow. (From Danielsen and Ottesen 2001.) The nonlinear ejection effect (Eq. 4.7d) tends to enhance the differences

for Eqs. 4.6c

$$E_v(t) = 2a|V_v - b| + cF_1$$

and 4.6d:

$$E_v(t) = 2a|V_v - b| + cF_2,$$

respectively.

Introduction of the ejection effect makes $E_v(t)$ asymmetric.

This description of the ventricle, or any cardiac chamber for that matter, contains 11 parameters, all of which have identifiable physiological meanings. The sizable number offers the flexibility to accommodate a number of different phenomena as follows: two parameters (a and b) for the characterization of the chamber's diastolic properties, four parameters τ_c, τ_r, τ_α, and t_d for crossbridge movement, two (c and d) for the magnitude of systolic pressure augmentation, and three (two k's and τ) for the characterization of the ejection effect.

To enable evaluation by parameter values for a particular ventricle, its volume and pressure must be measured throughout the heart cycle for both ejecting and isovolumic beats. The same approach, characterization based on parameters instead of variables, was recently advanced for muscle strip (Palladino and Noordergraaf 2007) and is

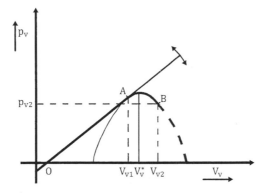

Fig. 4.26 This drawing details the procedure described in the text on how the downturn in the top curve of Fig. 9.1 may be introduced. Ventricular volume, V_v, and pressure, p_v, make up the axes. The active term in Eq. 4.7d is shown at one instant in time; it rotates around point O as time progresses. The downturn in pressure at high ventricular volume, or for a weakened heart, is part of the parabola depicted (Eq. 4.9). The heavy line identifies point A where the transition occurs

expected to yield a unifying theory for all ventricular properties. Utilization of variables invites nonuniqueness in the definition of properties.

The first term on the right of Eq. 4.6d is quadratic and indicates stiffening of the passive wall as volume increases. The second term needs adaptation to limit the range over which the active pressure–volume relation is approximately linear (Fig. 4.23). This modification may be achieved, e.g., as depicted in Fig. 4.26 by the heavy line, which attaches the linear function to part of a parabola. Both the function itself and its volume derivative should be continuous at the transition point A, where ventricular volume equals V_{v1}.

The parabola is described by

$$p_v = m_1 V_v{}^2 + m_2 V_v + m_3 \tag{4.8}$$

with the coefficients m_1, m_2, m_3, and the volume V_{v1} to be determined.

The directional coefficients at A, $2m_1 V_{v1} + m_2$ (from differentiating Eq. 4.8) and $cF_2(t)$ (from the time-variant linear function) must be equal

$$2m_1 V_{v1} + m_2 = cF_2(t) \tag{4.9a}$$

$V_v{}^*$, the volume at which the parabola peaks, is assumed to be known and independent of pressure. At this peak, the derivative of Eq. 4.8 equals zero

$$2m_1 V_{v1}{}^* + m_2 = 0 \tag{4.9b}$$

At point B, with known coordinates $[V_{v2}, p_{v2}]$ on the parabola, it holds that

$$p_{v2} = m_1 V_{v2}{}^2 + m_2 V_{v2} + m_3 \tag{4.9c}$$

Furthermore, point A must lie on both the quadratic and the linear graphs

$$m_1 V_{v1}^2 + m_2 V_{v1} + m_3 = (cV_{v1} - d)F_2(t) \tag{4.9d}$$

Equations 4.9 provide four algebraic equations in the four unknowns. The pressure $p_v(V_{v1})$ at any point in time during the heart beat follows directly. Further generalizations will appear in Sect. 8.2.

In the preceding approach the shape of the ventricle does not explicitly enter into the analysis. Knap et al. (2002) placed the emphasis primarily on shape, which refers to an observation first made by Harvey (1628). Harvey noted that the ejecting ventricle becomes smaller and more elongated. Nevertheless, the left ventricle was often considered to be spherical, especially after it had been pointed out that tangential stress in its (passive) wall is only half that in a cylinder for the same value of $(r/h)p_v$, where h denotes wall thickness (Laplace's law). Consideration of minimum values went through a popular period. Eventually, it was recognized that the spherical ventricle presents itself when it is in failure. Hence, the measurement of shape may yield clinical information. Ultrasound technology permits the collection of such information in a noninvasive procedure. Knap et al. proposed as a measure, or index, elongation (ELO), defined as

$$ELO = \frac{SLv_{exper} - SLv_{theor}}{SLv_{theor}} \tag{4.10}$$

where SLv_{exper} denotes the measured internal surface area of the left ventricle and SLv_{theory} that of an equivolumic sphere. Thus, ELO equals 0 for a spherical ventricle. The more elongated the ventricle the higher the value of the index becomes. Figure 4.27 displays ELOs for three groups of humans measured at end diastole and end systole, i.e., at maximum and minimum volumes. The results indicate that higher end-systolic values are associated with healthier conditions. Both more complex and simpler alternative indices and measurement techniques have been proposed in recent years.

During the second half of the twentieth century, numerous investigators became interested in the question whether measurement of pressure within the wall of the ventricle (intramyocardial pressure, IMP, or p_{im}) might give information about the contractile properties of the ventricle. This led to the employment of a wide variety of transducers, the sensitive element of which was imbedded in the wall. All investigators found that $p_{im} \geq 0$, while displaying a strong negative gradient in the direction of the pericardium. There was, however major disagreement on whether or not its systolic peak exceeds peak cavity pressure. Experimental results were about equally divided between the two possibilities. Further work resolved this issue: embedded sensors that made contact with contracting fibers recorded the high values, while those that did not recorded the low values (Rabbany et al. 1989).

The search for the origin of the measured intramyocardial pressure required the determination of wall stresses via

$$p_{im} = -\frac{\sigma_r + \sigma_t + \sigma_l}{3} \tag{4.11}$$

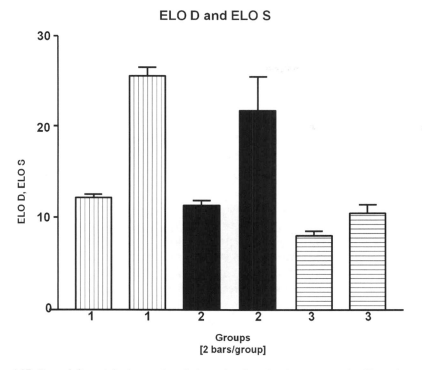

Fig. 4.27 From *left* to *right* three pairs of elongation bars for three groups, healthy volunteers ($N = 29$), patients with hypertension and occasional signs of heart failure ($N = 10$), patients in severe failure ($N = 10$). The *left* bar of each pair was measured at end-diastole and indicates a more spherical ventricle than its end-systolic companion. Vertical scale displays *ELO* in percentage values of Eq. 4.11 (From Knap et al. 2002)

where the indices refer to coordinates in the radial, tangential, and longitudinal directions in the tissue surrounding a small pocket of fluid within the wall (Sommerfeld 1947).

Computation of p_{im} in a thick-walled multilayered cylinder of solid material with a time varying elastic modulus $E(t)$, as well as in a similar sphere, showed it to be negative. Insertion of a fluid film between adjacent layers left the pressure in the tissue pocket negative, but made it positive in the fluid films, both exhibiting a radial gradient. These observations led to a fundamental change in the approach to modeling. Reasons for difficulties are that in many models, cause and effect are interchanged which proves to carry penalties. If cavity pressure is made the independent variable, systolic increase in cavity pressure then becomes responsible for negative pressure in a tissue pocket. Reduction of cavity pressure to zero reduces wall stresses to zero, meaning that coronary flow should not be impeded during systole, while intramyocardial pressure should remain at zero. Both are contradicted by the experiment. Consequently, contraction and relaxation of the wall material must be viewed as the cause, the rise and fall in ventricular pressure its effect. Commencing with the contracting and relaxing myocyte resolves the problems cited (Rabbany 1991; Rabbany et al. 2000). Robinson (1963), Chadwick (1982), and Hunter and Smaill (1988) took a broader approach by proposing left ventricular models in which the relaxed and the time-varying activated ventricular pressure–volume relations (Fig. 4.23) serve as independent variables.

Although much confusion, both experimental and conceptual, has been eliminated, the measurement of intramyocardial pressure has yet to achieve clinical status.

4.4   Coronary Blood Supply

The coronary vasculature provides the critical supply route for the heart muscle's needs. It is unique in the sense that it provides most of the requirements for the heart to pump against the load from which its own perfusion pressure derives. As such it has, for a long time, been scrutinized for its physiological properties, and then, beginning a century ago, became of interest to the clinician in tests for coronary flow obstruction in the human. More recently, when it became possible to bypass or remove partial or complete arterial obstructions, cardiovascular surgeons joined the interested parties.

The coronary bed presents a more sophisticated area for the determination of pressure–flow relations as a consequence of the fact that flow impedance is time varying. Flow through the coronary vessels is a function of the difference between upstream (root aortic) pressure and downstream (mostly atrial) pressure. As in other vascular beds, the diameter of the smaller arteries is subject to vasomotor changes induced by nervous and humoral, including autoregulatory, influences. The major variation, particularly for the left ventricle, is introduced by the rhythmic contraction and relaxation of the myocardium, in which an overwhelming number of the coronary vessels is embedded. As early as 1689, Scaramucci advanced the theory that coronary vessels are squeezed empty by the contraction of the heart and perfused again during diastole, but Ström (1679–1710) claimed that the aortic valve leaflets, when in the open position, obstruct coronary artery inflow. Bellhouse and Bellhouse (1969) focused attention on the location of the coronary ostia in relation to the formation of a vortex in the coronary sinuses, which invalidated Ström's anatomical interpretation at least for the normal aortic valve. It took until 1898 for Porter, in the premier volume of the American Journal of Physiology, to provide an experimental foundation for Scaramucci's theory. The changes in coronary flow imposed by this extravascular mechanical effect are large, depend on the systolic blood pressure level, which in turn depends on root aortic pressure (Anrep and Häusler 1928) and occur in the frequency of the heart beat.

Two major groups of theories may be recognized in the efforts to explain the observed reduction, or even reversal, of coronary arterial inflow and the simultaneous enhancement of venous efflux during ventricular systole. One is the so-called vascular waterfall concept (Sect. 3.3.2) introduced by Downey and Kirk (1975) to the analysis of the coronary circulation. Its inability to explain a number of well-established experimental observations led to its eventual demise in this area.

The second group of theories is referred to as the intramyocardial pump concept proposed by Spaan et al. (1981). This concept, clearly reminiscent of Scaramucci's and Porter's classical work, proved to be far more powerful, especially after the introduction of nonlinear features of compliance and resistance by making them dependent on prevailing transmural pressure of coronary vessels. Gordon (1974) generated the first model of the coronary circulation, which, though very simple, he found to offer a useful conceptual framework for interpreting or predicting responses of the coronary circulation. Kenner had shown earlier, on the basis of wave transmission considerations, that inflow of a vessel can be inhibited by time-varying changes of its peripheral resistance (1969).

All of these models suffer from severe lumping and the absence of a vascular network, which impede interpretation. A far more detailed, recent model will be found in Sect. 6.3.

4.5   Conclusions

The heart never relinquished its central role in the circulation despite extensive discussions of its characteristics. Contraction and relaxation are its two most conspicuous functions and should require two identifiable triggers. The unique second trigger required for relaxation has largely escaped resolution, even though there is no discussion about the fact that the heart relaxes.

The contraction and relaxation discussion exemplifies the requirement for a scientist to inspect and explore each separate aspect and function while retaining an overview of the circulation as a whole. This may result in a seemingly separate function becoming an instability caused by a prior activity.

4.6   Summary

The heart is the focus of this chapter. Torrent-Guasp's discovery of a band structure constituting the ventricular chambers, and subsequently for the atria as well, made it possible to formulate a detailed model to analyze contraction and relaxation phenomena for part of the ventricular walls. This large model contains around 5,000 bonds based on Huxley's crossbridge concept. Operation of this model yielded the, by that time, well-established experimental force–length relations. It also offered an explanation of why muscle, once stimulated, relaxes without requiring a long searched after provision of a separate trigger: contracted heart muscle is inherently unstable.

The insight gained afforded major reduction and reformulation of the cardiac chambers formulations to give them a workable size, first for a passive chamber, then generalized to include contraction and relaxation. This incorporated the ventricles' ejection effect and atrial suction, the latter at one time condemned by Harvey, while offering a method to quantify ventricular elastance for the full cardiac cycle.

References

Anrep, von G. and Häusler H.: The coronary circulation. I. The effect of changes of the blood-pressure and of the output of the heart. J. Physiol. 65: 357–373, 1928.

Arts T., Veenstra P.C. and Reneman R.S.: Epicardial deformation and left ventricular wall mechanics during ejection in the dog. Am. J. Physiol. 243 (Heart Circ. Physiol. 12): H379–H390, 1982.

Bellhouse B. and Bellhouse F.: Fluid mechanics of model normal and stenosed aortic valves. Circ. Res. 25: 693–704, 1969.

Brady A.J.: Time and displacement dependence of cardiac contractility: problems in defining the active state and force-velocity relations. Fed. Proc. 24: 1410–1420, 1966.

Braunwald E., Ross J. Jr. and Sonnenblick E.H.: Mechanism of Contraction in the Normal and Failing Heart. Little, Brown, Boston, Massachusetts, 1968.

Brutsaert D.L., Clerck De N.M., Goethals M.A. and Housmans P.R.: Relaxation of ventricular cardiac muscle. J. Physiol. 283: 469–480, 1978.

Buoncristiani J.F., Liedtke A.J., Strong R.M. and Urschel C.W.: Parameter estimates of a left ventricular model during ejection. IEEE Trans. Biomed. Eng. BME-20:110–114, 1973.

Burch G.E., Ray C.T., Cronvich J.A.: The George Fahr Lecture. Certain mechanical peculiarities of the human cardiac pump in normal and diseased states. Circulation V: 504–513, 1952.

Burger H.C.: Heart and Vector. Physical Basis of Electrocardiography. H.W. Julius, (ed.), Gordon & Breach, New York, 1968.

Burkhoff D., Tombe de P.P. and Hunter W.C.: Impact of ejection on magnitude and time course of ventricular pressure-generating capacity. Am. J. Physiol. 265 (Heart Circ. Physiol. 34): H899–H909, 1993.

Campbell K.B., Ringo J.A., Knowlen G.G., Kirkpatrick R.D. and Schmidt S.L.: Validation of optional elastance-resistance left ventricle pump models. Am. J. Physiol. 251 (Heart Circ. Physiol. 20):H382–H397, 1986.

Caulfield J.B. and Borg T.K.: The collagen network of the heart. Lab. Invest. 40: 364–372, 1979.

Chadwick R.S.: Mechanics of the left ventricle. Biophys. J. 39: 279–288, 1982.

Cyon E.: Über den Einfluss der Temperaturänderungen auf Zahl, Dauer und Stärke der Herzschläge. Berichte Ueber die Verh. der Königlich. Sächsischen Ges. der Wissenschaften zu Leipzig. Math.-Phys. Classe 18: 256–306, 1866.

Dalecki D., Keller B.B., Carstensen E.L., Neel D.S., Palladino J.L. and Noordergraaf A.: Thresholds for premature ventricular contractions in frog hearts exposed to lithotripter fields. Ultrasound Med. Biol. 17: 341–346, 1991.

Dalecki D., Raeman C.H., Child S.Z. and Carstensen E.L.: Effects of pulsed ultrasound on the frog heart: the radiation force mechanism. Ultrasound Med. Biol. 23: 275–285, 1997.

Danielsen M.: Modeling of Feedback Mechanisms which Control the Heart Function in a View to an Implementation in Cardiovascular Models. Ph.D. Dissertation, Roskilde Univ., 1998.

Danielsen M. and Ottesen J.T.: Describing the pumping heart as a pressure source. J. Theor. Biol. 212: 71–81, 2001.

De Pater L. and Berg van den J.W.: An electrical analogue of the entire human circulatory system. Med. Electron. Biol. Eng. 2: 161–166, 1964.

Downey J.M. and Kirk E.S.: Inhibition of coronary flow by a vascular waterfall mechanism. Circ. Res. 36: 753–760, 1975.

Durrer D., Dam van R.T.H., Freud G.E., Janse M.J., Meijler F.L. and Arzbaecher R.C.: Total excitation of the isolated human heart. Circulation 41: 899–912, 1970.

Einthoven W., Fahr G. und Waart de A.: Über die Richtung und die manifeste Grösse der Potentialschwankungen im menschlichen Herzen und Über den Einfluss der Herzlage auf die Form des Elektrokardiogramms. Pflügers Arch. gesamte Physiol. Menschen Tiere 150: 275–315, 1913.

Elliott G.F., Rome E.M., Spencer M.: A type of contraction hypothesis applicable to all muscles. Nature 226: 417–420, 1970.

Fick A.: Mechanische Arbeit und Wärmeentwickelung bei der Muskelthätigkeit. Brockhaus, Leipzig, 1882.

Frank O.: Die Grundform des arteriellen Pulses. Z. Biol. 37: 433–526, 1899.

Frank O.: Zur Dynamik des Herzmuskels. Z. Biol. (Munich) 32: 370–447, 1895. [English transl.: C.B. Chapman and E. Wasserman: Am. Heart J. 58: 282–317, 467–478, 1959.

Gasser H.S. and Hill A.V.: The dynamics of muscular contraction. J. Physiol. 96: 398–437, 1924.

Glitsch H.G.: Characteristics of Active Sodium Transport in Intact Cardiac Cells. Chapter 2 in: Excitation and Neural Control of the Heart. M.N. Levy and M. Vassalle (eds.), Amer. Physiol. Soc., Bethesda MD, 1982.

Goltz Fr. and Gaule J.: Über die Druckverhältnisse im Innern des Herzens. Archiv für die gesammte Physiologie 17: 100–120, 1878.

Gordon R.J.: A general mathematical model of coronary circulation. Am. J. Physiol. 226: 608–615, 1974.

Gordon A.M., Huxley A.F. and Julian F.J.: The variation in isometric tension with sarcomere length in vertebrate muscle fibers. J. Physiol. 184: 170–192, 1966.

Harvey G.: Exercitatio Anatomica, De Motu Cordis et Sanguiris in Animalibus, Frankford, 1628.

Heidenhain R.: Mechanische Leistung, Wärmeentwicklung und Stoffumsatz bei der Muskeltätigkeit. Ein Beitrag zur Theorie der Muskelkräfte. Breitkopf und Härtel, Leipzig, 1864.

Helmholtz H.: Über den Stoffverbrauch bei der Muskelaktion. Müller's Arch. Anat. Physiol. 72–83, 1845.

Helmholtz H.: Über die Wärmeentwickelung der Muskelaction. Müller's Arch. Anat. Physiol. 144–164, 1848.

Hill A.V.: The heat of shortening and the dynamic constants cf muscle. Proc. Roy. Soc. London, Sect. B 126:136–195, 1939.

Hoffman B.F.: Effects of Digitalis on Electrical Activity of Cardiac Fibers. In: Digitalis. C. Fisch and B. Surawicz (eds.), Grune and Stratton, New York, 1969.

Hunter P.J. and Smaill B.H.: The analysis of cardiac function: a continuum approach. Progr. in Biophys. and Mol. Biol. 52: 101–164, 1988.

Huxley H.E.: Structural arrangements and the contraction mechanism in striated muscle. Proc. Roy. Soc. Lond. B, 160:442–448, 1964.

Huxley H.E.: The mechanism of muscle contraction. Science 164:1356–1366, 1969.

Huxley A.F. and Simmons R.M.: Proposed mechanism of force generation in striated muscle. Nature (London) 233: 533–538, 1971.

Huxley A.F. and Simmons R.M.: Mechanical transients and the origin of muscular force. Cold Spring Harbor Symp. Quant. Biol. 37: 669–680, 1973.

Ingels N.P. Jr. and Thompson N.P.: An electrokinematic theory of muscle contraction. Nature 211:1032–1035, 1966.

Ingels N.B. Jr., Daughters G.T., Nikolic S.D., DeAnda A., Moon M.R., Bolger A.F., Komeda M., Derby G.C., Yellin E.L. and Miller D.C.: Left ventricular diastolic suction with zero left atrial pressure in open-chest dogs. Am. J. Physiol. 270 (Heart Circ. Physiol. 39): H1217–H1224, 1996.

Iwazumi T.: A New Field Theory for Muscle Contraction. Ph.D. Dissertation, Univ. of Pennsylvania, 1970.

Iwazumi T.: Molecular Mechanism of Muscle Contraction: Another View. Ch. 2 in: Cardiovascular System Dynamics, J. Baan et al. (eds.), MIT Press, Cambridge, 1978.

Kenner T.: The dynamics of pulsatile flow in the coronary arteries. Pflügers Arch. 310: 22–34, 1969.

Knap B., Juznic G., Bren A.F., Drzewiecki G. and Noordergraaf A.: Elongation as a new shape index for the left ventricle. Int. J. Cardiov. Imaging 18: 421–430, 2002.

Laulanié F.: Principes et problèmes de la thermodynamique musculaire d'après les récents traveaux de M. Chaveau. Rev. Vét. 15: 505–514, 1890.

Lev M. and Simkins C.S.: Architecture of the human ventricular myocardium. Lab. Invest. 5: 395–409, 1956.

Little R.C.: Volume elastic properties of the right and left atrium. Am. J. Physiol. 158: 237–240, 1949.

Lower R.: Tractatus de Corde. Elzevier, Amsterdam, 1669.

Mayow J.: 1674. English translation published as reprint no. 17 by the Alembic Club under the title: On Molecular Motion and Animal Spirits *in*: Medical-physical works, 1907.

Meyer K.H.: über Feinbau, Festigkeit und Kontraktilität tierischer Gewebe. Biochem. Zs. 214: 253–281, 1929.

Mulier J.P.: Ventricular Pressure as a Function of Volume and Flow. Ph.D. dissertation. Catholic Univ. of Leuven, 1994.

Nielsen P.M.F., le Grice I.J., Smaill B.H. and Hunter P.J.: Mathematical model of geometry and fibrous structure of the heart. Am. J. Physiol. 260 (Heart Circ. Physiol. 29): H1365–H1378, 1991.

Noble M.I.M. and Pollack G..H.: Molecular mechanisms of contraction. Circ. Res. 40: 333–342, 1977.

Noordergraaf A.: Circulatory System Dynamics. Academic Press, New York NY, 1978.

Palladino J.L.: Models of Cardiac Muscle Contraction and Relaxation. Ph.D. dissertation, Univ. of Pennsylvania, 1990.

Palladino J.L. and Noordergraaf A.: Muscle Contraction Mechanics from Ultrastructural Dynamics. Chapter 3 *in*: Analysis and Assessment of Cardiovascular Function. G.M. Drzewiecki and J.K-J. Li (eds.), Springer, New York NY, 1998.

Palladino J.L. and Noordergraaf A.: A paradigm for quantifying ventricular contraction. Cell. Mol. Biol. Letters 7: 331–335, 2002.

Palladino J.L. and Noordergraaf A.: Defining muscle elastance as a parameter. Proc. 29th Ann. Int. Conf. IEEE EMBS, pages 5315–5318, Lyon, France, 2007.

Palladino J.L., Rabbany S.Y., Mulier J.P. and Noordergraaf A.: A perspective on myocardial contractility. J. Techn. Health Care 5: 135–144, 1997.

Palladino J.L., Drzewiecki G.M. and Noordergraaf A.: Modeling Strategies in Physiology. Chapter 158 *in*: Biomedical Engineering Handbook. J.D. Bronzino, (ed.), CRC Press, Boca Raton FL, 2000a.

Palladino J.L., Ribeiro L.C. and Noordergraaf A.: Human Circulatory System Model Based on Frank's Mechanism. Pp. 29–40 *in:* Mathematical Modelling in Medicine, J.T. Ottesen and M. Danielsen (eds.), IOS Press, Amsterdam, 2000b.

Parmley W.W., Brutsaert D.L. and Sonnenblick E.H.: Effect of altered loading on contractile events in isolated cat papillary muscle. Circ. Res. 24: 521–532, 1969.

Patterson S.W. and Starling E.H.: On the mechanical factors which determine the output of the ventricles. J. Physiol. 48: 357–379, 1914.

Pettigrew J.B.: On the arrangement of the muscular fibres in the ventricles of the vertebrate heart, with physiological remarks. Philosophical Trans. 154: 445–500, 1864.

Polissar M.J.: Physical chemistry of contractile process in muscle. I. A physicochemical model of contractile mechanism. Am. J. Physiol. 168: 766–781, 1952.

Pollack G.H.: Muscles & Molecules. Ebner & Sons, Seattle WA, 1990.

Porter P.K., Ryan W.A. Jr., Melbin J. and Noordergraaf A.: Features of compliance pumping. *In*: Frontiers of Engineering in Health Care, A.R. and J.H. Potvin (eds.), IEEE Eng. Med. Biol. Soc., pp. 176–180, 1982.

Quick C.M., Li J.K-J. and Noordergraaf A.: The three element model approximated from myocyte properties. Thirteenth Southern Biomed. Eng. Conf., J. Vossoughi (ed.), Washington DC, pp. 816–819, 1994.

Quick C.M., Berger D.S., Stewart R.H., Laine G.A., Hartley C.J. and Noordergraaf A.: Resolving the hemodynamic inverse problem. IEEE Trans. Biomed. Eng. 53: 361–368, 2006.

Rabbany S.Y.: The Genesis of Intramyocardial Pressure. Ph.D. Dissertation, Univ. of Pennsylvania, Philadelphia PA, 1991.

Rabbany S.Y., Kresh J.Y. and Noordergraaf A.: Intramyocardial pressure: interaction of myocardial pressure and fiber stress. Am. J. Physiol. 257 (Heart Circ. Physiol. 26): H357-H364, 1989.

Rabbany S.Y., Kresh J.Y., Noordergraaf A.: Myocardial wall stress: evaluation and management. Cardiovasc. Engineering 5: 3–10, 2000.

Rabbany S.Y., Danielsen M. and Noordergraaf A.: A brief assessment of myocardial viability in surgically remodeled hearts. Cardiov. Engineering 1: 155–161, 2001.

Robinson D.A.: Ventricular Dynamics and the Cardiac Representation Problem. In: Circulatory Analog Computers. A. Noordergraaf, G.N. Jager, N. Westerhof (eds.). North-Holland Publ. Co., Amsterdam, 1963.

Roy C.S.: On the influences which modify the work of the heart. J. Physiol. 1: 452–496, 1879.

Roy C.S. and Adami J.G.: Remarks on failure of the heart from overstrain. Brit. Med. J. ii: 1321–1326, 1888.

Sagawa K., Suga H. and Nakayama K.: Instantaneous pressure-volume ratio of the ventricle versus instantaneous force-length relation of papillary muscle. In: Cardiovascular System Dynamics, J. Baan et al., (eds.), MIT Press, Cambridge MA, 1978.

Scher A.M.: Newer Data on Myocardial Excitation. In: Electrophysiology of the Heart. B. Taccardi and G. Marchetti (eds.), Pergamon Press, Oxford, 1965.

Shear D.B.: Electrostatic forces in muscle contraction. J. Theor. Biol. 28:531–546, 1970

Shoucri R.M.: Studying the mechanics of left ventricular contraction. The relation between the active force of the myocardium and the pressure-volume relation. IEEE Eng. Med. Biol. 17: 95–101, 1998.

Sommerfeld A.: Vorlesungen über Theoretische Physik. Band II, Dieterich'sche Verlagsbuch-handlung, Wiesbaden, 1947.

Sonnenblick E.H.: Force-velocity relations in mammalian heart muscle. Am. J. Physiol. 202: 931–939, 1962.

Spaan J.A.E., Breuls N.P.W. and Laird J.D.: Diasolic-systolic coronary flow differences are caused by intramyocardial pump action in the anesthetized dog. Circ. Res. 49: 584–593, 1981.

Spencer M. and Worthington C.R.: A hypothesis of contraction in striated muscle. Nature 187: 388–391, 1960.

Starling E.H.: The Linacre Lecture on the Law of the Heart. Delivered at St. John's College, Cambridge, 1915. Longmans, Green, London, 1918.

Streeter D.D., Powers W.E., Ross M.A. and Torrent-Guasp F.: Three-dimensional fiber orientation in the mammalian left-ventricular wall. In: Cardiovascular System Dynamics. J. Baan et al., (eds.) MIT Press, Cambridge MA, 1978.

Ström C.M.: Cited by A. von Haller in: Elementa Physiologicae Corporis Humani, Vol. I, Section V, p. 499. Bousquet, Lausanne, Switserland, 1762.

Suga H.: Theoretical analysis of a left-ventricular pumping model based on the systolic time-varying pressure/volume ratio. IEEE Trans. Biomed. Eng. 8: 47–55, 1971.

Suga H. and Sagawa K.: Instantaneous pressure-volume relationship and their ratio in the excised, supported canine left ventricle. Circ. Res. 35: 117–126, 1974.

Swammerdam J.: Biblia Nature. Severinus, Leiden, 1737 (Vols. 2 and 3).

Torrent-Guasp F.: La estructuracion macroscopia del miocardio ventricular. Revista Espanola de Cardiologia 33: 265–287, 1980.

Torrent-Guasp F.F.E.S.C., W.F. Whimster, K. Redmann: A silicone rubber mould of the heart. Technology and Health Care 5: 13–20, 1997.

Tsien R.W. and Hess P.: Excitable Tissues. The Heart. In: Physiology of Membrane Disorders, 2nd edition, T.E. Andreoli, J.F. Hoffman, D.D. Fanestil and S.G. Schultz (eds.), Plenum Medical Bock Co., New York, 1986.

Weber E.: Muskelbewegung. In: Handwörterbuch der Physiologie, Vol. 3. B. R. Wagner (ed.), Vieweg, Braunschweig, 1846.

Wilson L.G.: William Croone's Theory of Muscular Contraction. Notes and Records of the Royal Society of London, 16: 158, 1961.

Winegrad S.: Resting sarcomere length-tension relation in l ving frog heart. J. Gen. Physiol. 64:343–355, 1974.

Appendix

Questions

4.1 Tigerstedt, in his 1921 textbook, proposed an expression for the calculation of the total force F, also referred to as the total ventricular load, generated, or carried, by a spherical ventricle. This expression was given the form of $F = p_v S$, where p_v denotes ventricular pressure and S the ventricle's internal wall area. Burch et al. (1952) found that F may actually be smaller during systole than during diastole and called this a "unique characteristic for the cardiac pump." Is Burch's conclusion surprising, or is Tigerstedt's equation flawed?

4.2 Explain that there is a smooth transition of the left-hand side of Eq. 4.4b from finite to infinite values owing to the behavior of the second term on the right.

4.3 Cardiac chambers have been described as pumps consisting of a time-varying pressure source in series with a fixed value compliance. Such a combination operates indeed as a pump as shown, e.g., by De Pater and Van den Berg (1964). Is this a "model" or a "simulation"?

4.4 Develop an expression for the increase in external work done by the left ventricle under normal conditions above the level when the same stroke volume is ejected during the same time interval, but at a constant rate.

4.5 Does the opening of the pulmonary valve precede or follow (a) the first heart sound; (b) the R wave of the ECG; (c) the closure of the mitral valve; (d) maximum acceleration of blood into the pulmonary artery; (e).the instant that right ventricular volume is maximal?

4.6 When the phonocardiogram shows a murmur between the first and the second heart sounds, what are the possible diagnoses?

4.7 If left ventricular stroke volume exceeded that of the right ventricle by 0.5 ml at a heart rate of 70/min. (a) how long would it take to deplete the pulmonary vasculature; (b) what prevents this from occurring in a normal subject?

4.8 If the heart's pumping performance remained unchanged, and if the other vascular bed resistances were unaffected, how much would mean systemic arterial blood pressure change upon removal of one kidney?

4.9 The resistance of a vascular bed has been variously defined as $R_1 = (p_a - p_v)/Q$, or as $R_2 = d(p_a - p_v)/dQ$. Is $R_1 = R_2$? Arterial and venous pressures are denoted p_a and p_v, respectively; Q denotes bed perfusion.

4.10 Referring to Fig. 4.18, the Young's modulus of a sarcomere will increase from the relaxed state to the state in which the crossbridges are attached. What should happen to this modulus when the heads rotate?

4.11 During isovolumic contraction, the left ventricle modifies its shape and would change its volume by a virtual volume, if that were not prevented by the constant blood volume in it. What effect, if any, does this have on pressure build up in the ventricular cavity?

4.12 It has been proposed that average blood pressure, $\bar{p}$, be redefined as p°, with

$$p^\circ = \frac{\int p(t)Q(t)dt}{\int\limits_T Q(t)dt}$$

Determine whether or not $\bar{p} = p^\circ$

4.13 If the ventricles become passive, as they may as the result of a heart attack, how do internal ventricular pressure and external compression pressure, imposed by cardiopulmonary resuscitation, operate on coronary flow?

4.14 During space flights, the heart was observed to become smaller and stroke volume decreased. These observations were originally interpreted as deterioration of cardiac muscle in the space environment, analogous to skeletal muscle and bone structure. Is an alternative interpretation imaginable for the heart?

4.15 To consider the ventricle as a pressure source is popular among numerous investigators. Formulate the definition of a pressure source. Does the ventricle meet the requirement(s)? If not, does it qualify as a flow source?

4.16 Identify a physiologic mechanism causing disqualification of the ventricles as pressure sources.

Answers

4.1 The proposed equation is actually a vector equation, not a scalar one. If $\overrightarrow{F} \neq 0$, this force would operate to move the ventricle within the chest cavity. Burch's conclusion is derived from a faulty equation.

4.2 Ejection flow decreases from a finite value to zero at the end of ejection.

4.3 A simulation. There is no attempt to describe how the heart actually works.

4.4 Under normal conditions, the external work, W, during one heart cycle of duration T equals Eq. 4.2a

$$W = \int_T p_{ao}(t) Q_{ej}(t) \tag{4.12}$$

with

$$p_{ao}(t) = \bar{p} + \sum_n p_n sin(n\omega t + \phi_n) \tag{4.13}$$

and

$$Q_{ej}(t) = \bar{Q} + \sum_n Q_n sin(n\omega t + \psi_n) \tag{4.14}$$

substitution, multiplication, and integration yields

$$W = \bar{p}\bar{Q}T + \sum \frac{p_n Q_n}{2} T \cos(\phi_n - \psi_n) \tag{4.15}$$

The second term on the right is the increase; it tends to be small compared to the first term on the right. In not a few publications, the cosine factor is omitted, which may induce surprising conclusions.

Alternatively, W may be related to the input impedance of an arterial system (Eq. 5.27e) as

$$W = \bar{p}\bar{Q}T + T \sum \frac{|Q_n|^2}{2} Re[Z_{in}] \tag{4.16}$$

Re $[Z_{in}]$ indicates the real part of the input impedance.

4.5 All but (d) follow; (d) precedes.

4.6 Leakage of one (two) atrioventricular valve(s) and/or one (two) stenotic outflow valve(s).

4.7 (a) If the pulmonary vasculature contains 14% of 5 l of blood, its volume equals 700 ml. Exsanguination would take 20 min. (b) As the pulmonary blood volume decreases, the filling pressure for the left ventricle drops as well. Consequently, left ventricular stroke volume becomes smaller.

4.8 Assuming mean arterial, p_a, and venous, p_v, pressures 110 and 10 mmHg, respectively and cardiac output at 5,000 cm^3/min prior to kidney removal, the total systemic peripheral resistance R_s equals 1.2 mmHg cm^{-3} s. The peripheral resistance of one kidney, R_k, assuming 11% of cardiac output for its perfusion, equals 10.9. Removal of the kidney makes the new total peripheral, R_s' higher, owing to their parallel arrangement. Hence,

$$\frac{1}{R_s'} + \frac{1}{R_k} = \frac{1}{R_s} \tag{4.17}$$

which yields $R_s' = 1.35$. Thus $p_a - p_v$ will augment to 113, and if venous pressure remains unchanged, arterial pressure will rise to 123 mmHg.

4.9 The definition for R_1 implies the assumption that R_1 is a constant, independent of prevailing pressures and flow; the definition for R_2 does not imply such an assumption. If linearity applies $R_1 = R_2$; if it does not, they may be different.

4.10 The modulus remains unchanged, though the contractile force builds up.

4.11 If the virtual volume change is positive, wall muscle will shorten to compensate and the rate of cavity pressure rise will be smoother.

4.12 The numerator in this new definition equals work. The expression for this is given in the answer to Question 4.4. Hence,

$$p^\circ = \bar{p} + \sum \frac{p_n Q_n}{2\bar{Q}} \cos(\phi_n - \psi_n) \tag{4.18}$$

The cosines lie in the first or the fourth quadrants for most, if not all values of n and are, therefore, generally positive. This tends to make $p^\circ > \bar{p}$

4.13 Internal ventricular pressure jointly with externally imposed pressure compress the myocardium resulting in reduced coronary perfusion.

4.14 Yes, if the filling of the heart slips to a lower level, as it appears to do in space, stroke volume will automatically decrease. This phenomenon is viewed as adaptation to the microgravity environment and is not considered to be caused by deteriorations of the cardiac musculature.

4.15 A pressure source is, by definition, insensitive to outflow, but a ventricle is, as shown by the ejection effect; analogous considerations disqualify it as flow sources as well.

4.16 Loss of crossbridges, when muscle shortens (rather than viscous effects (Hill 1939)).

Chapter 5
Transmission of Arterial Signals, Venous Nonlinearity, and Body Movement

> *[...] les conduits de l'homme sont pour chaque endroit de son corps et il est de fait avéré qu'il (= le coeur) parle devant les conduits appartenant à chaque endroit du corps.*
>
> — The Ebert papyrus (Bardinet's 1995 translation from the Egyptian).

Digest: Arteries are shown to serve at least four different functions. First, they provide functional pressure reservoirs, which furnish blood supplies far steadier in time than the intermittent pumping of the ventricle. Second, they generate companion pressure and flow waves that deliver pulsatile pressure and flow to most of the peripheral organs. Third, the interplay between outgoing and reflected pressure and flow waves is such as to reduce strongly the input impedance as seen by the ventricle for all but the lowest frequency components, which significantly reduces the amount of physical work required from the ventricle to generate stroke volume. Fourth, they accommodate changing demands by the peripheral organs for oxygen supply, carbon dioxide washout, metabolic supply, etc. by regional alteration of peripheral resistance, primarily through adjustment of arteriolar diameters. As a feature of great practical value, the elaborate array of arteries, formulated mathematically, is amenable to reduction in size under certain circumstances. A canon is developed for the description and analysis of pressure and flow phenomena that is to be used in several subsequent chapters until, in Chap. 8, it is adapted to accommodate the generalization of Harvey's teaching. The canon promotes the careful balancing of compromises in selecting approximations.

Wave transmission studies provide attractiveness. Long term studies yield theories that meet at the heart rate.

5.1 Functions

The arteries provide a transport system of which, in view of the above quote, the Egyptians had already some basic awareness (Chap. 2). Since the anatomical arrangement of the arteries is such as to reach every peripheral organ, blood is furnished to each of them, to most directly (Fig. 2.7). Material carried by the

A. Noordergraaf, *Blood in Motion*, DOI 10.1007/978-1-4614-0005-9_5,
© Springer Science+Business Media, LLC 2011

blood is made available to answer local needs via the capillary extensions of the arteries, while breakdown products can be unloaded by the peripheral tissues via the same channels.

The mammalian cardiovascular system embodies two arterial pressure reservoirs, one in the systemic, and the other in the pulmonary vasculature. The term reservoir is a functional one, since from an anatomical point of view the reservoirs are comprised of a number of arteries in which blood pressure is maintained at a level significantly above atmospheric. These pressure reservoirs serve a number of functions, all realized by basically simple arrangements.

Maintenance of the pressure in the reservoirs is due to two features. The ventricles pump blood into the reservoirs, which, when the aortic and pulmonary valves operate normally, is prevented from returning to the ventricles to within a few percent of the ventricles' output, while the rate of outflow is restricted by the presence of high arteriolar resistances at the numerous peripheral ends. These outflows qualify under impedance-defined flow as will be explained in Sect. 8.3.

Reservoir pressures display a steady as well as a pulsatile component. The steady (or mean) component, obtained as the time-averaged value of the recorded reservoir pressure, is of virtually the same magnitude throughout the larger arteries of either arterial system and carries primary responsibility for perfusion of its periphery. Under normal conditions, the steady component ($\bar{p}_{ao}$ for the systemic and $\bar{p}_{pul}$ for the pulmonary system) is larger than the pulsatile component, the sums being usually characterized by their maximum and minimum values ($p_{s(ystolic)}$ and $p_{d(iastolic)}$, respectively). Steady values may be quickly estimated from

$$\bar{p} = \frac{2}{3}p_d + \frac{1}{3}p_s \tag{5.0}$$

for each of the reservoirs.

The steady components are used to calculate the value of the peripheral resistances, R_s and R_p, of the systemic and pulmonary systems:

$$R_s = \frac{(\bar{p}_{ao} - \bar{p}_{sv})}{\bar{Q}} \tag{5.1a}$$

$$R_p = \frac{(\bar{p}_{pa} - \bar{p}_{pv})}{\bar{Q}} \tag{5.1b}$$

where $\bar{Q}$ denotes average blood flow around the cardiovascular system and $\bar{p}_{sv}, \bar{p}_{pv}$ the steady (or mean) values of systemic and pulmonary venous pressures. Since the latter are normally much lower than arterial pressures, they are often omitted from Eqs. 5.1.

The brief duration of ventricular ejection in conjunction with the elastic (recoil) properties of the arteries generate traveling pairs of pressure and flow pulses. The second function, therefore, is to generate pressure and flow pulses that reach into the peripheral organs. This wave propagation feature looks impressive owing to the modest speed of the wave transmission (in the aorta and its branches 6–12 m/s; in the pulmonary arteries even lower, 0.5–4 m/s, resulting in local differences in the timing of, for instance, peak pressures by up to 0.3 s).

A fraction of the waves caused by the intermittent ventricular pumping is reflected, primarily by the arterioles, small muscular arteries situated between the larger arteries and the capillaries. The design of the arterial systems is such that of the reflected waves, only the low frequency components actually reach the ventricles; this may be viewed as a feedback system. At the ventricle, these low frequency components may become subject to re-reflection toward the periphery, as happens to the higher frequency components at the multiple branching sites encountered while on their way to the heart. This feature is responsible for lowering the input impedance of the arterial systems, making it easier for the ventricles to inject blood into the arteries, a third function. As a consequence, the energy required per beat by the ventricles to perform their external work, shifting blood out of the ventricles and into the reservoirs, is primarily set by the steady components of the pressures in the reservoirs multiplied by the stroke volumes, thus easily outweighing that of the pulsatile contributions.

The pressure in the systemic reservoir is monitored continuously by the baroreceptors and reported to the central nervous system. This allots the nervous system a degree of central control over this pressure. The response of the baroreceptors is strongly frequency dependent, ignoring in the long run the pressure's steady component. The responsibility for controlling the steady component is assigned primarily to the kidneys (Sect. 9.2.1).

In addition to the presence of central control, the peripheral organs exercise strong local control to accommodate changing needs, a fourth function. This local control is achieved by altering the contractile state of the smooth muscle in the walls of the local arterioles (Chap. 9).

5.2 Pulse Transmission

5.2.1 The Moens-Korteweg Formula

Predicting the speed of propagation of the disturbance, the pulse wave velocity, generated by the ventricles has been experienced as a major challenge in the spirit of Descartes. The method of approach was outlined by Euler as early as 1776, but Thomas Young (1809) provided the first of many derivations of such a formula for the pulse wave velocity in a passive vessel. In view of its relative lucidity, Resal's derivation (1816) will be summarized here.

Considering a nonviscous fluid in a purely elastic, uniform artery of radius r, cross-sectional area S and infinite length, the Weber brothers (1850, 1866) had applied Newton's second law of motion, force equals mass times acceleration, to a segment of artery with axial length dz (Fig. 5.1) resulting in

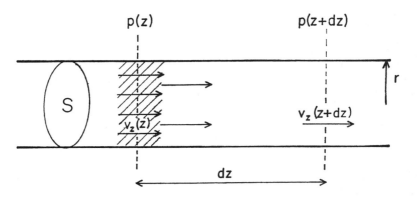

Fig. 5.1 Segment of artery with pressures and particle velocities at neighboring sites as marked S = cross-sectional area. See text for further explanation

$$Sp(z) - Sp(z + dz) = \pi r^2 dz \rho \frac{dv_z}{dt} \qquad (5.2a)$$

or

$$-S \frac{\partial p}{\partial z} dz = \pi r^2 dz \rho \frac{\partial v_z}{\partial t} \qquad (5.2b)$$

leading to

$$-\frac{\partial v_z}{\partial t} = \frac{1}{\rho} \frac{\partial p}{\partial z} \qquad (5.2c)$$

where $p(z)$ denotes the blood pressure at axial location z, v_z the velocity component in the axial direction, ρ the density of blood, and t time. To this, Resal added his own expression for the equation of continuity (i.e., conservation of mass: inflow minus outflow equals the rate of change in volume V of the segment under consideration)

$$Sv_z(z) - Sv_z(z + dz) = \frac{dV}{dt} \qquad (5.3a)$$

Hence

$$-S \frac{\partial v_z}{\partial z} = \frac{\partial S}{\partial t} dz \qquad (5.3b)$$

Or

$$-\frac{\partial v_z}{\partial z} = \frac{1}{S}\frac{\partial S}{\partial t} \tag{5.3c}$$

Equations 5.2c and 5.3c form two equations in three unknowns p, v_z, and S. Resal then took steps to express S in p for the elastic vessel by dividing tangential stress on the wall σ_t, from what is popularly called Laplace's law

$$\sigma_t = \frac{pr}{h} \tag{5.4a}$$

where h denotes wall thickness, by tangential strain, ε_t

$$\varepsilon_t = \frac{dr}{r} \tag{5.4b}$$

and put their ratio equal to the elastic modulus E (named after Young), yielding

$$S = \pi r^2 + \frac{2\pi p}{Eh}r^3 \tag{5.5a}$$

the last term on the right being the change in area dS. Taking only p in this term to be time dependent, it follows

$$\frac{\partial S}{\partial t} = \frac{2\pi}{Eh}\frac{\partial p}{\partial t}r^3 \tag{5.5b}$$

Substitution of S and $\partial S/\partial t$ in Eq. 5.3c and assuming that $dS \ll S$ leads to

$$-\frac{\partial v_z}{\partial z} = \frac{2r}{Eh}\frac{\partial p}{\partial t} \tag{5.6}$$

resulting in two equations in two unknowns.

Differentiation of Eq. 5.2c with respect to z and of Eq. 5.6 with respect to t yields the wave equation

$$\frac{\partial^2 p}{\partial t^2} = \frac{Eh}{2\rho r}\frac{\partial^2 p}{\partial z^2} \tag{5.7}$$

providing the propagation velocity of the pressure pulse, also called the pulse wave velocity, or the phase velocity, c_{ph}, as the square root of the coefficient on the right-hand side

$$c_{ph} = \left(\frac{Eh}{2\rho r}\right)^{1/2} \tag{5.8a}$$

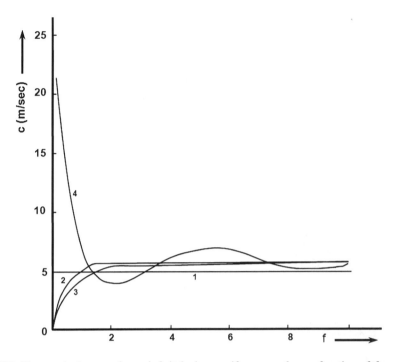

Fig. 5.2 Phase velocity, c_{ph}, in an infinitely long uniform vessel as a function of frequency $f (=\omega/2\pi)$; graph marked 1 displays the Moens-Korteweg approximation (Eqs. 5.8) in which blood viscosity is set to 0; graph marked 2 includes blood viscosity (Eqs. 5.8i); graph marked 3 is based on a more general theory (Eqs. 5.12b or 5.13c); graph marked 4 represents experimentally obtained wave velocity in man

This is the Moens-Korteweg formula for the pulse wave velocity, which continues to enjoy widespread popularity. It is often written as

$$c_{ph} = \sqrt{\frac{V}{\rho}\frac{dp}{dV}} = \sqrt{\frac{S}{\rho}\frac{dp}{dS}} \qquad (5.8b, c)$$

where V denotes the volume of a short segment of artery Sdz (line 1 in Fig. 5.2). The transition from Eq. 5.8a to 5.8c may be made with the aid of Eq. 5.5a. In view of its experimental support for higher frequency components in the in vivo system, the Moens-Korteweg formula established pulse wave propagation in larger arteries as a passive phenomenon, rather than an active one as thought originally, thereby effacing a mystery. At one time or another, all vessels were assumed to be passive.

The Moens-Korteweg formula may be extended to incorporate the viscous properties of the fluid. For a segment of vessel of unit length, the equation of motion becomes

$$-\frac{\partial p}{\partial z} = L'\frac{\partial Q}{\partial t} + R'Q \qquad (5.8d)$$

and the equation of continuity

$$-\frac{\partial Q}{\partial z} = \frac{C'\partial p}{\partial t} \qquad (5.8e)$$

where $L' = \frac{\rho}{\pi r^2}, R' = \frac{8\mu}{\pi r^4}, C' = \frac{dS}{dp}$, (called area compliance), the $'$ indicates the value of the parameter per unit axial length and Q denotes volume flow. In the first term on the right of the equation of motion the inertia of the fluid is accounted for in a fashion similar to that in the above derivation of the Moens-Korteweg formula (Eq. 5.8a), and assumes a flat velocity profile. The second term covers the viscous effect and assumes a parabolic velocity profile, thus the Hagen–Poiseuille equation. The inertial and viscous effects are simply summed, i.e., assumed not to interact.

Partial differentiation of these equations and a few substitutions lead to the wave equation in p of the form

$$\frac{\partial^2 p}{\partial z^2} = L'C'\frac{\partial^2 p}{\partial t^2} + \frac{R'C'\partial p}{\partial t} \qquad (5.8f)$$

with as solution in an infinitely long vessel

$$p(z,t) = p_0 e^{-\gamma z + j\omega t} \qquad (5.8g)$$

in which

$$\gamma = \alpha + j\frac{\omega}{c_{ph}} \qquad (5.8h)$$

In general, γ is a complex number, the real part of which, α, defines wave attenuation owing to heat exchange. The phase velocity, c_{ph}, becomes frequency dependent, (line 2 of Fig. 5.2) which is not in Eq. 4.8a,

$$c_{ph} = \omega\left[\frac{\omega^2 L'C'}{2} + \frac{\omega}{2}\left[\omega^2 L'^2 C'^2 + R'^2 C'^2\right]^{\frac{1}{2}}\right]^{-\frac{1}{2}} \qquad (5.8i)$$

Elimination of the viscous properties makes $R' = 0$, and Eq. 5.8i reduces to

$$c_{\mathrm{ph}} = [L'C']^{-\frac{1}{2}} \tag{5.8j}$$

which is equivalent to Eq. 5.8c.

5.2.2 Refined Studies of Pulse Wave Velocity in Infinitely Long Vessels

Beginning with the studies by Witzig (1914), scholars have made great strides toward a more consistent and more thorough analysis of wave propagation through infinitely long elastic tubes, as well as through a vessel with finite length, while taking into account wave reflection. Karreman (1952) generalized Witzig's work. Womersley (1957) extended Karreman's work by laying the foundation for subsequent analysis of arterial systems. The preoccupation with pulse wave velocity was replaced by the formulation of a broader set of questions. Further generalized development for passive vessels by Jager (1965) will be summarized here. (Active vessels and chambers will appear in Chap. 8.)

The approach requires the formulation of three aspects of the events in arteries.

1. The Navier–Stokes equation, restricted to streamline flow, to relate blood pressure, p, to blood particle velocity, v, often referred to as the equation of motion for the fluid.
2. An expression stating that blood is considered an incompressible fluid.
3. Since arterial walls are elastic, an equation of motion for the wall.

In cylindrical coordinates, z (axial), and r (radial) and assuming rotational symmetry, the Navier–Stokes equations read:

$$-\frac{\partial p}{\partial z} = \rho \left[\frac{\partial}{\partial t} v_z + v_r \frac{\partial}{\partial r} v_z + v_z \frac{\partial}{\partial z} v_z \right] - \mu \left[\frac{\partial^2}{\partial r^2} v_z + \frac{1}{r} \frac{\partial}{\partial z} v_z + \frac{\partial^2}{\partial z^2} v_z \right] - \rho g \tag{5.9a}$$

$$-\frac{\partial p}{\partial r} = \rho \left[\frac{\partial}{\partial t} v_r + v_r \frac{\partial}{\partial r} v_r + v_z \frac{\partial}{\partial z} v_r \right] - \mu \left[\frac{\partial^2}{\partial r^2} v_r + \frac{1}{r} \frac{\partial}{\partial r} v_r + \frac{\partial^2}{\partial z^2} v_r - \frac{v_r}{r^2} \right] \tag{5.9b}$$

The incompressibility of blood is expressed by the equation of continuity, also in cylindrical coordinates:

$$\frac{1}{r} \frac{\partial}{\partial r} r v_z = -\frac{\partial}{\partial z} v_z \tag{5.10}$$

The quantities t denotes time, ρ blood density, μ its viscosity, and g the acceleration of gravity. In Weber's original plan $\mu = 0$, thereby only recognizing the inertial property of blood.

Proposals to characterize the (visco)elastic properties of the wall abound. Here, the dynamic (Navier) equation for the thick wall is used. It reads, for wall displacements u, again in cylindrical coordinates:

$$\rho_0 \frac{\partial^2}{\partial t^2} u_z = -\frac{\partial \pi}{\partial z} + \mu_0 \left[\frac{\partial^2}{\partial r^2} u_z + \frac{1}{r} \frac{\partial}{\partial r} u_z - \frac{\partial^2}{\partial z^2} u_z \right] \tag{5.11a}$$

$$\rho_0 \frac{\partial^2}{\partial t^2} u_r = -\frac{\partial \pi}{\partial z} + \mu_0 \left[\frac{\partial^2}{\partial r^2} u_r + \frac{1}{r} \frac{\partial}{\partial r} u_r + \frac{U_r}{r^2} u_r \right] \tag{5.11b}$$

where $\pi = -\lambda_0 \, \mathrm{div}\, u$, λ_0 and μ_0 are Lamé constants, while ρ_0 denotes the density of the wall material.

After application of appropriate boundary conditions, the most significant of which is longitudinal constraint (most arteries are tethered along their longitudinal axis), neglecting the nonlinear terms as well as the second derivatives with respect to z in the Navier–Stokes equations and assuming that the wall is incompressible in the Navier equation, this set of five simultaneous partial differential equations can be solved in closed form. The most interesting parts are, for the steady state:

$$p(z,t) = p_a e^{-\gamma z} e^{j\omega t} \tag{5.12a}$$

which signifies a single pressure wave traveling away from the source through the infinitely long vessel. Its amplitude is p_a at the origin. Its frequency of oscillation is f, with $\omega = 2\pi f$. The wave propagation constant, γ is predicted as:

$$\gamma = j\omega \left[\frac{3\rho[r+h]^2}{Eh[2r+h][1 - F_{10}]} \right]^{\frac{1}{2}} \tag{5.12b}$$

for a thick-walled vessel. In this equation

$$F_{10}(\alpha) = \frac{2J_1\left(\alpha j^{\frac{3}{2}} \right)}{\alpha j^{\frac{3}{2}} J_0\left(\alpha j^{\frac{3}{2}} \right)} \tag{5.12c}$$

and

$$\alpha = r \sqrt{\frac{\omega \rho}{\mu}} \tag{5.12d}$$

where J_0 and J_1 are Bessel functions of the zeroth and first order, respectively (line 3 in Fig. 5.2 [line 4 is discussed in Sect. 5.3.1]), while the parameter α, which measures the ratio between inertial and viscous effects, is called the Womersley parameter, though it was introduced earlier by Witzig. E denotes the elastic modulus of the wall material and h the wall thickness.

At the same time solutions are obtained for v_z and v_r. Integration of v_z over the vessel's cross-sectional area, S, yields volume flow Q:

$$Q(z,t) = \frac{p_a S_\gamma}{jp\omega(1 - F_{10})e^{-\gamma z}e^{j\omega t}} \tag{5.12d}$$

which represents the flow wave that accompanies the pressure wave in Eq. 5.12a.

These considerations can be generalized further by making the wall material viscoelastic instead of elastic (Jager 1965) and by including non-Newtonian aspects of blood viscosity (Jager et al. 1965).

The quantities pressure $p(z, t)$, and flow $Q(z, t)$ emerge as the fundamental variables. Their expressions (Eqs. 5.12a, e) witness dependence on the parameters of the vessel (radius, compliance, etc. of the vessel), while the frequency is set by the ventricle. The factor $e^{-\gamma z}$ in Eqs. 5.12a, d, contains γ, often erroneously referred to as the propagation "constant."

Of particular interest for the characterization of a segment of the infinitely long vessel are the quantities Z_l' and Z_t', the longitudinal impedance per length and the transverse impedance times length, which are defined as:

$$Z_l' = -\frac{\frac{\partial p}{\partial z}}{Q} \quad \text{and} \quad Z_t' = -\frac{p}{\frac{\partial Q}{\partial z}} \tag{5.12e}$$

Substitution of the partial derivatives from Eqs. 5.12e yields

$$Z_l' = \frac{j\omega\rho}{S(1 - F_{10})} = j\omega L'(\alpha) + R'(\alpha) \tag{5.13a}$$

and

$$Z_t' = \frac{1}{j\omega}\frac{hE(2r + h)}{3S(r + h)^2} = \frac{1}{j\omega C'} \tag{5.13b}$$

While

$$\gamma = \left[\frac{Z_l'}{Z_t'}\right]^2 \tag{5.13c}$$

as an alternate to Eq. 5.12b.

Equations 5.13a, b may be rewritten formally as

$$-\frac{\partial p}{\partial z} = L'(\alpha)\frac{\partial Q}{\partial t} + R'(\alpha)Q \tag{5.14a}$$

and

$$-\frac{\partial Q}{\partial z} = C' \frac{\partial p}{\partial t}$$ (5.14b)

where, with $F_{10} = M_{10}\, e^{j\varepsilon 10}$,

$$L'(\alpha) = \frac{\rho}{SM_{10}} \cos \varepsilon_{10}$$ (5.15a)

and

$$R'(\alpha) = \frac{\pi \mu \alpha^2}{S^2 M_{10}} \sin \varepsilon_{10}$$ (5.15b)

Womersley (1957) tabulated the function $(1 - F_{10})$ for frequencies of cardio-vascular interest.

Equations 5.14 proved to furnish a powerful tool in the resolution of a multitude of cardiovascular problems.

Instead of starting with the Navier–Stokes equation, other approaches have been proposed, e.g., the application of the Lagrange equation, which deals with consideration of potential and kinetic energies.

In Resal's derivation $C' = \frac{2\pi r_0^3}{hE}$ (from Eq. 5.5a) one elastic parameter was used, while two were utilized in the derivation of the expression for C' in Eq. 5.13b. These expressions assume strongly simplified descriptions, because even for a linear, anisotropic (which arterial wall material is), solid material 21 independent parameters may be recognized, more if actual behavior is better approximated (Sommerfeld 1947; Fung 1997). Few of these perplexing parameters have been measured. Some of the theoretical and experimental difficulties encountered were exposed by Weizsäcker et al. (1984, 1996; Weizsäcker and Pinto 1988), Weizsäcker (2000). Residual stress, observed by Bergel (1960), subsequently quantified by Vaishnav and Vossoughi (1983) and many others, is also not taken into account.

5.2.3 Wave Travel in a Vessel of Finite Length

In the two preceding sections wave propagation in an infinitely long vessel was formulated. To move closer to reality, waves propagating along a vessel of finite length will be considered in this section. Equations (5.13a, b) provide convenient tools to achieve this purpose. These equations are repeated here, without indicating the dependence of some of the coefficients on the parameter α (Eq. 5.12d):

$$-\frac{\partial p}{\partial z} = L' \frac{\partial Q}{\partial t} + R'Q$$ (5.16a)

and

$$-\frac{\partial Q}{\partial z} = \frac{C'\partial p}{\partial t} \qquad (5.16b)$$

The former equation relates the pressure gradient along the vessel to flow through it, while the latter relates the flow gradient along the vessel to pressure. The reason for using partial derivatives is that both pressure and flow depend on the location where they are observed as well as the moment in time when they are observed. Written formally, $p = p(z, t)$ and $Q = Q(z, t)$. A uniform vessel will be assumed, making L', R', and C' practically independent of both z and t.

To obtain a solution for pressure, flow must be eliminated from Eqs. 5.16a, b. This can be achieved by differentiating Eq. 5.16a partially with respect to z and Eq. 5.16b partially with respect to t. The result is:

$$\frac{\partial^2 p}{\partial z^2} = L'C'\frac{\partial^2 p}{\partial t^2} + \frac{R'C'\partial p}{\partial t} \qquad (5.17a)$$

The same procedure, but reversing the order of taking derivatives, permits elimination of pressure, resulting in:

$$\frac{\partial^2 Q}{\partial z^2} = L'C'\frac{\partial^2 Q}{\partial t^2} + \frac{R'C'\partial Q}{\partial t} \qquad (5.17b)$$

Equations 5.17a, b constitute the wave equations for pressure and flow, respectively. They have the same form, suggesting that their solutions will be of similar form also. It may be noted that Eq. 5.17a is different from Eq. 5.7 because, in the latter, blood was considered nonviscous ($\mu = 0$, making $R' = 0$). To obtain steady state periodic solutions the propagation constant γ must meet the following condition

$$\gamma^2 = (j\omega L' + R')j\omega C' \qquad (5.18)$$

Since there are two solutions for γ, equal except for sign, the solution for the wave equations contains two waves instead of one, as was the case in the preceding section. One set of solutions, named after J.-B. L. d'Alembert (1717–1783), reads:
for p:

$$p(z, t) = [p_a e^{-\gamma z} + p_r e^{\gamma z}]e^{j\omega t} \qquad (5.19a)$$

and similarly for Q:

$$Q(z, t) = [Q_a e^{-\gamma z} + Q_r e^{\gamma z}]e^{j\omega t} \qquad (5.19b)$$

In words, both the pressure and the flow signals consist of the sum of an antegrade (i.e., forward) traveling wave and a retrograde (i.e., backward) traveling wave, the amplitude of each varying periodically with time. The two antegrade waves are companions, as are the two retrograde ones. All four propagate at the same speed (Eq. 5.18), the phase velocity, c_{ph}, though, in general, the sums do not. Their speed is denoted the apparent wave velocity, c_{app}. Karreman (1952), whose interest was stimulated by his suffering from coarctation of the aorta, was the first to emphasize reflection of pressure waves.

Any vessel of finite length terminates in a load. In general, the antegrade pressure and flow waves will be transmitted through the load in part, and be reflected in part. The reflected waves appear in the solutions above with a plus γz exponent. If conditions are such that the reflected waves travel the total distance back to the origin and are, in part, reflected there again, they become new antegrade waves traveling in the direction of the termination and the process may be repeated again. The solutions in Eqs. 5.19a, b may be viewed as lumping together all antegrade waves in a single term; similarly for all retrograde waves. The individual waves may, however, be recognized separately in view of the fact that B_i times the solutions in Eqs. 5.19 are also solutions. In general, B_i is a complex number, with $i = 1,2,...,n$. With identification of the individual waves, Eqs. 5.19 becomes (Berger et al. 1993):

$$p(z,t) = \sum_{i=1}^{n} B_i[p_a e^{-\gamma z} + p_r e^{\gamma z}]e^{j\omega t} \tag{5.20a}$$

$$Q(z,t) = \sum_{i=1}^{n} B_i[Q_a e^{-\gamma z} + Q_r e^{\gamma z}]e^{j\omega t} \tag{5.20b}$$

The special case of all B_i's $= 0$, except $B_1 = 1$, reduces Eqs. 5.20 to Eqs. 5.19.

For a distributed, though simplified, model of the systemic arterial system, Berger et al. demonstrated that the reflected pressure and flow signals (a) contain primarily low frequency harmonics, (b) which reduce rapidly in amplitude with each round trip. This phenomenon is stronger, the lower the peripheral resistance, i. e., the lower the peripheral reflection coefficient. For each selected value of n in Eqs. 5.20, a unique solution can be obtained for the individual pressure and flow signals. Figure 5.3 reproduces an example for pressure with $n = 5$, separately for antegrade (P_{ant}) and retrograde components (P_{ret}).

5.2.4 Concepts in Linear Wave Propagation

Pressure and flow in an artery are related through the parameters of the system in which they occur. Ultimately, system parameters, some time-varying, determine not only their relation, but also pressure and flow themselves.

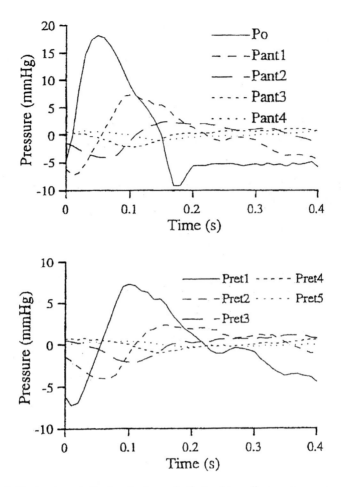

Fig. 5.3 Individual antegrade (*top*) and retrograde (*bottom*) traveling pressure waves in a model featuring reflection at both ends. The actually recorded pressure in a dog, p_o, is the sum of all 10 signals (5 round trips) shown (Eqs. 5.20) (Adapted from Berger et al. 1993)

Substitution of the appropriate derivatives of the expressions for pressure and flow of Eqs. 5.19 into Eq. 5.16b, and substitution of one γ (Eq. 5.18) in the result yields

$$p_a e^{-\gamma z} + p_r e^{\gamma z} = \left(\frac{j\omega L' + R'}{j\omega C'}\right)^{\frac{1}{2}} [Q_a e^{-\gamma z} - Q_r e^{\gamma z}] \qquad (5.21)$$

The coefficient on the right-hand side is determined by frequency, viscous and inertial properties of blood, and the vessel's compliance and thus by the system. Consequently, it acquired a name, the characteristic impedance of the vessel of interest. Its common symbol is Z_0. Comparison of right and left sides in Eq. 5.21 leads to the relations

$$Z_0 Q_a = p_a \qquad (5.22a)$$

And

$$-Z_0 Q_r = p_r \qquad (5.22b)$$

Therefore,

$$p(z,t) = Z_0 [Q_a e^{-\gamma z} - Q_r e^{\gamma z}]_2 e^{j\omega t} \qquad (5.23a)$$

and likewise

$$Q(z,t) = \frac{1}{Z_0}[p_a e^{-\gamma z} - p_r e^{\gamma z}]e^{j\omega t} \qquad (5.23b)$$

Hence, the characteristic impedance permits expressing pressure in terms of flow and vice versa.

If Z_0 is a real number, which closely applies in large vessels, Eq. 5.22a insists that antegrade pressure and flow waves have identical shapes and signs. The identity applies to reflected waves as well, though the latter display opposite signs (Eq. 5.22b).

In passing, it may also be noted that

$$\gamma^2 = \frac{Z_1'}{Z_t'} = -\frac{\omega^2}{c^2} \qquad (5.24a)$$

while

$$Z_0^2 = Z_1' Z_t' \qquad (5.24b)$$

where c denotes the complex phase velocity

$$c = j\omega \left[\frac{Z_t'}{Z_1'}\right]^{\frac{1}{2}} \qquad (5.24c)$$

For the special case of $\omega = 0$, γ goes to zero and Z_0 to infinity. Equation 5.23b shows that $Q(z,t) = 0$: the d'Alembert solution degenerates for $\omega = 0$. Steady flow and pressure issues can be solved by considering viscous effects only.

As early as 1892, Von Kries pointed out that measured pressures at two points along a single vessel permit resolution of the antegrade and retrograde pressure waves in Eq. 5.19a (Question 5.5) (1892). Westerhof et al. (1972) developed a variation based on pressure and flow signals measured at a single point, permitting the separation of both pressure and flow signals.

Another relevant impedance is the input impedance Z_{in}. Like Z_0, it is generally a function of frequency and is defined as the ratio of corresponding pressure $p(\omega_i)$ and flow $Q(\omega_i)$ harmonics ($i = 1,2,...$) at the same location z in a vessel:

$$Z_{in} = \frac{p(\omega_i)}{Q(\omega_i)} \tag{5.25}$$

where, in keeping with tradition, venous pressure is considered small compared to arterial pressure.

Input impedance can be related to properties of the system in several ways depending on the researcher's interest. Examples include:

$$Z_{in} = \frac{p_a(\omega_i)e^{-\gamma z} + p_r(\omega_i)e^{\gamma z}}{Q_a(\omega_i)e^{-\gamma z} + Q_r(\omega_i)e^{\gamma z}} = Z_0 \frac{p_a(\omega_i)e^{-\gamma z} + p_r(\omega_i)e^{\gamma z}}{p_a(\omega_i)e^{-\gamma z} - p_r(\omega_i)e^{\gamma z}} \tag{5.26a}$$

which expresses Z_{in} in pressure and characteristic impedance at any arbitrary point along the vessel. The last transition was made with the aid of Eq. 5.23b. If Eq. 5.23a is applied instead, Z_{in} is related to flow and Z_0 as:

$$Z_{in} = Z_0 \frac{Q_a(\omega_i)e^{-\gamma z} - Q_r(\omega_i)e^{\gamma z}}{Q_a(\omega_i)e^{-\gamma z} + Q_r(\omega_i)e^{\gamma z}} \tag{5.26b}$$

Specifically at $z = L$ where the vessel terminates in an impedance Z_L, from Eq. 5.26a:

$$Z_L = Z_0 \frac{p_a(\omega_i)e^{-\gamma L} + p_r(\omega_i)e^{\gamma L}}{p_a(\omega_i)e^{-\gamma L} - p_r(\omega_i)e^{\gamma L}} \tag{5.27}$$

Multiplication of numerator and denominator with $e^{\gamma L}$ and solving for $\frac{p_r}{p_a}$ yields:

$$\frac{p_r}{p_a} = \frac{Z_L - Z_0}{Z_L - Z_0} e^{-2\gamma L} \tag{5.28}$$

The global reflection coefficient, Γ_g, is defined as the ratio between the magnitude of the total reflected wave and that of the total outgoing one at any location z as

$$\Gamma_g(z) = \frac{p_r e^{\gamma z}}{p_a e^{-\gamma z}} = \frac{p_r}{p_a} e^{2\gamma z} \tag{5.29a}$$

The global reflection coefficient takes into account all reflected waves that contribute to wave pattern formation at location z (Eqs. 5.20).

Hence, at the entrance

$$\Gamma_g(0) = \frac{p_r}{p_a} \qquad (5.29b)$$

The global reflection coefficient incorporates local reflection coefficients. Γ_1, as they apply at a single branching site, or at a lumped termination, e.g.,

$$\Gamma_1(L) = \frac{Z_L - Z_0}{Z_L + Z_0} \qquad (5.29c)$$

In particular, $\Gamma_1 = 0$, if $Z_L = Z_0$, i.e., if the load impedance equals the characteristic impedance, referred to as impedance matching. At any point $z < L$ in a single uniform vessel, it is then impossible to conclude whether the vessel is of finite or infinite length. For this value of Γ_1, $p_r = 0$, meaning the absence of a reflected wave. From Eq. 5.26a, if $p_r = 0$, $Z_{in} = Z_0$. Likewise for flow (Eq. 5.26b).

Returning to input impedance once more, Eq. 5.25a gives at the entrance of the vessel ($z = 0$)

$$Z_{in} = Z_0 \frac{1 + \frac{p_r}{p_a}}{1 - \frac{p_r}{p_a}} \qquad (5.26c)$$

With Eq. 5.27 and substituting $\frac{j\omega_i}{c}$ for γ, results in

$$Z_{in} = Z_0 \frac{Z_L + Z_0 + (Z_L - Z_0)e^{-j\frac{2\omega_i L}{c}}}{Z_L + Z_0 - (Z_L - Z_0)e^{-j\frac{2\omega_i L}{c}}} \qquad (5.26d)$$

A simpler expression for input impedance at the entrance is obtained from Eq. 5.26c by substituting p_r/p_a for $z = 0$ from Eq. 5 29b. This results in:

$$Z_{in} = Z_0 \frac{1 + \Gamma_g(0)}{1 - \Gamma_g(0)} \qquad (5.26e)$$

The input impedance of the arterial systems carries the major responsibility for making the pulsatile work of the ventricles a small fraction of the steady work, thereby reducing by a substantial factor, the total amount of work required to eject the stroke volume.

5.2.5 Nonlinear Pressure–Flow Relation in a Collapsible Vessel Such as a Vein

Wiggers offered a conceptual model that includes the venous return system (1954); it is reproduced as Fig. 2.5. Eventually, this inspired the formulation of detailed electrical (De Pater and Van den Berg 1964) and mathematical (Attinger and Anné 1966; Wiener et al. 1966) models of the closed circuit in which veins were treated as arteries with enhanced compliant properties. These gave way to descriptions in which local deviations from the circular cross section were permitted (Snyder and Rideout 1969; Moreno et al. 1969).

The volume, V_i, in a segment of vein within the thorax may be computed from

$$V_i = V(0) + C_i(t)p_{tr}(t) \qquad (5.30)$$

where the transmural pressure, $p_{tr}(t)$, equals $p_i(t) - p_e(t)$, i.e., internal (blood) pressure minus external (air) pressure, such as could be imposed by the respiratory system, and $V(0)$ the volume at zero transmural pressure. In general, the latter two pressures will vary with time, hence their difference, p_{tr}, will also. The change in volume, i.e., the flow, Q_i, into or out of the segment is obtained by differentiating Eq. 5.30, which yields a nonlinear relation for soft vessels like veins (and in principle for arteries as well)

$$Q_i(t) = C_i(t)\frac{dp_{tr}}{dt} + p_{tr}(t)\frac{dC_i}{dt} \qquad (5.31)$$

The variation in the value of C_i can be obtained with the aid of Eq. 5.5a, and recalling that $C_i = C_i' \times \Delta z$. Since $p_e(t)$ can be included or excluded, this approach permits quantitative evaluation of the respiratory influence on venous return and cardiac output, which in Fig. 10.8 will be shown to be significant, particularly during exercise, thus supporting Donders' ideas.

The more recent approach, presented here, follows that utilized in the development of a distributed model of the arterial system (Sects. 5.2 and 5.3). Thus, the nonlinear terms in the Navier–Stokes equations (Eqs. 5.9) will be neglected to preserve the impedance characterization developed in this chapter, while accommodating the key nonlinearities of shape and elastic properties. Accordingly, a uniform, partially collapsed, segment of vessel of length Δz will be considered and its longitudinal impedance per length, Z_l', and transverse impedance times length, Z_t', determined.

If the cross-sectional area of this segment is denoted S, the effective radius of a circle with the same area will be r. The cross-sectional shape was described by a "shape factor," denoted γ' and defined as

$$\gamma' = 2 - \sqrt{\frac{y_i}{r}} \qquad (5.32a)$$

with

$$1 \leq \gamma' \leq 2 \qquad (5.32b)$$

and y_i, an intercept as marked in Fig. 3.6b.

The longitudinal impedance per length, Z_l', retains the form in Eq. 5.13a with the expression for $L'(\alpha)$ unchanged from Eqs. 5.15, while the numerator of $R'(\alpha)$ in Eq. 5.15 must be multiplied by γ' of Eqs. 5.32. This transforms both L' and R' into nonconstant parameters and the properties into nonlinear ones, unlike for their arterial counterparts. The expression for the transverse impedance times length (Eq. 5.13b) remains unchanged (Kresch and Noordergraaf A 1969). In summary:

$$L' = \frac{\rho}{S} \tag{5.33a}$$

$$R' = \frac{8\pi\eta\gamma'}{S^2} \tag{5.33b}$$

$$C' = \frac{dS}{dp_{tr}} \tag{5.33c}$$

For *negative* transmural pressure ($p_{tr} < 0$), computer generated families of graphs for S and dS/dp_{tr} as a function of p_{tr} and of k, the eccentricity for $p_{tr} = 0$, are given in Figs. 3.3 and 3.5 in normalized form. Figure 3.4 provides an additional family of curves for y_i (Eq. 3.3), also normalized. The multiplication factors required to make the transition to an actual segment of vein are contained in the captions of Figs. 3.3–3.5.

For *zero* and *positive* transmural pressure ($p_{tr} \geq 0$), the segment of vein was treated as a thin-walled artery with a circular cross section. In view of the highly distensible nature of venous wall material, significant modulation of the radial dimension may be expected. To accommodate the main features of this, wall thinning and wall stiffening (Attinger and Anné 1966; Anliker et al. 1969), when distended, were incorporated.

Application of the thin-walled version of Eq. 5.13b yields for the radial compliance of a vessel with radius r_i

$$\frac{dr_i}{dp_{tr}} = \frac{3r_i^2}{4h_iE_t(r_i)} \tag{5.33d}$$

Allowing for constant wall volume

$$h_i = \frac{h(0)r(0)}{r_i} \tag{5.33e}$$

and a strongly nonlinear tangential wall modulus

$$\frac{E_t(r_i)}{E_t(r(0))} = \left[\frac{r_i}{r(0)}\right]^5 \tag{5.33f}$$

the derivative becomes

$$\frac{dr_i}{dp_{tr}} = \frac{3r(0)^4}{4h(0)E_t(r(0))r_i^2} = \frac{K}{r_i^2} \tag{5.33g}$$

where (0) denotes at $p_{tr} = 0$.

Integration yields

$$r_i = \left[r(0)^3 + 3Kp_{tr}\right]^{\frac{1}{3}} \tag{5.34a}$$

indicating that the rate of increase in r_i is less than that of p_{tr}, due to stiffening, while

$$\frac{dr_i}{dp_{tr}} = K\left[r(0)^3 + 3Kp_{tr}\right]^{-\frac{2}{3}} \tag{5.34b}$$

which is always positive, and

$$C_i' = 2\pi K\left[r(0)^3 + 3Kp_{tr}\right]^{-\frac{1}{3}} \tag{5.35}$$

which imposes a reduction on C_i' as transmural pressure climbs, all three (Eqs. 5.34 and 5.35) as dictated by experiments on veins. It may be noted that there appears to be a tendency among vessels to increase nonlinear elastic properties from systemic arteries to pulmonary arteries to veins. For veins, this stiffening should promote filling of the atria with increased venous volumes in a disproportional fashion (Sect. 10.2).

Kresch and Noordergraaf A (1969) also derived an expression for the phase velocity, c_{ph}, for uniformly collapsing vessels of various shapes. They found that the Moens-Korteweg formula (Eq. 5.8a) holds by approximation. This prediction was tested by Brower and Scholten with the result reproduced in Fig. 3.12. It is of interest to observe that the phase velocity exhibits a minimum around zero transmural pressure where the compliance, dS/dp_{tr}, tends to be very large. In this range, flow velocity may easily exceed phase velocity. Griffiths (1971) as well as Brower and Scholten (1975) maintain that the transitions between supersonic and subsonic flow are responsible for the generation of instabilities in the flow, which occasionally have been observed in collapsible tubes though not in veins in vivo.

Measurements of wave speed at high frequencies were carried out by Anliker et al. (1969) in the abdominal vena cava of dogs. Velocities were found to increase from 2 to 6 m/s when the transmural pressure was stepped up from 5 to 25 cm H_2O, indicating that the effect of increasing diameter is outweighed by wall stiffening. Ultrasonic measurement of wave velocity in human veins at physiologic pressure, but using a two-point measurement, indicate 1–3 m/s, depending on the size of the vein and on whether breathing was normal or held (Nippa et al. 1971).

5.2.6 Body Movement

In the equation of motion (Eq. 5.16a), it was assumed that the vessel is fixed in its spatial location and that the heart is the sole source of pressure and flow in blood vessels. This equation, together with a statement concerning the incompressibility of the fluid, yielded the Moens-Korteweg formula (Eq. 5.8a). There are, however, other reasons why pressure and flow phenomena in the arteries may be generated, such as walking and running. Formulated more generally, since most of the arteries are tethered to the body frame, the vessel wall participates in the movement of the body. Such conditions are therefore more normal than lying quietly in the horizontal position with the skeletal musculature relaxed. Most, though not all, clinical examinations are performed under such restrictive conditions, adhering to ideas that go back at least to Harvey. This poses a new challenge of designing and applying transducers, themselves insensitive to acceleration and deceleration, for measurement under conditions where motion alters events in the cardiovascular circuit. It has been reported, for instance, that hoof beats are recognizable in running giraffes' arterial pressure. Under specialized conditions, as in a plane flying sequential Keplerian and non-Keplerian trajectories (Sect. 10.2.5), or in BASH experiments (Sect. 9.4), body acceleration and deceleration may reach significant magnitudes. In these early experiments regarding the effect of motion on pressure and flow, little attention was paid to sensor artifacts.

For the elementary case of a uniform elastic vessel with inflow $Q(t) = Q_0 e^{j\omega t}$ at one end, while terminating in its characteristic impedance, Z_0, at the other, both pressure and flow will be pulsatile throughout the length of the vessel. Introduction, in addition, of a sinusoidal vessel wall displacement $D(t) = D_0 e^{j\omega t}$ along the z-axis (the longitudinal axis) only will modify both pressure and flow as a consequence of the blood's inertial and viscous properties.

It would be attractive to modify the analysis in section 5.2 above to allow for the inclusion of vessel motion. Instead of following this complex route, externally induced vessel wall motion will be approximated by the simple expedient of adding a dimensionally compatible term to the equation of motion, in the form of Eq. 5.16a to become

$$-\frac{\partial p}{\partial z} = L'\frac{\partial Q}{\partial t} + R'Q - \rho\frac{d^2 D(t)}{dt^2} \tag{5.36a}$$

while leaving Eq. 5.16b unchanged

$$-\frac{\partial Q}{\partial z} = \frac{C'\partial p}{\partial t} \tag{5.36b}$$

Development of the wave equations following the procedures described in Sect. 5.2.3 above yields

$$\frac{\partial^2 p}{\partial z^2} = \frac{L'C'(\partial^2 p)}{\partial t^2} + \frac{R'C'\partial p}{\partial t} \qquad (5.37)$$

And

$$\frac{\partial^2 Q}{\partial z^2} = L'C'\frac{\partial^2 Q}{\partial t^2} + R'C'\frac{\partial Q}{\partial t} - \frac{\rho C'(\mathrm{d}^3 D)}{\mathrm{d}t^3} \qquad (5.38)$$

The solution for p remains of the same form as in Eq. 5.19a

$$p(z,t) = [p_a e^{-\gamma z} + p_r e^{\gamma z}]e^{j\omega t} \qquad (5.39a)$$

while that for Q becomes

$$Q(z,t) = [Q_a e^{-\gamma z} + Q_r e^{\gamma z}]e^{j\omega t} + k\frac{\mathrm{d}^2}{\mathrm{d}t^2}D(t) \qquad (5.39b)$$

where k is a constant to be determined. Retention of the requirement for γ^2 (Eq. 5.18), also requires that

$$k = \frac{\rho}{Z_1'(\omega)} \qquad (5.40)$$

It should be noted that k contains the inertial and viscous properties of blood (Eq. 5.13a).

Equations 5.39a, b contain four unknown coefficients: p_a, p_r, Q_a, and Q_r that need to be evaluated to make computation of $p(z, t)$ and $Q(z, t)$ feasible. Since the relations in Eqs. 5.22a, b remain valid, p_a and p_r can be expressed in Q_a and Q_r, or vice versa, respectively. The two remaining coefficients can be evaluated from two boundary conditions. Selecting entrance flow $Q(0, t)$ as $Q_0 e^{j\omega t}$, and the load impedance (at $z = L$) as the characteristic impedance, Z_0, it follows after some manipulation that

$$Q_a = \frac{2[Q_0 + k\omega^2 D_0]e^{\gamma L} - k\omega^2 D_0}{2e^{\gamma L}} \qquad (5.41a)$$

and

$$Q_r = \frac{k\omega^2 D_0}{2e^{\gamma L}} \qquad (5.41b)$$

This simple example, in which entrance flow and vessel displacement occur at the same frequency, as was applied in BASH (Sect. 9.4), serves to illustrate the havoc played by the extra term in Eq. 5.39b, compared to Eq. 5.19b, with the elegant expressions for Z_{in} in Eqs. 5.26–5.29 above. It originates from body shaking and vanishes when the body stops moving ($D_0 = 0$). Changes in pressure and flow may induce apparent modification in parameter values.

The example also demonstrates that both pressure and flow can be altered significantly under the influence of movement. For an aortic size vessel, acceleration with a magnitude <0.5 g can easily add a multiple of the original magnitude of flow at the distal end. In simpler terms: blood in larger vessels is "loose." This furnishes an example of impedance-defined flow, in which acceleration and deceleration provides the mechanism. Even a person lying quietly in bed is accelerated and decelerated by the heart beat (with an amplitude in the milli-g range, Starr and Noordergraaf A (1967)).

Pressure and flow modification are sensitive to the phase relation between cardiac pumping and body movement. For example, when the phase of the last term in Eq. 5.36a is inverted, the sign of k (in Eq. 5.39b) inverts also. In the example, entrance flow is defined as independent of body motion. In reality, left ventricular outflow is sensitive to root aortic pressure (Sect. 4.3). Hence, cardiac pumping performance will tend to alter with body movement as well.

The illustrated approach may be generalized to a network of blood vessels of any complexity, as well as to body oscillation frequencies different from heart rate.

Earlier, Belardinelli et al. (1991) analyzed the effect of transient body acceleration and deceleration on pressure in the dog's carotid artery and reported gratifying agreement with experimental observations.

5.3 Interpretation and Reduction

5.3.1 Interpretation of Experimentally Observed Phenomena; Their Expansion

Normal arterial systems, during rest in the horizontal position, display a number of dynamic properties that have been confirmed over and over again. The first is that the pressure pulse gains in magnitude as it travels away from its source, a ventricle, to the periphery. Spengler (1843) may well have been the first to observe this. Most of the scientific community dismissed his observations originally as artifact, probably attributable to poor instrumentation, reasoning that because a wave propagating through a viscous fluid contained in an artery with probably a viscoelastic wall would exchange energy (heat) with its environment and thus would be expected to lose, rather than gain, amplitude as actually happens in the tiny vessels. The second property seemed to lend support to this argument, when later, as it became possible to measure volume flow, it was found that the amplitude of this signal indeed decreased during its entire travel to the periphery (Fig. 5.4).

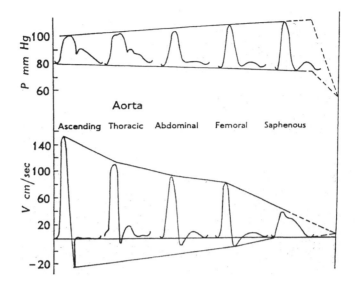

Fig. 5.4 Pressure and flow velocity pulses as a function of location. Volume flow pulses reduce slower in amplitude than velocity pulses, since individual arterial cross-sectional area decreases as well (From McDonald 1960)

The preoccupation with the prediction of the pulse wave velocity was noted above. Porjé (1946) eventually compared Fourier transforms of recorded pressure pulses in humans to predicted values and found agreement for high frequency components and major discrepancies for low frequency components, thus complicating the picture further (graph 4 in Fig. 5.2).

Randall and Stacy (1956) pioneered the introduction of a fourth feature by borrowing the input impedance concept (Eq. 5.25) from electrical engineering. From simultaneous measurements of pressure and flow at the entrance of the aorta and computing the ratio of pressure and flow by harmonic, the magnitude of the ratio identified the value of the peripheral resistance at zero frequency, while for higher frequencies the magnitude fell sharply to a weak minimum after which it leveled off to form a plateau (Fig. 5.5). Deeper into the system, input impedance of a more peripheral part of the system tends to be less smooth.

The new challenge became not just to predict pulse wave velocity, but to explain all four broadly accepted phenomena on the basis of a single theory.

Several investigators have put their shoulders to the wheel by developing quantitative models of the circulatory system or of a part thereof. Examples of the former are De Pater and Van den Berg's model consisting of passive electrical lines for arteries and veins with pressure generators to represent the four cardiac chambers (1964), and Attinger and Anné's model (1966) with a similar approach containing less detail, but solving the equations on a digital computer. The emphasis in these works was primarily to ascertain whether or not a model could mimic what was known about the behavior of the real system at the time when not a few educated people, for philosophical/religious reasons, felt that even raising such a "validation"

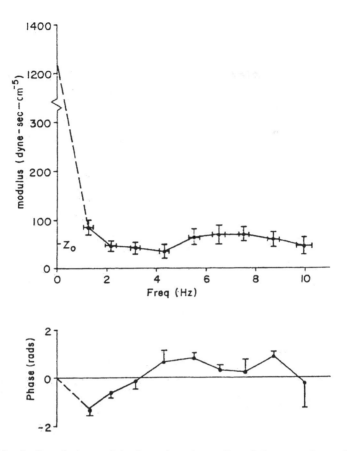

Fig. 5.5 Magnitude and phase of the input impedance, Z_{in}, of the systemic arterial system averaged over five normal men (Courtesy of Nichols et al. 1977)

question meant downgrading respect for the living organism. Another example belonging to the digital catagory was provided by Taylor's studies (1966) of a generalized description of the systemic arterial system alone. The emphasis here was on answering the question what requirements the description must satisfy to yield results similar to those observed experimentally (e.g., for input impedance). Taylor found that the architecture of the arterial system was a key element of the answer.

Cardiovascular investigators believed for a long time that vascular trees incorporating multiple branching sites should display strong reflection of antegrade (i.e., toward the periphery) waves, though designers of telephone cable transmission systems had known for some time that this could be, but was not necessarily, valid (Eq. 5.29c).These researchers did not appreciate the significance of the increase in cross-sectional area at branch points. Karreman (1952, 1954), as well as many others, on the basis of experimental studies by Hamilton and Dow (1939) and Hamilton (1944), tended to believe that reflection in the systemic arteries was strong enough for the system to resonate. Womersley (1957) pursued this idea in more detail and found that, for realistic conditions, impedance matching was approximated and hence, reflection coefficients were small; this finding reduced the likelihood of resonance to occur and appeared to rule out the possibility to explain pressure pulse peaking and flow pulse flattening on the basis of reflection at branching sites encountered during antegrade propagation.

The meticulously chronicled book by Wetterer and Kenner (1968) analyzed the considerable body of available experimental evidence. It including flow measurement, as well as the mathematical analyses carried out up to what might be called the transition period. This later led to the integration of the various pieces into a single theory. Thus the book reviews critically the applicability of Frank's windkessel theory (Sect. 5.3.2), treats wave propagation and reflection for both pressure and flow pulses in vessels of finite length, develops and analyzes the beginnings of their own distributed model, while identifying errors and misunderstandings in earlier publications. McDonald's 1974 book emphasizes anatomical and physiological properties of arteries in detail, making it a classic reference document for such data, while ignoring the newer insights that had become available since the publication of the first edition.

To deal with a branching system of arteries with individually different geometric and elastic properties, the larger arteries were thought of as subdivided into short uniform sections of 5–10 cm in length. The very large number of tiny vessels were lumped and considered resistive. These resistive elements were distributed according to the radius of the arteries feeding the various peripheral beds in such a way that their parallel combination accounted for the total peripheral resistance of the arterial system of interest. Each segment was characterized by a longitudinal and a transverse impedance (Eqs. 5.13a, b), taking into account its own properties. Such a characterization is insensitive to the presence or absence of reflected waves. This resulted in a set of several hundred differential equations, requiring simultaneous solution. Since the digital computer had not been developed at the time (the project was initiated in 1956) to a level sufficiently powerful to complete such a task successfully, an adjustable hard wired analog computer was designed and built, including the Bessel functions in Eq. 5.13a (Jager et al. 1965). It incorporated time transformation and solved the set of equations in a few milliseconds. The four properties of the system, referred to above, manifested themselves promptly (Westerhof et al. 1969; Westerhof and Noordergraaf A 1970). A similar analog was developed for the study of the pulmonary arterial system (Pollack et al. 1968). They provided tools to pinpoint the mechanisms responsible for the four phenomena.

Measurements on the electrical analogs of the systemic and pulmonary arterial systems revealed that the arterial systems are endowed with considerably more sophistication than originally appreciated. Antegrade pulses experience little reflection until they reach the arteriolar regions, where significant reflection usually occurs. Since arterioles control blood flow into the microcirculation their impedances are subject to local and neural influences, which override impedance matching requirements. Peripheral vasodilatation causes strong reduction of reflection as shown in dogs (Li et al. 1982). Unless the peripheral impedances are exceptionally small, pressure waves encounter positive, and flow waves negative reflection coefficients. Thus, retrograde waves are generated. During their return to the ventricles they encounter some of the same branching sites, which in the direction of their advance exhibit significant impedance mismatches (Hardung 1952; Li et al. 1984). As a result, a fraction of the reflected waves is reflected again and become antegrade waves. The considerable number of such sites together act as a reflector that prevents most of these waves to return to their ventricle. This reflector mechanism loses its effectiveness for the low frequency components of the signals when the wave lengths tend to exceed the length of the system. From the point of view of each of the ventricles, it appears that its arterial system is virtually reflection-free for high frequency components while displaying identifiable reflected waves for low frequency components. The transition is gradual in nature; this is relevant because it occurs around the heart frequency.

Since most reflection coefficients are complex numbers, phase shifts are introduced at reflection sites. This phenomenon, in conjunction with the differences in distance traveled by reflected waves, tends to promote their destructive addition upon arrival at the branching site.

Recognition of the effects imposed by the architecture of arterial systems makes it possible to interpret the four observed phenomena summarized above. Addressing the discrepancy between predicted and measured pulse wave velocity first (Fig. 5.2), it was noted that the deviation is most spectacular in the range of the low harmonics. This is the range where reflected waves reach the ventricle. Consequently, the velocity observed experimentally in the central region is the apparent velocity, which can exceed the phase velocity (Question 5.1), while for higher frequencies the phase velocity is measured in good approximation. The interpretation of the input impedance is very similar. At low frequencies it is influenced by the presence of reflected waves, which are nearly absent for higher frequencies. Therefore, in this higher range, the input impedance lies around the characteristic impedance (Eq. 5.26e).

With respect to pressure and flow pulses, it should be remembered first, that the presence of reflected waves is more abundant in distant arteries than in central ones. Second, it should be recalled that when the peripheral reflection is positive for pressure signals, which is commonly the case, that for flow signals will be negative (Eq. 5.22). Consequently, addition of antegrade and retrograde pressure signals will tend to be constructive, while for flow signals it will tend to be destructive. Thus, it can be expected that the pressure signal gains amplitude while advancing in the peripheral direction, while the flow signal loses amplitude in the same direction, which is what has been observed on innumerable occasions (Kuhn 1962).

Viscous losses in larger arteries, whether originating in the viscous properties of blood or in the viscoelastic properties of the wall, were found to play a small role (Westerhof and Noordergraaf A 1970). Also, due to the effect of reflection at branching sites, the arterial systems do not manifest any significant degree of resonance, despite the minute influence of damping.

Both input impedance and wave velocity were found to be strongly frequency dependent, which raised the question whether the system's compliance and peripheral resistance as viewed from the site of the ventricle could be as well. To answer these questions, the long tradition of considering these quantities as constants must be set aside, at least temporarily. Starting with Frank's equation describing conservation of mass (1899)

$$Q_{in} = Q_{stored} + Q_{out} \tag{5.42}$$

where Q_{in} denotes flow into the arterial system, Q_{out} its outflow into the veins, and Q_{stored} the flow that changes the volume of blood, V, in the arteries. Quick et al. (1998) defined the storage capacity, i.e., the compliance, C_{app}, and peripheral resistance, R_{app}, by linear frequency-dependent transfer functions as

$$C_{app} = \frac{dV}{dp_{in}}(\omega) = \frac{V(\omega)}{p_{in}(\omega)} \tag{5.43a}$$

and

$$R_{app} = \frac{P_{in}(\omega)}{Q_{out}(\omega)} \tag{5.43b}$$

in which $p_{in}(\omega)$ represents a harmonic of the input pressure; similarly for the other quantities. The subscript "app" is in analogy to "apparent" as in apparent wave velocity, c_{app}. The transfer function permits a phase difference between input pressure and arterial volume. (In the windkessel theory, this difference is set at zero). An explicit expression for C_{app} may be derived:

$$C_{app} = \frac{R_{app} - Z_{in}}{j\omega R_{app} Z_{in}} \tag{5.44}$$

It can be argued that R_{app} ranges from the value at zero frequency, traditionally called peripheral resistance, to infinity at a very high frequency. Substitution of either extreme in Eq. 5.44 has little impact on the frequency dependence of magnitude and phase angle of C_{app}. As the example in Fig. 5.6 shows, C_{app} is also a strong function of frequency. Its magnitude approaches the total compliance in the arterial system, while its phase angle goes to zero, as the frequency approaches zero. At higher frequencies, the magnitude of C_{app} drops precipitously, meaning that the ventricle sees an increasingly stiff system. The reason for this may be visualized as inertial and viscous effects shielding from view, by the ventricle, the more distant compliances.

The time-varying part of the volume stored in the arterial system, $V(t)$, i.e., the total arterial volume minus end diastolic volume, may be computed in the time domain with the aid of Eqs. 5.30 and 5.31

$$V(t) = \int_{t_{ED}}^{t} \left[Q_{in} - \frac{P_{in}}{R_{app}} \right] dt \tag{5.45}$$

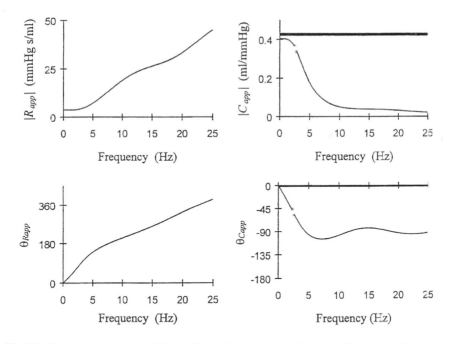

Fig. 5.6 Magnitude and phase of R_{app} (*left*) and C_{app} (*right*) as a function of frequency of the same model as used in Eqs. 5.19 and 5.20. The heavy horizontal line represents the actual compliance in this model (Adapted from Quick et al. 1998)

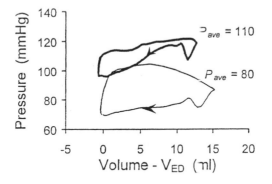

Fig. 5.7 Systemic arterial pressure-volume ($V(t)$) loops in two dogs with different mean arterial pressures (Adapted from Quick 1999)

where t_{ED} denotes the instant when end diastole occurs ($V(t) = 0$). Figure 5.7 illustrates an example for a dog in which R_{app} is replaced by R_s (Quick 1999). The dependence of pressure on $V(t)$ is not a straight line as often assumed, but a loop owing to the frequency dependence of the apparent compliance. The loop is traversed in clockwise direction as distinct from the ventricular pressure–volume loop (Sect. 4.3).

In an arterial system a number of complexities must be faced. A selection follows.

The Moens-Korteweg formula in a vessel free of reflection, and ignoring viscous effects, makes the phase velocity independent of frequency (Eq. 5.8a). When viscous effects are incorporated, it becomes frequency dependent (Eqs. 5.8h and 5.12b). This change is attributable to wave transmission. If wave reflection is incorporated as well, the term apparent wave velocity is employed because the observed velocity may deviate strikingly from the phase velocity in the range of the lower harmonics of the cardiovascular system (Eq. 5.18).

The characteristic impedance, Z_0, forms the frequency dependent input impedance of a vascular system totally free of reflected waves. If it is a real number, pressure and flow at the entrance to the system have identical wave forms. In the presence of reflection, it is converted into the input impedance, Z_{in}, which, in the cardiovascular system, tends to exceed Z_0, especially for low frequencies (Eq. 5.26e). Arterial compliance, C_{app}, as sensed by the ventricle, is another quantity influenced by transmission properties joined by the presence of reflected waves. These two effects tend to make the compliance, as observed, smaller than the total compliance present in the system, except in the very low frequency range (Eqs. 5.26), while R_{app} tends to fall to the value of the traditional peripheral resistance R_s or R_p as frequency approaches zero.

As more data on arterial properties continue to become available, the original distributed analog model could be updated and refined, e.g., by the introduction of nonlinear wall properties. Advances in digital hardware and software permitted transfer to the digital computer (Li et al. 1990; Stergiopulos et al. 1992 and several other investigators) and enhanced flexibility. Such refinements have not significantly affected the interpretation of the basic phenomena.

5.3.2 Reduced and Simplified Small Models

Small models may be obtained sometimes by a process of reasoned reduction in the size of larger ones (Sect. 1.2, Level 7). Simplified models can be formulated through a basically arbitrary reduction in the size of larger ones, or by simple definition of a small one. It is often profitable to make this distinction in the evaluation of small models with respect to their realistic applicability.

It occurred to the Reverend Stephen Hales (1733) to compare the systemic arterial system with the reservoir used in contemporary fire engines, as well as in pipe organs, to convert intermittent inflow into steady outflow. This idea and Hales' development of the precursor of the catheter-manometer system were to have enduring influence.

Otto Frank (1899) and his school adopted Hales' concept and renamed it the windkessel. Frank became fascinated by the idea of establishing a measure of cardiac performance for which he selected cardiac output, CO. Since pulsatile flow measurement had not yet become feasible, the windkessel theory was developed in terms of pressure. Considering a reservoir in which the pulse wave velocity approaches infinity, the governing equation became:

$$Q(t) - \frac{p}{R_s} = \frac{1}{E'}\frac{dp}{dt} \qquad (5.46)$$

in which $Q(t)$ denoted instantaneous ventricular ejection flow, reservoir pressure, p, divided by peripheral resistance, R_s, outflow, with the right-hand side representing the variation in volume stored by the reservoir, dV/dt, expressed in terms of pressure via

$$\frac{dV}{dt} = \frac{dV}{dp}\frac{dp}{dt} \qquad (5.47)$$

where dp/dV was defined as the modulus of elasticity E' of the reservoir, a property of the system. In the steady state, total ejection flow into the windkessel equals total outflow from the windkessel, making the right-hand side vanish. The quantity of interest follows from $CO = fV_s$, $f =$ measured heart rate, with $1/f = T$, $t_s =$ the duration of ejection, $V_s =$ stroke volume, and, hence

$$V_s = \int_0^{t_s} Q(t)\,dt = \int_0^{T} Q(t)\,dt = \frac{1}{R_s}\int_0^{T} p(t)\,dt \qquad (5.48)$$

The variable $p(t)$ is measured on any given subject or patient and taken to be the solution of the differential equation (5.46). R_s requires separate estimation (Noordergraaf A 1978).

Comparison with available methods for the measurement of cardiac output, such as the Fick method (1870) or the Stewart principle (1897) exposed differences with a large unpredictable scatter, the cause of which proved difficult to identify with any of the methods applied, but the ease with which the windkessel approach could be used in the clinic, noninvasively and repeatedly, enhanced its stature immensely. The twentieth century literature reports a wide variety of attempts to improve the theory aimed at making cardiac output estimates more accurate.

Although these efforts were doomed, the windkessel concept has retained its position as the simplest model of the systemic arterial system with a realistic touch. Landes (1943) attempted to improve the windkessel by bringing in a low level of distributed properties and found that the result compared poorly to windkessel behavior, which struck him as "paradoxical." The windkessel is often referred to as a two-element (resistive-capacitive) model. (The even simpler one-element [resistive] models (Hill et al. 1958; Vadot 1962) failed to achieve popularity). A century later, the windkessel concept found its way into the venous side of the peripheral vasculature (Mandeville et al. 1999).

Across the fence, researchers with a primary interest in models based on wave transmission concepts have searched for their own small models. A model representing a single uniform or nonuniform artery tends to display strong

Fig. 5.8 Two-element
(without Z_0) and three-
element (with Z_0) arterial
models, drawn with electrical
symbols. The former was
conceived by Frank (1899)
and is traditionally referred to
as the windkessel model, the
latter was designed by
Westerhof and Noordergraaf A
(1969) and is usually referred
to as the modified windkessel,
occasionally as the westkessel

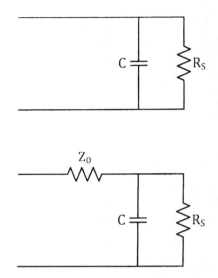

resonance, unlike the real system. Ways to avoid resonance are discussed in
Sect. 5.2 above. One is to employ the infinitely long uniform vessel that served as
a vehicle in the detailed studies to enable prediction of pulse wave velocity. The
alternative is to employ a uniform vessel of finite length that terminates in the
vessel's characteristic impedance, Z_0, reducing the terminal reflection coefficient to
zero (Eq. 5.29c). The actual arterial system manifests reflection, however, though it
is weak in magnitude and strongly frequency dependent in the larger arteries.

Combination of these observations offers an alternative approach, which
resulted in the so-called three-element, or modified windkessel model (Fig. 5.8):
at low frequencies peripheral reflection is observed, the pulse wave velocity is high
(Fig. 5.2) and to the ventricle the system behaves like a windkessel. At high
frequencies, the ventricle sees a system virtually free of reflection, similar to an
infinitely long vessel, and thus an input impedance, approximately equal to the
characteristic impedance. In between, around a frequency equal to the heart rate,
the system changes smoothly from one mode of behavior into the other (Fig. 5.9).
The series combination of the vessel's characteristic impedance and a windkessel
proved to handle the entire input impedance spectrum surprisingly realistically for
such a simple model.

This finding implies that the long-standing conflict between investigators
supporting the windkessel theory and those favoring the wave transmission theory
was misdirected. It is not a question of either or, since one theory works well in the
lowest frequency range while the other offers a good approximation in the highest
frequency range, without overlapping each other. Quick et al. (2006) offered a
method to determine a value for "high" and "low" for any given arterial system.

The three-element model can be easily converted into its fluid-mechanical
equivalent and has found extensive application in experiments where the ventricle
must be provided with a realistic vascular load in fluid-mechanical form, such as in

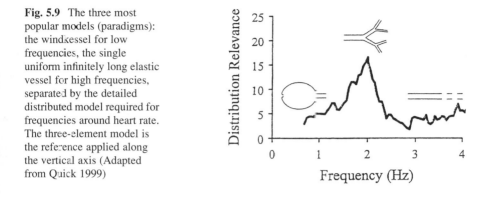

Fig. 5.9 The three most popular models (paradigms): the windkessel for low frequencies, the single uniform infinitely long elastic vessel for high frequencies, separated by the detailed distributed model required for frequencies around heart rate. The three-element model is the reference applied along the vertical axis (Adapted from Quick 1999)

testing artificial valves, or artificial hearts (Westerhof et al. 1971). The three-element model has also been applied in its original form to reduce the size of a fully distributed model to represent the impedance of one or more peripheral parts of an arterial system when wave transmission in those parts is of no interest to the subject of study (Westerhof and Noordergraaf A 1969). It gradually loses its attractiveness if it is used in more peripheral parts since the presence of reflected waves becomes more dominant further away the heart.

Inasmuch as both the two-element and the three-element windkessels contain a compliance, popularly denoted as the total arterial system compliance, they were seized upon to obtain clinical estimates of this quantity, an extension of these models beyond their original purpose. The numerical values of the elements for the three-element windkessel may be estimated from measurement of pressure and flow in the root of the aorta which yield the input impedance, Z_{in}. Its magnitude at zero frequency defines the peripheral resistance, the average value for the high frequency magnitudes is taken to be the characteristic impedance, Z_0, while the compliance, C, may be obtained as the best fit of the input impedance of the three-element model to its experimentally derived counterpart. Several variations on this theme are available as well. For the two-element windkessel there is no call for a Z_0 estimate. The resultant values for arterial compliance were inconsistent as shown, e.g., by Stergiopulos et al. (1995), who compared the results of seven different techniques against its known value in a distributed model of the arterial system.

As suggested by the three-element model, the actual arterial compliance was considered to be a constant. Quick et al. (1998) demonstrated, however, that, like C_{app}, compliance as seen by the ventricle is dependent on frequency. In this instance, that stems from shielding by inertial and viscous effects. In addition, C_{app}, also like c_{app}, is sensitive to the presence of reflected waves. Hence, the ventricle sees only a frequency-dependent fraction of the total compliance. This was deemed to be the cause of the earlier inconsistent findings. It is possible, nevertheless, to extract the total compliance, C_{tot}, fairly accurately by calculating its value at a frequency low enough to, in fact, eliminate most of the effect of shielding and of the phase difference between pressure and flow in the root of the aorta (Fig. 5.6). This frequency may fall below the heart rate, but can be furnished by natural or induced irregular heartbeats (e.g., sinus arrhythmia, Quick et al. 2000).

Modification of apparent compliance may be applied to quantify alteration in arterial system properties via characterization of reflection as a feedback control (Quick et al. 2002).

First introduced by Otto Frank, the concept of an effective length, L, of an arterial system gained popularity. The purpose here was to simplify the description of a branching system of arteries feeding individual peripheral organs, which, in the systemic system, are located at very different distances from the ventricle, ranging from the coronary circulation to the feet. Each artery that reaches a peripheral organ may be expected to generate a reflected wave at the level of the arterioles which control blood flow through that particular organ. This means that reflected waves originate over a large spectrum of distances. The effective length of the system or the effective lengths of parts of the system, if the system is so subdivided, are the lengths measured from the ventricle to the location where all reflected waves from that part, or from the whole, appear to originate. On the basis of intuition, Frank (1905) suggested first that the iliac bifurcation might qualify as the effective reflection site for the entire system ($L \sim 50$ cm). Subsequent analytically based studies led to the common conclusion that L exists, though investigators arrived at widely different values for the distance of the effective reflection site from the ventricle; Burattini and Di Carlo offered a summary (1988).

Campbell et al. (1989) elucidated this problem by showing from the wave equations for a single uniform viscoelastic vessel (Eqs. 5.17) that there is an infinite number of solutions for L, and for the effective terminal impedance as well, if the input impedance of the single vessel is exactly to match the measured input impedance of an arterial system. A fortiori, one can design reflection sites at an infinite number of downstream locations, all of which produce a given reflected pressure wave at the entrance. If an effective reflection site exists indeed, it has not been found. Characterizing the transmission properties over a well-defined length of distensible vessel has been more rewarding (Burattini and Campbell 2000).

The absence of a unique solution haunts the applicability of the asymmetric T model. The concept of two reflection sites, also introduced by Frank (1905), was rediscovered by McDonald (1965; 1974). This simple model recognizes the ascending aorta as the vertical part of the T. At its upper end two (usually uniform) vessels branch off, one in the cephalic direction, the other in the caudal direction, each terminating at its own effective length. The model is called asymmetric since the effective length of the caudal branch is usually taken to be longer than that of its cephalic counterpart.

The source of such problems is found in the change of the questions offered for solution. Thus far, the emphasis was on solving forward problems: given an arterial system, can measurable quantities, like pulse wave velocity or input impedance, be interpreted on the basis of the known architecture and the properties of the individual vessel making up the system. Most of the questions of this type have been answered. In the process, investigators turned to the inverse problem: given one or more measured quantities, can estimates be made of features internal to the system, such as the location of a reflection site or the compliant properties of selected vessels. Quick et al. (2001a) illustrated the gravity of the problems encountered by showing that there is an infinite variation in arterial properties possible within an arterial system, all of them displaying the exact same input impedance.

On the other hand, the solution of forward problems identified a modest number of solutions to inverse problems. Examples are: peripheral resistance, regional pulse wave velocity, total compliance, and characteristic impedance of the aorta. Such quantities can serve to interpret differences in measured input impedances (Quick et al. 2006).

Many other simple models have been presented. Most of them were validated on the basis of the argument that they were able to reproduce the transformation of the pressure pulse, while ignoring the flow pulse. This affords the designer extra leeway not available to the real system. For example, the magnitude of a pressure pulse propagating through a single vessel, modeled as narrowing away from the ventricle, will tend to increase in the same direction. This overlooks the well-established fact that the actual system gains in cross-sectional area owing to the presence of branches. Reallocation of flow will occur as a result (Melbin and Noordergraaf A 1983).

5.4 Conclusions

The arterial systems have captured the interest of numerous investigators. The focus shifted often: originally whether the living system could be modeled at all, to whether current models of the system are accurate enough even when smaller details are incorporated. This discussion detracted attention from the early discovery of their special properties and their physiological significance such as facilitation of ventricular ejection. It also postponed the analysis of large nonlinear phenomena in other parts of the cardiovascular system, especially of the venous vasculatures. Properties of arteries could be formulated by longitudinal and transverse impedances derived for thick walled vessels via a set of five simultaneous differential equations, solved in closed form.

The evolution of thinking about the arterial system offers the bioscientist potential for insight. Originally thought to be only a plumbing feature to reach every organ, it has been confirmed that it, in fact, is what it seemed to be, a plumbing system, though one with highly sophisticated properties.

5.5 Summary

This chapter is the longest one, as a result of enduring interest by scientists for more than two centuries. For most of this period the interest was narrowly focused on the analytical prediction of pulse wave velocity. Eventually, it matured to the quest for a single theory to interpret all well-established arterial phenomena. As it turned out, arterial systems possess a far more sophisticated design than just a combination of branching vessels that reach every location of the body, as originally proposed in the Ebert papyrus. A sizable model with distributed properties greatly facilitated the pinpointing of the critical features in nature's arterial arrangements. It also illustrates the prevailing approach in this book: model design starts with the development of a set of equations, i.e., a mathematical model. The equations may be solved with an analog computer through the application of equivalent circuits, or by a digital computer in which the equations themselves are programmed. In both, the expanded concept of impedance plays a key role. This philosophy carries over to the analysis of pressures and flows in veins, lymphatics, and impedance-defined flow, and may include nonlinear phenomena, where deemed valuable.

Concurrently, an array of simple models had been developed. The comparison between these, mostly intuitive, models and the one derived by logical reduction of the much larger one with distributed properties, made most of the intuitive models obsolete. Only two survived, namely, Otto Frank's classical two-element model and its three-element more accurate variation, which derived from logical reduction. There is some discernable activity in expanding the three-element model again.

Arterial models have achieved a level of refinement that created a canon on how such studies can be performed successfully.

This chapter offers two additional features. One is an extension of the material discussed in Chap. 2 in which the nonlinear wall properties of venous walls are incorporated under conditions of various transmural pressures. The other treats a simple example of what happens to arterial pressure and flow when the whole body is shaken. Especially the second case opens new vistas.

References

Anliker M., Wells M.K. and Ogden E.: The transmission characteristics of large and small pressure waves in the abdominal vena cava. IEEE Trans. Biomed. Eng. 16: 262–274, 1969.

Attinger E.O. and Anné A.: Simulation of the cardiovascular system. Ann. New York Acad. Sc. 128: 810–829, 1966.

Belardinelli E., Ursino M. and Fabbri G.: A linear propagation model adapted to the study of fast perturbations in arterial hemodynamics. Comput. Biol. Med. 21: 97–110, 1991.

Bergel D.H.: The Visco-Elastic Properties of the Arterial Wall. Ph.D. Diss., Univ. of London, 1960.

Berger D.S.: Repeated Reflections and the Effects of Wave Reflections on Arterio-Ventricular Function. Ph.D. Dissertation, Rutgers Univ., New Brunswick NJ, 1993.

Berger D.S., Li J.K-J., Laskey W.K. and Noordergraaf A.: Repeated reflection of waves in the systemic arterial system. Am. J. Physiol. 264 (Heart Circ. Physiol. 33): H269-281, 1993.

Brower R.W. and Scholten C.: Experimental evidence on the mechanism for the instability of flow in collapsible vessels. Med. Biol. Eng. 13: 839–845, 1975.

Burattini R. and K.B. Campbell: Physiological relevance of uniform elastic tube-models to infer descending aortic wave reflection: a problem of identifiability. Ann. of Biomed. Eng. 28:512–523, 2000.

Burattini R. and Di Carlo S.: Effective length of the arterial circulation determined in the dog by aid of a model of the systemic input impedance. IEEE Trans. Biomed. Eng. 35:53–61, 1988.

Campbell K.B., Lee L.C., Frasch H.F. and Noordergraaf A.: Pulse reflection sites and effective length of the arterial system. Am. J. Physiol. 256 (Heart Circ. Physiol. 25):H1684-H1689, 1989.

De Pater L. and Berg van den J.W.: An electrical analogue of the entire human circulatory system. Med. Electron. Biol. Eng. 2: 161–166, 1964.

Drzewiecki G.M., Melbin J. and Noordergraaf A.: The Korotkoff sound. Ann. Biomed. Eng. 17: 325–359, 1989.

Fick A.: Über die Messung des Blutquantums in den Herzventrikeln. Sitzungsber. Phys.-Med. Ges. Würzburg, p. 16, 1870.

Frank C.: Die Grundform des arteriellen Pulses. Z. Biol. 37: 483–526, 1899.

Frank O.: Der Puls in den Arterien. Z. Biol. 46: 441–553, 1905.

Fung Y.C.: A first course in continuum mechanics 2nd ed. Prentice-Hall, Englewood Cliffs, NJ, 1977.

Griffiths D.J.: Steady flow through veins and collapsible tubes. Med. Biol. Eng. 9: 597–602, 1971.

Hales S.: Statical Essays: Containing Haemostaticks, or an Account of some Hydraulick and Hydrostatical Experiments made on the Blood and Blood-Vessels of Animals; etc., Vol. 2. Innys and Manby, London, 1733.

Hamilton W.F.: The patterns of the arterial pressure pulse. Am. J. Physiol. 144: 235–241, 1944.

Hamilton W.F. and Dow P.: An experimental study of the standing waves in the pulse propagated through the aorta. Am. J. Physiol. 125: 48–59, 1939.

Hardung V.: Zur mathematischen Behandlung der Dämpfung und Reflexion der Pulswellen. Arch. Kreislaufforsch. 18: 167–172, 1952.

Hill W.S., Polleri J.O. and Matteo A.L.: Essay on a Hydrodynamic Analysis of the Blood Circulation. Univ. of Montevideo. ANCAP, Ministerio de Salud Poeblica, Montevideo, Uruguay, 1958.

Jager G.N.: Electrical Model of the Human Systemic Arterial Tree. Ph.D. Dissertation, Univ. of Utrecht, 1965.

Jager G.N., Westerhof N. and Noordergraaf A.: Oscillatory flow impedance in electrical analog of arterial system: representation of sleeve effect and non-newtonian properties of blood. Circ. Res. 16: 121–133, 1965.

Karreman G.: Some contributions to the mathematical biology of blood circulation. Reflections of pressure waves in the arterial system. Bull. Math. Biophysics 14: 327–350, 1952.

Karreman G.: The resonance of the arterial system. Bull. Math. Biophysics 16; 159–170, 1954.

Kresch E. and Noordergraaf A.: A mathematical model for the pressure-flow relationship in a segment of vein. IEEE Trans. Bio-Medical Eng. BME-16: 296–307, 1969.

Kries J von.: Studien zur Pulslehre. Akad. Verlagsbuchshandlung, Freiburg i. B., 1892.

Kuhn T.S.: The Structure of Scientific Revolutions. The University of Chicago Press, Chicago IL, 1962.

Landes G.: Einige Untersuchungen an elektrischen Analogieschaltungen zum Kreislaufsystem. Z. Biol. 101: 418–429, 1943.

Li J.K-J., Melbin J. and Noordergraaf A.: Evidence for pulse reflection in the dog femoral artery. 35th Ann. Conf. Eng. Med. Biol., Philadelphia PA, 1982.

Li J.K-J., Melbin J. and Noordergraaf A.: Directional disparity of pulse reflection in the dog. Am. J. Physiol. 247: H95-H99, 1984.

Li J.K-J., Cui T. and Drzewiecki G.M.: A nonlinear model of the arterial system incorporating a pressure-dependent compliance. IEEE Trans. Biomed. Eng. 37: 673–678, 1990.

Mandeville J.B., Marota J.J.A., Ayata C., Zaharchuck G., Moskowitz M.A., Rosen B.R. and Weisskoff R.M.: Evidence of a cerebral postarteriole windkessel with delayed compliance. J. Cerebral Blood Flow and Metabolism 19: 679–689, 1999.

McDonald D.A.: Wave propagation in the arterial tree. Proc. 18th Ann. Conf. Eng. in Med. Biol., Philadelphia PA, p.1, 1965.

McDonald D.A.: Blood Flow in Arteries. Arnold, London. 1st ed., 1960, 2nd ed., 1974.

Melbin J. and Noordergraaf A.: Pressure gradient related to energy conversion in the aorta. Circ. Res. 52: 319–327, 1983.

Moreno A.H., Katz A.I. and Gold L.D.: An integrated approach to the study of the venous system with steps toward a detailed model of the dynamics of venous return to the right heart. IEEE Trans. Biomed. Eng. 16: 308–324, 1969.

Nichols W.W., Conti C.R., Walker W.E. and Milnor W.R.: Input impedance of the systemic circulation in man. Circ. Res. 40: 451–458, 1977.

Nippa J.H., Alexander R.H. and Folse R.: Pulse wave velocity in human veins. J. Appl. Physiol. 30: 558–563, 1971.

Noordergraaf A.: Circulatory System Dynamics. Academic Press, New York NY, 1978.

Noordergraaf A.: Compliance in cardiovascular function. Medicinsky Razgledi 30, suppl. 1: 3–13, 1991.

Pollack G.H., Reddy R.V. and Noordergraaf A.: Input impedance, wave travel, and reflections in the pulmonary arterial tree: Studies using an electrical analog. IEEE Trans. Biomed. Eng. BME 15: 151–164, 1968.

Porjé I.G.: Studies of the arterial pulse wave, particularly in the aorta. Acta Physiol. Skand. 13, Suppl. 42: 1–68, 1946.

Quick C.M.: Reconciling Windkessel and Transmission Descriptions of the Arterial System and the Stability of Muscular Arteries. Ph.D. Dissertation, Rutgers Univ., New Brunswick NJ, 1999.

Quick C.M., Berger D.S. and Noordergraaf A.: Apparent arterial compliance. Am. J. Physiol. 274 (Heart Circ. Physiol. 43): H1393-H1403, 1998.

Quick C.M., Berger D.S., Hettrick D.A. and Noordergraaf A.: True arterial system compliance estimated from apparent arterial system compliance. Ann. Biomed. Eng. 28:291–301, 2000.

Quick C.M., Young W.L. and Noordergraaf A.: Infinite number of solutions to the hemodynamic inverse problem. Am. J. Physiol. 280: H1472-H1479, (2001a).

Quick C.M., Berger D.S. and Noordergraaf A.: Constructive and destructive addition of forward and reflected arterial pulse waves in the arterial system. Am. J. Physiol. 280: H1519–H1527, (2001b).

Quick C.M., Berger D.S. and Noordergraaf A.: Arterial pulse wave reflection as feedback. IEEE Trans. Biomed. Eng. 49: 440–445, 2002.

Quick C.M., Berger D.S., Stewart R.H., Laine G.A., Hartley C.J. and Noordergraaf A.: Resolving the hemodynamic inverse problem. IEEE Trans. Biomed. Eng. 53: 361–368, 2006.

Randall J.E. and Stacy R.W.: Mechanical impedance of the dog's hind leg to pulsatile blood flow. Am. J. Physiol. 187: 94–98, 1956.

Resal H. Note: sur les petits movement d'un fluide incompressible dans un tuyau élustique. J. Math pures et appliqués, 3rd series, 2: 342–344, 1816.

Snyder M.F. and Rideout V.C.: Computer simulation studies of the venous circulation. IEEE Trans. Biomed. Eng. 16: 325–334, 1969.

Sommerfeld A.: Vorlesungen über Theoretische Physik. Band II, Dieterich'sche Verlagsbuch-handlung, Wiesbaden, 1947.

Spengler L.: Symbolae ad Theoriam de Sanguinis Arteriosi Flumine. Dissertation, Marburg, 1843.

Starr I. and Noordergraaf A.: Ballistocardiography in Cardiovascular Research. Lippincott Co., Philadelphia PA, 1967.

Stergiopulos N., Young D.F. and Rogge T.R.: Computer simulation of arterial flow with applications to arterial and aortic stenoses. J. Biomech. 25: 1477–1488, 1992.

Stergiopulos N., Meister J.J. and Westerhof N.: Evaluation of methods for estimation of total arterial compliance. Am. J. Physiol. 268 (Heart Circ. Physiol. 37); H1540-H1548, 1995.

Stewart G..N.: Researches on the circulation time and on the influences which affect it: IV. The output of the heart. J. Physiol. 22: 159–183, 1897.

Taylor M.G.: The input impedance of an assembly of randomly branching elastic tubes. Biophys. J. 6: 29–51, 1966.

Vadot L.: Examen des problèmes d'hémodynamique au moyen d'une analogie électrique. Application particulière aux malformations cardiaques. Pathol. Biol. Semaine Hop., 10: 1499–1509, 1962

Vaishnav R.N. and Vossoughi J.: Estimation of Residual Strains in Aortic Segments. In: Biomedical Engineering II, Recent Developments, C.W. Hall (ed.), Pergamon Press, New York, 1983.

Weber E.H.: Ueber die Anwendung der Wellenlehre auf des Lehre from Kreislaufe des Blutes und ins besondere auf die Pulslehre. Ber. Verh. Kgl. Saechs. Ges. Wiss., Math. Phys. Kl., 1850.

Weizsäcker H.W.: Beschreibung und Messung der Arteriene astizität. In: Physiologie an der Schwelle zum 21. Jahrhundert, H. Hinghofer-Szalkay (ed.), Blackwell, Wien, 2000.

Weizsäcker H.W. and Pinto J.G.: Isotropy and anisotropy of the arterial wall. J. Biomech. 21: 477–487, 1988.

Weizsäcker H.W., Pascale K., Kenner T.: Elasticity of rat thoracic aortas in simple elongation. Biomedizinische Technik 29: 30–38, 1984.

Weizsäcker H.W., Holzapfel G.A., Desch G.W. and Pinto J.G. Constitutive Equation for Elastic and Muscular Arteries. In: Advances in Physiological Fluid Dynamics. M. Singh, V.P. Saxena (eds.). Narose Publ. House, New Delhi, 1996.

Westerhof N. and Noordergraaf A.: Arterial viscoelasticity: a generalized model. J. Biomech. 3: 357–379, 1970.

Westerhof N. and Noordergraaf A.: Reduced models of systemic arteries. Proc. Int. Conf. Med. Eng., 8th, Chicago, Session 6–2, 1969.

Westerhof N., Elzinga G. and Sipkema P.: An artificial arterial system for pumping hearts. J. Appl. Physiol. 31: 776–781, 1971.

Westerhof N., Sipkema P., Bos van den G.C. and Elzinga G.: Forward and backward waves in the arterial system. Cardiovasc. Res. 6: 648–656, 1972.

Wetterer E., Kenner Th.: Grundlagen der Dynamik des Arterienpulses. Springer-Verlag, Berlin, Heidelberg, New York, 1968.

Wiener F., Morkin E., Skalak R. and Fishman A.P.: Wave propagation in the pulmonary circulation. Circ. Res. 19: 834–850, 1966.

Wiggers C.J.: Physiology in Health and Disease. Lea & Febiger, Philadelphia PA, 1934, 1954.

Witzig K.: Über erzwungene Wellenbewegungen zäher, inkompressibler Flüssigkeiten in elastischen Röhren. Ph.D. Dissertation, Univ. of Bern, Bern, 1914.

Womersley J.R.: An Elastic Tube Theory of Pulse Transmission and Oscillatory Flow in Mammalian Arteries. WADC Technical Report TR 56–614, 1957.

Young T.: On the function of the heart and arteries: The Croonian lecture. Phil. Trans. Roy. Soc. 99: 1–31, 1809.

Appendix

Questions

5.1 The sum of two pressure signals (e.g., of an outgoing wave and its reflected part) may travel at a speed different from their phase velocities. This velocity is referred to as the apparent velocity, c_{app}, of the sum. Show that c_{app}/c_{ph} is sensitive to the magnitude and the sign of the reflected wave. Possible examples are the following sets $\{p_a = 1;\ p_r = 0.9;\ \omega z = 75;\ c_{ph} = 500\}$, $\{p_a = 1;\ p_r = 0.1;\ \omega z = 75;\ c_{ph} = 500\}$, $\{p_a = 1;\ p_r = -0.1;\ \omega z = 75;\ c_{ph} = 500\}$. Assume that fluid viscosity equals zero.

5.2 Argue that a reflected sine wave is less filtered by a discontinuity, the lower its frequency.

5.3 Can a composite (i.e., containing more than one harmonic) pressure wave and its companion flow wave move at different speeds?

5.4 Resolve a pressure and a flow signal, measured at the same site, z_0, in a single vessel into its antegrade and retrograde components.

5.5 Express output pressure, p_2, and flow, Q_2, at the end of a uniform vessel of length L, in the entrance pressure, p_1, and flow, Q_1, with the aid of the three parameters shown in Fig. 5.10 (below).

5.6 Show that two vessels in parallel cannot, in general, be replaced by a single vessel that manifests the same pressures and the same total flow as the parallel combination (Fig. 5.11).

5.7 Consider two elastic vessels in series, the first characterized by L_1, γ_1, and Z_1, the second by $L_2 = \infty$, γ_2, and Z_2 (Fig. 5.11) see below. Can the pressure and flow pulses in vessel 2 be larger or smaller than in vessel 1?

5.8 Figure 5.12 shows four junctions marked with the characteristic impedances for each of the vessels involved. The arrowhead defines the entry site for pressure and flow pulses. For simplicity, set the magnitude of the input signals arriving at the junction at 1 (arbitrary units). In each case, the vessel(s) beyond the junction is (are) taken to be infinitely long to avoid reflected waves originating from other sites. Determine pressures and flows.

5.9 Two popular models to describe viscoelastic material are the Voigt and Maxwell's models discussed in Westerhof and Noordergraaf A (1970). In Laplace notation, the complex Young modulus, E_c, for the Voigt model is $E_c(s) = (c_0 + c_1 s)/d_0$, for the Maxwell model $E_c(s) = c_1 s/(d_0 + d_1 s)$. The c's and d's are constants, while s denotes the Laplace operator. Show that for a step increase in length, the Voigt model predicts a brief unbounded force to appear, while for a step increase in force, the Maxwell model predicts an eventually unbounded length.

5.10 Is it possible for the antegrade and retrograde terms in the flow signal of Eq. 5.23b to cancel each other?

5.11 Is it possible to recognize reflected waves in (a) the two-element windkessel as defined by Frank, and (b) the three-element (modified) windkessel?

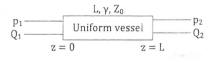

Fig. 5.10 Pertains to Question 5.5

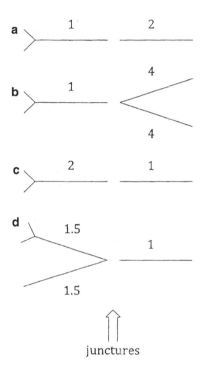

junctures

Fig. 5.11 Pertains to Question 5.8

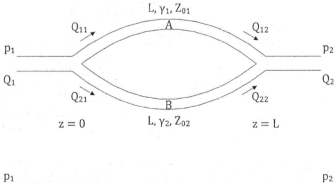

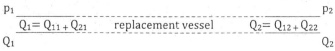

Fig. 5.12 Pertains to Question 5.6

5.12 A measured pressure or flow pulse can be separated in its antegrade and retrograde traveling components. In the process of carrying out this separation, is the mean pressure also broken up into two parts?

5.13 Input impedance is generally expressed as a complex number $Z_{in} = -Z_{in}|e^{j\theta}$. In research reports, frequently the absolute value alone is applied to calculate work. Correct?

5.14 Consider two points A and B along a stretch of a branchless uniform artery in vivo. The pressure $p_A(t)$ is measured and all properties of the artery between A and B are known. Compute $p_B(t)$.

5.15 Does the transfer function between the pressure in the root of the aorta and in a digital artery remain unchanged for the same person at different times? Is it invariant among different persons at the same time?

5.16 In the simple case that an artery splits up into two equal branches, it can be shown easily that impedance matching can, in principle, be achieved by adapting the elastic properties of the branches, or by adapting primarily their geometric properties. In mammalian arteries, adaptation is primarily achieved through changes in radii. Identify the physiological implication if the major alternative had been selected (Noordergraaf A 1991).

5.17 In the systemic arterial system, does the following equation apply: $p_{ao}(t) = p_{end\ diastolic} + Q_{ej}(t)R_s$?

5.18 Explain why the input impedance of the three-element windkessel matches reality better than that of the two-element windkessel.

5.19 A number of investigators measure flow velocity instead of volume flow (convenient when using ultrasound sensors), then define impedance as pressure divided by flow velocity instead of volume flow. (a) Do these two definitions of impedance have the same dimension? (b) Researchers in the field of acoustics define impedance as $\rho_c ph$. What is its dimension? (c) What is the dimension of cardiac output normalized by body surface area?

5.20 Applying the boundary conditions that led to Eqs. 5.41a, b, develop the full expressions for $p(z, t)$ and $Q(z, t)$, and show that $p(L, t) = Z_0 Q(L, t)$.

5.21 Is it possible, in principle, to model a systemic arterial system by representing individually all vessels up to and including the capillary level? If so, could all local reflection coefficients be determined along the paths from the left ventricle to the capillaries?

5.22 When feeling the arterial pulse, while increasing the pressure exerted by the finger, the initial signal perceived yields information about the stiffness of the arterial wall, subsequently about the pressure of the blood inside. Provide an explanation. Hint: see Drzewiecki et al. (1989).

5.23 Some investigators concluded from their analyses of distributed arterial models that significant reflection takes place wherever branch points are found. Could this be a modeling artifact?

5.24 A fluid-filled, infinitely long, uniform elastic tube will not show flow when a constant pressure is applied at its entrance. Show this mathematically.

5.25 Could the philosophical/religious objections, mentioned in Sect. 5.3 be advanced as an excuse to not proceed from duplication refinement to interpretation?

5.26 The wide and ever-expanding variety of closed loop cardiovascular models necessitates the use of keywords/expressions to distinguish their pros and cons.

A number of such terms are listed below: (1) the model is small, (2) one dimensional, (3) linear, (4) lumped, (5) no heart, (6) no valves, (7) blood viscosity $= 0$, (8) blood density $= 0$, (9) significant wave reflection occurs at every arterial branching site, (10) the total cross-sectional area of arteries away from the heart tapers down, (11) elastic properties of veins and arteries are equal, and (12) all parameter values are constant.

On the basis of your judgment, separate the 12 pros and cons into two groups: desirable and undesirable.

Answers

5.1 The relation between an antegrade wave, a retrograde wave, and their sum, propagating through an inviscid medium, may be written as

$$p_a e^{j\left(\omega t - \omega \frac{z}{c_{ph}}\right)} + p_r e^{j\left(\omega t + \omega \frac{z}{c_{ph}}\right)} = p_{sum} e^{j\left(\omega t - \omega \frac{z}{c_{app}}\right)} \tag{5.49}$$

which simplifies to

$$p_a \cos \omega \tfrac{z}{c_{ph}} - jp_a \sin \omega \tfrac{z}{c_{ph}} + p_r \cos \omega \tfrac{z}{c_{ph}} + jp_r \sin \omega \tfrac{z}{c_{ph}}$$
$$= p_{sum} \cos \omega \tfrac{z}{c_{app}} - jp_{sum} \sin \omega \tfrac{z}{c_{app}} \tag{5.50}$$

Sorting by real and imaginary parts and division yields

$$\frac{-p_a + p_r}{p_a + p_r} \tan \omega \tfrac{z}{c_{ph}} = - \tan \omega \tfrac{z}{c_{app}} \tag{5.51}$$

And

$$p_{sum} = \frac{(p_a + p_r) \cos \omega \tfrac{z}{c_{ph}}}{\cos \omega \tfrac{z}{c_{app}}} \tag{5.52}$$

The solutions are $c_{app} = 9500, 610, 411$ (i.e., less than c_{ph}), and $p_{sum} = 1.9$. 1.1, 0.9, respectively.

5.2 With the aortic and the pulmonary valves closed and the heart frequency low, the longitudinal impedances that define the details of the architectural arrangements (Fig. 11.1) tend to disappear with respect to the peripheral resistances. This applies more rigorously the lower the frequency and, hence the longer the wavelength, λ ($c_{app} = n\lambda$), $n =$ frequency of interest. Long waves do not recognize local or regional details, they only perceive an arterial reservoir.

5.3 Yes, they could. For a single harmonic, let the antegrade signals be p_a and Q_a, both positive. If the reflection coefficient is such that p_r is positive as well, then Q_r will be negative. Their compositions will progress at different velocities (Question 5.1). If the same conditions were to apply to all harmonics in the signals, the composite waves would behave likewise. Such conditions are unlikely to prevail.

5.4 After Fourier transformation of the measured signals, for harmonic ω_i, and setting $z_0 = 0$, addition of Eq. 5.19a and Z_0 times Eq. 5.23b yields $p(\omega_i) + Z_0 Q(\omega_i) = 2p_a(\omega_i)$, or $p_a = [p(\omega_i) + Z_0 Q(\omega_i)]/2$. Subtraction yields $p_r = [p(\omega_i) - Z_0 Q(\omega_i)]/2$. A similar procedure applied to Eqs. 5.19b and 5.23a gives $Q_a = [p/Z_0 + Q]/2$ and $Q_r = [p/Z_0 - Q]/2$.

5.5 Figure Q. 5.10 defines a uniform vessel characterized by its length, L, propagation constant, γ, and characteristic impedance, Z_0. Equations 5.19a and 5.24b, evaluated at the entrance ($z = 0$), yield the coefficients p_a and p_r as: $p_a = [p_1 + Z_0Q_1]/2$, and $p_r = [p_1 - Z_0Q_1]/2$. Evaluating the same equations at the exit ($z = L$) and substituting for p_a and p_r leads to

$$p_2 = \frac{1}{2}\left[e^{-\gamma L} + e^{\gamma L}\right]p_1 + \frac{Z_0}{2}\left[e^{-\gamma L} - e^{\gamma L}\right]Q_1 \tag{5.53}$$

and

$$Q_2 = \frac{1}{2Z_0}\left[e^{-\gamma L} - e^{\gamma L}\right]p_1 + \frac{1}{2}\left[e^{-\gamma L} + e^{\gamma L}\right]Q_1 \tag{5.54}$$

Rewritten in standard form: $p_2 = A_{11}p_1 + A_{12}Q_1$ and $Q_2 = A_{21}p_1 + A_{22}Q_1$, with $A_{11} = A_{22}$. This is called the two-port approach. It is easily generalized to apply to nonuniform vessels.
5.6 Figure Q. 5.12 shows two uniform vessels A and B in parallel, characterized by L, γ_1, Z_{01} and by L, γ_2, Z_{02}. Further, $Q_1 = Q_{11} + Q_{21}$, and $Q_2 = Q_{12} + Q_{22}$. As in the answer to Q. 5.5, exit pressure and flows are expressed in entrance pressure and flows separately for vessels A and B. Written in the simple form, it follows that
for vessel A:

$$p_2 = A_{11}p_1 + A_{12}Q_{11}, \tag{5.55}$$

and

$$Q_{12} = A_{12}p_1 + A_{22}Q_{11}, \tag{5.56}$$

with

$$A_{11} = A_{22} \tag{5.57}$$

for vessel B:

$$p_2 = B_{11}p_1 + B_{12}Q_{21} \tag{5.58}$$

and

$$Q_{22} = B_{21}p_1 + B_{22}Q_1 \tag{5.59}$$

with

$$B_{11} = B_{22} \tag{5.60}$$

for the replacement vessel C (bottom):

$$p_2 = C_{11} p_1 + C_{12}[Q_{11} + Q_{21}] \tag{5.61}$$

and

$$Q_2 = C_{21} p_1 + C_{22}[Q_{11} + Q_{21}] \tag{5.62}$$

By analogy:

$$C_{11} = C_{22} \tag{5.63}$$

For the replacement vessel not to change pressures or flows, it must be true from the sum of the p_2's of vessels A and B that:

$$p_2 = \frac{1}{2}[A_{11} + B_{11}]p_1 + \frac{A_{12}}{2}Q_{11} + \frac{B_{12}}{2}Q_{21} \tag{5.64}$$

equals p_2 of the replacement vessel; similarly for Q_2. This, in turn, requires that

$$C_{11} = \frac{A_{11} + B_{11}}{2} \tag{5.65}$$

$$C_{21} = A_{21} + B_{21} \tag{5.66}$$

$$2C_{12} = \frac{A_{12}Q_{11} + B_{12}Q_{21}}{Q_{11} + Q_{21}} \tag{5.67}$$

$$C_{22} = \frac{A_{22}Q_{12} + B_{22}Q_{22}}{Q_{12} + Q_{22}} \tag{5.68}$$

However, the requirement that $C_{11} = C_{22}$ can only be satisfied if vessels A and B are identical, or when either Q_{11} or Q_{21} equals zero, the latter of which is trivial. Hence, it may be concluded that the number of nonidentical parallel vessels can be reduced or augmented only by allowing alteration of pressure and/or flow, which would provide a signal to its environment.

Taking into consideration the text following Eqs. 5.24a, b, any set of parallel vessels carrying steady flow only ($\omega - 2\pi = 0$) can be replaced by a single vessel. This is the likely origin of the assumption that replacement by a single vessel can be executed under all circumstances.

5.7 Starting from Eqs. 5.19a and 5.23b, with the coordinate dependent parts only,

$$p(z) = p_a e^{-\gamma_1 z} + p_\gamma e^{+\gamma_1 z} \tag{5.69}$$

and

$$Q(z) = \frac{1}{Z_1}\left[p_a e^{-\gamma_1 z} - p_\gamma e^{\gamma_1 z} \right] \tag{5.70}$$

at $z = 0$

$$p_a + p_r = p_0 \tag{5.71}$$

at $z = L_1$

$$\frac{Z_1 \left[p_a e^{-\gamma L_1} + p_r e^{y_1 L_1} \right]}{p_a e^{-y_1 L_1} - p_r e^{y_1 L_1}} = Z_2 \tag{5.72}$$

or denoting

$$\frac{p_a}{p_r} = \frac{Z_2 e^{y_1 L_1} + Z_1 e^{y_1 L_1}}{Z_2 e^{-y_1 L_1} - Z_1 e^{-y_1 L_1}} = A \tag{5.73}$$

one finds that $p_a = \frac{A p_0}{1+A}$, and $p_r = \frac{p_0}{1+A}$. The pressure pulse, $p(L_1)$, and the flow pulse, $Q(L_1)$, at the end of the first vessel, which are also the entrance pressure and flow pulses of the second vessel are found by substituting for p_a and p_r, as well as for A in the expressions for $p(z)$ and $Q(z)$ above. It will be seen that for $Z_2 \gg Z_1$ the pressure pulse at the entrance of the second vessel is higher than at the entrance of the first and that the situation is the other way around for the flow pulse.

For $Z_2 \ll Z_1$, pressure and flow pulses change place in the preceding sentence. This implies that it is no difficult matter to design a number of vessels in series in which either the pressure or the flow keeps increasing over some distance.

5.8 Figure 5.13 shows the answers. In the first column, the local reflection coefficient, Γ_1, is shown for each case. To illustrate for the second case

$$\Gamma_1 = \frac{2-1}{2+1} = 0.33 \tag{5.74}$$

The pressure amplitude at the junction thus becomes 1(antegrade) + 0.33 (retrograde) = 1.33. The same number applies to the entrance pressure ampli-tude of the branches. The reflection coefficient for flow has the opposite sign (Eqs. 5.22). The flow amplitude arriving at the junction equals 1 − 0.33 = 0.67; this flow distributes over the branches as dictated by the ratio of their input impedances.

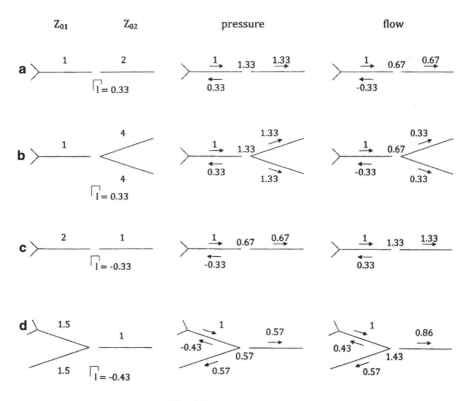

Fig. 5.13 Solutions belonging to Fig. 5.11

Pressure	Flow
Incoming pressure signal p_a set at 1 at juncture	Incoming flow signal Q_a set at 1 at juncture
Local reflection coefficients for pressure	Local reflections coefficient for flow
(a) 0.33; (b) 0.33; (c) −0.33; (d) −0.43	(a) −0.33; (b) −0.33; (c) 0.33; (d) 0.43
Magnitude p_r of reflected pressure signal	Magnitude Q_r of reflected flow signal
(a) 0.33; (b) 0.33; (c) −0.33; (d) −0.43	(a) −0.33; (b) −0.33; (c)0.33; (d); 0.43
Magnitude of transmitted pressure wave(s)	Magnitude of transmitted flow wave(s)
(a) 1.33; (b) 1.33; in both branches;	(a) 0.67; (b) 0.33 in each branch;
(c) 0.67; (d) 0.57	(c) 1.33; (d) 0.86 and 0.57

5.9 For the Voigt model, a unit step increase in length $\varepsilon(s) = 1/s$, the stress $\sigma(s)$ becomes $\sigma(s) = (c_0 + c_1 s)/d_0 s$, which, transformed back into the time domain, contains a delta function. For the Maxwell model, $\varepsilon(s) = (d_0 + d_1 s)/c_1 s^2$. Transformation yields a step plus a term proportional to time. These difficulties disappear if the complex Young modulus is written with an equal number of nonvanishing terms in numerator and denominator. Inclusion of nonlinear features requires further extension.

5.10 Starting with Eqs. 5.19a and 5.23b, let the boundary condition at $z = 0$ be $p_0 = p_a + p_r$ and Eq. 5.27 at the end L of a uniform vessel. From these two equations p_a and p_r can be determined. After some manipulation, it follows that

$$p_a = p_0 \frac{e^{\gamma L}[Z_0 + Z_L]}{Z_L[e^{-\gamma L} + e^{\gamma L}] - Z_0[e^{-\gamma L} - e^{\gamma L}]} \tag{5.75}$$

and

$$p_r = p_0 \frac{e^{-\gamma L}[Z_L - Z_0]}{same} \tag{5.76}$$

Substitution of p_a and p_r in Eq. 5.23b transforms the original question into: is it possible that the following equality

$$e^{2\gamma[L-z]} = \frac{Z_L - Z_0}{Z_L + Z_0} \tag{5.77}$$

applies? The answer is yes, when $z = L$ and $Z_L = \infty$. The physical meaning of this answer is when the far end is closed and total flow at that point therefore vanishes.

5.11 (a) Frank defined his two-element windkessel by setting $c_{ph} = \infty$, which, by Eq. 5.12a, eliminates the transmission feature and makes $\gamma = 0$. As Eq. 5.18 shows, reduction of γ to zero may be achieved in two ways: $L' = R' = 0$, or $C' = 0$. Frank chose the former option, thus retaining a distensible reservoir. The answer to question (a) is therefore: no
(b) Yes, see Question 5.4.

5.12 Mean pressure means that $\omega = 0$, hence $\gamma = 0$ (Eq. 3.18) and pulse analysis does not apply to mean pressure (the reason is cited in the text following Eq. 5.24a, b). Not realizing this, in quite a few reports in the literature it is concluded that a reflected pressure signal always enlarges the (measured) amplitude of antegrade plus retrograde signals. Therefore, as emphasized by Berger (1993), the separation should be performed only on the oscillatory part of the measured pressure and flow. These signals oscillate around zero values, as do their antegrade and retrograde components. The error may seriously have clouded the evaluation of the effect of reflection (Sect. 5.2.3, above; Berger 1993; Quick 1999).

5.13 No, part of the information was ignored.

5.14 Network theory teaches that only a limited range of questions is answerable. For a network of vessels of which all properties are known and possess a single entrance and a single exit, any two of the four quantities – input pressure and flow, output pressure and flow – must also be known to permit computation of missing pressures and flows. Specifically, for a single vessel with given input pressure $p_A(0, t)$ and output flow $Q_B(L, t)$, p_a and p_r can be determined with the aid of Eqs. 5.19a and 3.23b for each of the harmonic components ω. Once p_a and p_r have been obtained, a host of other pressures and flows may be computed. Alternatively, the same solutions can be obtained if, instead of $Q_B(L, t)$, the load impedance at B were known. In Question 5.14 neither requirement is satisfied, and the question is not answerable.

5.15 No, it is not; multiple parameters unrelated to the two vessels may alter transmission characteristics in the same person with time. Among different people these characteristics tend to be different also.

5.16 For illustrative purposes, let the main artery (characteristic impedance Z_0) divide into two identical branches (characteristic impedance Z_1). A perfect match requires that $\Gamma_1 = 0$ (Question 3.8), which applies when $Z_1 = 2Z_0$. Equation 3.25b states that $Z_0 = \sqrt{Z_1'Z_t'}$. This value may be doubled for the branches by increasing E in Eq. 3.13b by a factor of four, making the branches stiffer, or by lowering S in Eqs. 3.13a, b, i.e., by a primarily geometric change in properties. The latter implies that the branches are narrower than the main artery, though their combined cross-sectional area is larger than that of the main artery. Nature prefers the latter approach, thereby preventing peripheral arteries from being extremely stiff.

5.17 Rewriting the equation yields $[p_{ao}(t) - p_{ed}]/R_s = Q_{ej}(t)$. The bracketed term is the pressure pulse. Since p_{ed} and R_s are fixed numbers for a given heart beat, the pressure pulse and the ejection flow should have the same shape, which is not the case even allowing for a benevolent approximation.

5.18

$$\Gamma = \frac{R_s - j\omega Z_0 R_s C_s}{R_s + j\omega Z_0 R_s C_s} \tag{5.78}$$

hence, $\lim \Gamma = 1$ for $\omega = 0$ and -1 for $\omega = \infty$, with a minimum in between. The minimum value for $|\Gamma|$ occurs as a result of the minimum value for $Z_{in} = Z_0$ for the three-element model, while it equals 0 for the two-element model, both at the higher end of the frequency range of interest.

5.19 (a) no: m l^{-2} t^{-1} and m l^{-4} t^{-1}, respectively, (b) m l^{-2} t^{-1} (i.e., the same dimension as when flow velocity is used), and (c) l t^{-1}.

5.20 With Eqs. 5.22, $p_a = Z_0 Q_a$ and $p_r = -Z_0 Q_r$, $p(z, t)$ (Eq. 5.32a) and $Q(z, t)$ (Eq. 5.32b) become

$$p(z,t) = Z_0 \left[\frac{2[Q_0 + k\omega^2 D_0]e^{\gamma L} - k\omega^2 D_0}{2e^{\gamma L}} e^{-\gamma z} - \frac{k\omega^2 D_0}{2e^{\gamma L}} e^{\gamma z} \right] e^{j\omega t} \tag{5.79}$$

and

$$Q(z,t) = \left[\frac{2[Q_0 + k\omega^2 D_0]e^{\gamma L} - k\omega^2 D_0}{2e^{\gamma L}} e^{-\gamma z} - \frac{k\omega^2 D_0}{2e^{\gamma L}} e^{\gamma z} \right] e^{j\omega t} - k\omega^2 D_0 e^{j\omega t} \tag{5.80}$$

Replacement of the coordinate z by L and sorting of terms leads directly to $p(L, t) = Z_0 Q(L, t)$, with

$$Q(L,t) = \frac{2[Q_0 + K\omega^2 D_0] - K\omega^2 D_0[e^{-\gamma L} + e^{\gamma L}]}{2e^{\gamma L}} e^{j\omega t} \tag{5.81}$$

which, for $D_0 = 0$ reverts to the classical wave transmission expression for an antegrade wave in a reflection-free system: $Q(L,t) = Q_0 e^{-\gamma L}$.

5.21 In principle, yes. In practice, no, the number of vessels is too large.

5.22 The compliance of the artery itself increases initially with increasing deformation. For a venous example, see Fig. 3.5. At the appropriate level of deformation, primarily blood pressure is sensed during palpation.

5.23 Yes, it could. Simply putting together a branching system on the basis of measured or interpolated anatomical and elastic data tends to generate abnormal pressure and flow curves as compared to their experimentally obtained counterparts. This is attributed to the generation of local reflection coefficients. Improvement of matching improves wave patterns and reduces reflection coefficients.

5.24 The input impedance for this kind of elastic tube is given by the characteristic impedance Z_0. In Z_0, the frequency of the input signal appears in the denominator. Hence, for $\omega = 0$, Z_0 will tend to infinity and no flow will occur in response to a constant pressure.

5.25 Expressed in broader terms, it has been.

5.26 Desirable: 1,3

Undesirable: all others.

Chapter 6
The Microcirculation

Magnum certè opus oculis video

— Marcello Malpighi, describing his discovery of the
pulmonary capillaries in two publications dated 1661,
dedicated not to his Grand Duke, but to the mathematician
Giovanni A. Borelli, co-designer of several of Malpighi's
fundamental experiments.

Digest: Malpighi recognizes the unique function of the capillaries. The sheet model. Capillary exchange measured indirectly and directly. Wave transmission through 28 generations of vessels. Pressure-flow relations in glass capillaries and in vivo. Muscular small vessels may become unstable. A section of the coronary vasculature modeled in detail leads to the conclusion that cardiac contraction impedes coronary perfusion. Vasomotion, venomotion influence hematocrit in capillaries.

Venomotion promotes venous return.

6.1 Overt and Covert Mission

6.1.1 Mission

The Hippocratic Corpus recognized the necessity of breathing and of transportation through blood vessels. Galenus, adding more detail, embedded this in his theory of the circulation (Sect. 2.4.1). Caesalpinus and Harvey revolutionized Galenus' theory by introducing recirculation (Sect. 2.4.2). Malpighi (1661) furnished the copestone by his discovery, made possible by the microscope, that capillary vessels provide a direct connection between arteries and veins, thereby replacing Harvey's pores in the periphery. Van Leeuwenhoek, using a microscope of his own secret construction, rather promptly provided a method to measure red blood cell velocity in 1688. He derived the flow velocity from red blood cell travel over a measured

A. Noordergraaf, *Blood in Motion*, DOI 10.1007/978-1-4614-0005-9_6,
© Springer Science+Business Media, LLC 2011

distance during the time interval in which a person can distinctly pronounce a four-syllable (Dutch) word.

Initiated by Malpighi in 1666, the microcirculation came to be recognized as the essential exchange station of the circulatory system: an organ of interchange of substances between blood and tissue, primarily occurring through the walls of the capillaries.

6.1.2 Representation of the Microvasculature

In studies of the circulatory system, e.g., as embodied in the windkessel theory (Sect. 5.3), the properties of the microvasculature have classically been lumped together in the notion of total peripheral resistance, on the basis of the concept that the lion's share of the resistance to blood flow can be associated with the small blood vessels, primarily the arterioles. This is in spite of the fact that their prolific branching pattern provides a multitude of parallel pathways. The total peripheral resistance is, in analogy to Ohm's law, defined as the ratio between the arteriovenous pressure difference across the microvasculature and the flow through it, yielding a one-element model characterization.

In investigations that concentrated on a specific region of the circulatory apparatus, such as the brain or the kidneys, or on wave transmission in an arterial tree (Chap. 5), a more detailed breakdown was often required. Regional peripheral resistances were then introduced following the same definition but only applied to the microvasculature of interest to the segment of the microvasculature of interest. The parallel combination of all such regional resistances then forms the total peripheral resistance. This has proven a useful approach in characterizing and analyzing a number of aspects of circulatory function. Figure 6.1 illustrates the uneven distribution of resistance among the vascular beds.

To account for the dynamic behavior of the coronary circulation, where the tissue pressure surrounding the arteries, the microvessels, and the veins rises and falls in time with the heartbeat, it became desirable to allow for the possibility of flow out of the veins into the arteries at the time tissue pressure is climbing. Frasch et al. (1998) designed a five-element windkessel model to meet this need. It eliminates the asymmetry in the structure of the three-element model (Sect. 5.3) as shown in Fig. 6.2.

Starting from self-described morphologist Weibel's (1963) statement that the air–blood barrier in the lung is a sheet, Sobin and Tremor (1966) and Fung and Sobin (1969) proposed a model describing the alveolar capillaries as two endothelial sheets held apart and supported by septal tissue in the form of posts. These researchers developed a geometric model for the lung, determined the characteristic dimensions for the cat's lung according to the model, and presented a detailed theory of blood flow in the proposed alveolar sheet. Guntheroth et al. (1974), using a dog model and availing themselves of scanning electron microscopy instead of ordinary light microscopy, criticized the sheet model on the basis of their observation of a significant gradient in capillary density in the direction perpendicular to the

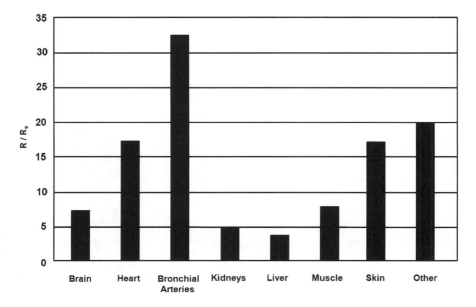

Fig. 6.1 The ratio between resistances R of specific systemic beds and the total systemic peripheral resistance R_s. The sum of their inverses yields $R/R_s = 1$

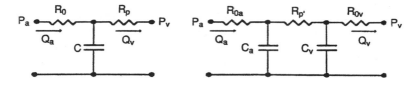

Fig. 6.2 *Left*: The three-element model discussed in Sec. 5.3, terminates in a peripheral resistance. *Right*: The five-element model, on the other hand, features a symmetric structure through individual recognition of arterial and venous compliances (From Frasch et al. 1998)

alveolar wall. They favored a tubular model, as originally described by Malpighi. Such a model has yet to be developed with a mathematical finesse comparable to that of the sheet flow model.

6.2 Properties of Small Vessels

6.2.1 Capillary Exchange, the Filtration Coefficient and Its Expansion

When traversing the vasculature, from the main artery that receives blood from the heart to the veins that return it to the heart, one finds that several characteristics change along the chosen pathway. In the first place, the branching is such that initially, as the branching order increases, the number of vessels in each order also increases, while their lengths and radii decrease. Subsequently, the inverse takes place. The maximum in the number per order is reached at the level of the narrowest vessels, the capillaries. In the second place, the composition of the walls changes. While arterial and venous walls consist of layers of elastic and fibrous tissue interwoven with smooth muscle elements which are separated from the blood they contain by a sheath of endothelium, the capillary wall virtually consists of endothelium only. In mammals, the endothelium is built up out of polygonal cells which are not considered to have contractile properties, although Krogh thought they had, owing to the cells of Rouget (Krogh 1922). Flow control activities were subsequently identified with precapillar sphincters (Nicoll and Webb 1946) or thoroughfare channels (Chambers and Zweifach 1946), both of which contain smooth muscle.

The main mechanism for the transfer of material across the capillary wall and its distribution in the tissues is considered to be diffusion. It is driven by concentration gradients and aided by the smallness of most diffusion distances. These have been estimated to range from a few microns (e.g., in active muscle) to an average of 50 mm (e.g., in resting muscle, when many capillaries are not perfused). The basic diffusion law that governs this economic form of transport was formulated by Fick more than a century ago (Fick 1855). Lipid soluble materials, which include O_2 and CO_2, pass readily through capillary endothelium and thus have a large area available.

Another mechanism is given by filtration of water soluble particles through pores in the capillary wall (Pappenheimer et al. 1951). It is driven by pressure differences which may be positive or negative. Some of these pressures have been identified and were stated in Starling's hypothesis (1985–1986) for the equilibrium, i.e., the no net flow condition, which may be formulated as

$$p_c = \pi_{pl} \tag{6.1}$$

This equality indicates that the fluid pressure in the capillary (p_c) equals the osmotic pressure in the capillary plasma (π_{pl}). The right-hand term arises from the fact that capillary endothelium has a low permeability to the colloidal constituents of blood plasma. The quantities in Eq. 6.1 may vary continuously and rapidly with circulatory adjustments to rest, exercise, changes in posture, etc. Landis (1927) generalized Eq. 6.1 by including the corresponding quantities for the surrounding tissue to introduce an expression for the quantification of fluid movement through filtration and reabsorption

$$Q = L_p S\big[(p_c - p_{ti}) - (\pi_{pl} - \pi_{ti})\big] \tag{6.2a}$$

where Q denotes capillary filtration flow through its wall, S the available capillary wall area, and L_p the capillary filtration coefficient. Setting $Q/S = J_v$ to normalize flow, it follows that

$$J_v = L_p\big[(p_c - p_{ti}) - \sigma(\pi_{pl} - \pi_{ti})\big] \tag{6.2b}$$

which also takes into account the finding that the capillary membrane is not totally impermeable to plasma proteins by the introduction of a solute reflection coefficient σ (Kedem and Katchalsky 1958). The reflection coefficient equals zero for solute permeability equal to that of water and one for total impermeability. The value of σ tends to increase with molecular size.

Landis (1927) developed a method for the estimation of the capillary filtration coefficient L_p in vivo. Reasoning that if the capillary's three port system (inflow at one end, outflow at the other, and transmural flow), were reduced to a two port system by occluding the outflow end, inflow would be equal to filtration flow. Their magnitude could then be estimated by observing red blood cell displacement in time, provided the capillary wall is rigid. This rigidity was considered a fact for a number of years. Landis applied his micro-occlusion method to capillaries in frog mesentery with different values of p_c in Eq. 6.2a. Assuming that the other pressures in this equation were independent of p_c, it then applies, for the collection of measurement points, each reading taken at the moment of occlusion (t_0), that

$$L_p = \frac{dJ_v}{dp_c}\bigg|_{t_0} \tag{6.3}$$

Since there are four pressures in Eqs. 6.2a, b, three other derivatives of the type specified in Eq. 6.3 are available and were applied as well. Capillary compliance caused the estimation of L_p to be subject to large errors, which were reduced significantly by measurement of red blood cell velocity relative to another red cell instead of with respect to the occluding needle (Zweifach and Intaglietta 1968; Muscarella et al. 1993; Fig. 6.3).

The value of L_p was found to increase from the arterial to the venous end of the capillary (Zweifach and Intaglietta 1968). An early model comprising 22 simultaneous equations argued for a broader inclusion of microvascular features (Wiederhielm 1979).

Some tissues have capillaries with assumed large clefts between their endothelial cells. Macromolecules are thought to be able to exit through them (Chambers and Zweifach 1947). As an alternate, exit may occur through "assisted" pathways provided that activation is achieved.

The relationship between flow and planar area of tissue serviced was found to be a linear one by Zweifach and Lipowsky (1977) for cat mesentery and rabbit omentum modules.

The measurement of transcapillary flow by micro-occlusion techniques was expanded by tagging blood constituents to permit tracing their movement by optical means, also pioneered by Landis in 1927 (Wiederhielm et al. 1973; Wayland and Fox 1978). Such measurements have cast doubts on the validity of the older concept that filtration and reabsorption are in balance over the length of the capillary. They indicate that filtration outweighs reabsorption in the capillary, which implies that reabsorption can occur in the venules. It also implies the availability of a larger area

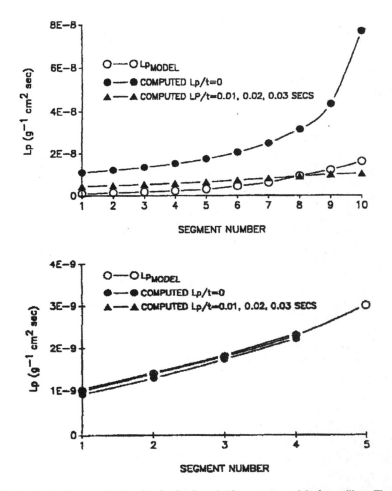

Fig. 6.3 Analysis of errors with the aid of a distributed, 10 segment, model of a capillary. The focus here is on the accuracy of measurement of L_p on the basis of two micro-occlusion methods. *Top*: The method applied by Landis (1927) and by Michel et al. (1974); *Bottom*: By Zweifach and Intaglietta (1968). L_p as incorporated in the model (*open circles*) and determined from the model by the above two methods on the same capillary (*filled circles*) at $t = 0$ as defined in Eq. 6.3 (From Muscarella 1990)

for exchange than was classically conceived and places more emphasis on the lymphatic system (Chap. 7) for tissue drainage (Chen et al. 1976), and opened the field for quantitative clinical endeavors (Baxter and Jain 1989).

6.2.2   Wave Transmission and Rheology

Each of the above one-element representations of the microvasculature, regional or global, shares lumping of large numbers of small vessels. In fact, a single capillary is not identifiable. For negligibly small reflection of antegrade pressure waves in a relaxed arterial system (Sect. 5.2), Salotto et al. (1986) computed a number of

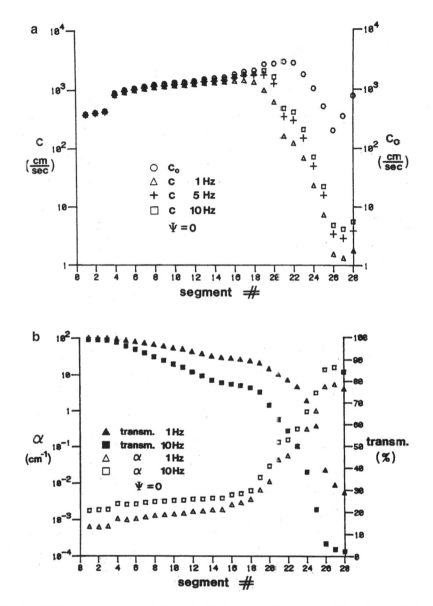

Fig. 6.4 (**a**) Computed values of the inviscid phase velocity c_0 and of the phase velocity c for purely elastic wall material throughout the hierarchy of 28 generations for three frequencies. (**b**) The attenuation constant α, computed for each generation and for two frequencies, and the cumulative effect of attenuation on the magnitude of a propagating antegrade pressure pulse (From Salotto et al. 1986)

features of wave transmission through a system of 28 generations of vessels, ranging from the aorta to a venule. The results show that phase velocity in the smaller vessels is reduced significantly by the viscous properties of blood (Fig. 6.4a) and that the aortic pressure pulse reaches the capillaries, especially for low frequencies (Fig. 6.4b). The stronger damping for high frequency components causes the smoother appearance of the pressure pulse in microvessels. The presence of reflection could tend to sustain the pressure pulse more effectively, though at the expense of the flow pulse.

Fåhraeus and Lindqvist reported in 1931 that the viscosity of blood drops below the value of arterial or venous blood when flowing through glass capillaries with a lumen diameter less than 0.3 mm. They also observed that the presence of red blood cells raises whole blood viscosity well above that of normal blood plasma. Consequently, the anomalous behavior of blood in narrow capillaries was attributed to dilution of blood, in turn ascribed to red cells being carried by the faster axial stream, while the slower marginal stream is free of red cells. The applicability to blood carrying capillaries of Poiseuille's law, dating from the 1840s, became seriously suspect.

When experiments employing glass capillaries could be replaced by experiments in vivo, Lipowsky et al. (1978) found that the flow resistance per unit length, denoted R' in Chap. 5 (e.g., Eq. 5.15), obeyed the fourth power of the radius in Poiseuille's law closely throughout the cat's mesentery microcirculation. These researchers suggested that this striking observation may be attributable to two opposing effects operating simultaneously. One, that the shear stress τ proved to be a nonlinear ascending function of average blood velocity $\bar{v}$, describable by

$$\tau^{0.5} = t_1 + t_2 \bar{v}^{0.5} \tag{6.4a}$$

and two, that the viscosity η could be represented by a nonlinear descending function, also of the Casson type, as

$$\eta^{0.5} = e_1 + e_2 \bar{v}^{-0.5} \tag{6.4b}$$

where the t's and the e's are empirical constants.

Murray argued in 1926 that for economic reasons (i.e., minimum expenditure of energy) blood flow, Q, through a vessel should be proportional, on mathematical grounds, to the radius cubed:

$$Q = kr^3 \tag{6.5}$$

This idea was tested experimentally by Mayrovitz and Roy (1983) in the rat cremaster muscle and found to apply on average. These theoretical and experimental results do not necessarily contradict the Poiseuille expression

$$Q = \frac{\pi r^4 \Delta p}{8\eta l}, \tag{6.6}$$

for

$$k = \frac{\pi r \Delta p}{8\eta l}, \tag{6.6a}$$

if, as the authors suggest, $\frac{\Delta p}{l}$, the average pressure gradient in a network of vessels, relates inversely to the radius. Pressure gradients in these experiments could not be measured accurately owing to equipment limitations.

The values for hematocrit (the fraction of blood occupied by red cells) in arterial and venous blood have been found to be equal. It would, therefore, be tantalizing to expect that the capillary hematocrit should be measured at the same level, since the same blood passes through it, except where shunts are available bypassing the capillaries. Yet, many years of experimental determinations yielded lower values, sometimes down to a small fraction of the values in large vessels. Several mechanisms, often related to the studies by Fåhraeus, later expanded with macromolecules forming an endothelial layer (Secomb et al. 2001), were proposed to explain such low values in narrow capillaries. It was argued, e.g., that wall exclusion of red cells leads to underestimation of hematocrit. Although this type of reasoning can account for the observation of a lower hematocrit in small capillaries, it fails to explain how the bulk of the red cells reach the veins (Duling and Desjardins 1987). In Sect. 6.3, a simple solution is offered for this problem.

6.2.3 Instability of Blood Vessels

The small vessels in the terminal arterial beds with a recognizable smooth muscle layer embedded in their walls have been shown to receive direct efferent innervation. In the smaller vessels with scattered muscle cells, innervation has not been demonstrated, though these cells respond to humoral substances. The picture that has developed indicates that neurogenic control loses significance as the vessels become smaller, while humoral and local control gain significance in the same direction up to the capillary. On the venous side the same hierarchy may apply, though this needs much more clarification.

The forces generated by smooth muscle contraction in minute vessels of certain kinds of tissues may be considerable when strongly stimulated, as Wiederhielm's (1969) experiments demonstrated. For constant intraluminal pressure, this leads to contraction, as may be seen by integrating (from Laplace's law, Eq. 5.4a after differentiation with respect to p)

$$\frac{\Delta r}{\Delta p} = \frac{r_0^2}{hE} \tag{6.7}$$

It follows that

$$\frac{1}{r_0^{\circ}} - \frac{1}{r_0} = \frac{p}{hE} \tag{6.8}$$

where r_0° is the radius for transmural pressure $p = 0$. Muscle contraction may be taken as equivalent to an increasing value of E. Hence, for constant pressure the

Fig. 6.5 (a) Path followed by a strongly stimulated vessel as the independent variable pressure is increased from A to E and decreased back to A. The *broken line* from C to D denotes the range of radii over which dilation is uncontrollable, that from F to B uncontrollable contraction (From Quick et al. 1996). (b) Predicted region of uncontrollable vessel radii for a strongly stimulated blood vessel (From Quick et al. 1996)

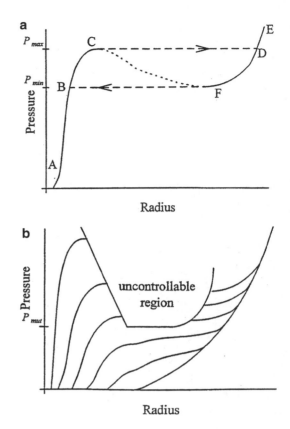

radius will tend to decrease. If irregularities occur in the geometry or in the mechanical properties of the vessel wall, the wall will eventually develop inward folds and the lumen will be filled in, provided the smooth muscle develops enough force. Diminution of blood pressure accelerates this process. The obvious way to ward off closure of the lumen is to keep the pressure sufficiently high. Assuming that active muscle tension remains constant with respect to radius, Burton concluded that the vessel will close completely for sufficiently low pressure. The highest value of pressure below which closure occurs was called the "critical closing pressure" by Burton (1951). However, Speden and Freckelton (1970) observed experimentally that complete closure does not occur, though strongly stimulated vessels are unable to maintain an equilibrium radius in a range of radii. In this range, they contract or dilate uncontrollably. This is schematically displayed in Fig. 6.5a. The vessel's pressure–radius relation is computed from the combined passive and (radius dependent) active wall properties under strong stimulation. The relation assumes a shape resembling the letter N (ABCFDE in the figure). For ascending pressure, the path actually followed is ABCDE, containing CD as the segment of uncontrollable dilation; for descending pressure it is EDFBA, containing FB as the segment of uncontrollable constriction (Quick et al. 1996).

They occur at different pressure levels as the experiment shows. Figure 6.5b outlines the region of instability. Weak or absent stimulation exhibits no instabilities. In these studies, pressure was altered slowly. Dynamic effects, if any, remain to be analyzed.

Uncontrollable dilation and constriction permit major changes in the perfusion (augmentation and reduction, respectively), of the vascular bed downstream of the unstable region, owing to the induced flow impedance changes. In a subsequent chapter (Sect. 10.4) this instability will appear as an extreme form of impedance-defined flow.

6.3 Microcirculatory Beds and Peripheral Micropumps

6.3.1 Analysis of the Coronary Circulation

Frasch (1993) and Frasch et al. (1998) employed in their analysis morphometric data of a part of the wall of the coronary casculature of the pig, assembled by Kassab (1990). This resulted in a total of over 200 arterial and venous branches in the selected part of the conorary vascular subsystem (Fig. 6.6). Each of the 58 terminal arterial segments (T shaped in Fig. 6.6) was connected to the corresponding terminal venous segments by a five-element windkessel model (Fig. 6.2) to account for microvascular dynamics.

Each vascular segment is characterized by an equation of motion and an equation of continuity (Eqs. 5.14) which form a nonlinear coupled set. The cross-sectional shape of each vessel was assumed to remain circular, with the area itself a function of transmural pressure, p_{tr}, both for positive and negative values of p_{tr}. Boundary conditions consisted of arterial inlet pressure, venous outlet pressure, as well as extravascular pressure depending on the radial location of the vessel segment and on ventricular pressure. Extravascular pressure through the wall was assumed to be a linear function of instantaneous ventricular pressure on the basis of experimental data, though not implied to be the generator of intramural pressure (Sect. 3.3). The equations were solved for the volumes of all segments, which permitted computation of their resistances and transmural pressures as a function of time. In turn, this permitted flow into and out of each segment to be computed. A particular set of results is reproduced in Fig. 6.7 for arterial and venous segments at three radial levels. Coronary pressures, flows, and volumes are strongly influenced by alternate compression and release. These studies provided insight into the mechanisms that underlie a significant range of experimental observations, previously controversial or poorly understood. An example is depicted in Fig. 6.8, in which experimental observations and theoretical results based on principles are compared. The comparison indicates that no vascular waterfall mechanism needs to be invoked. This figure also shows that vessel compression, occurring particularly

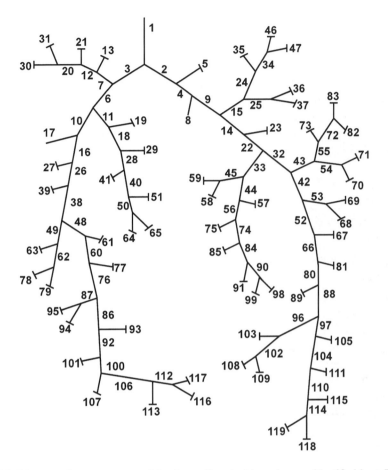

Fig. 6.6 Diagram of a coronary arterial subtree. Terminal branches are identified by a T. The venous counterpart is treated as its mirror image, with double the diameter at zero transmural pressure. The 58 terminal branches are each connected to their venous counterpart by five-element windkessels drawn in Fig. 6.2 (From Frasch et al. 1998)

on the venous side (Fig. 6.7), inhibits coronary perfusion. The control aspect of this will be discussed in Sect. 10.2.

Proposed reduced models for the entire coronary system may be found in Sect. 11.4.8.

6.3.2 Vasomotion, Venomotion, and Hematocrit

At first sight, viewed through a microscope, microcirculatory phenomena that impress the observer as lacking any organizational aspect are vasomotion (so-called for arterial vessels) and venomotion (in venous vessels). Both small arterioles and

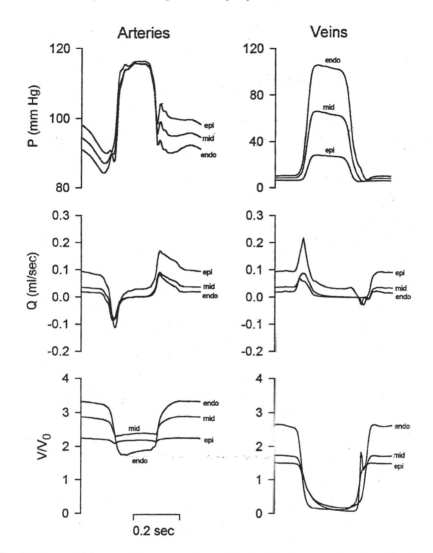

Fig. 6.7 Computed transmural pressures, flows, and normalized segmental volumes in selected arteries (*left*) and veins (*right*) from subepicardial (epi), mid wall (mid), and subendocardial (endo) regions . Selected vessels are major conduits along the principal pathway of the vascular tree. Input pressure is normal aortic pressure. Normalized volumes are phasic volumes divided by the segmental volumes at zero transmural pressure (From Frasch et al. 1998)

muscular venules exhibit contraction and dilation with irregular periods ranging from a few seconds to a few minutes. For the postcapillary vessels, this phenomenon was first reported by Jones (1852). The intermittent activity does not appear to bear any relationship to periodic phenomena elsewhere in the cardiovascular system.

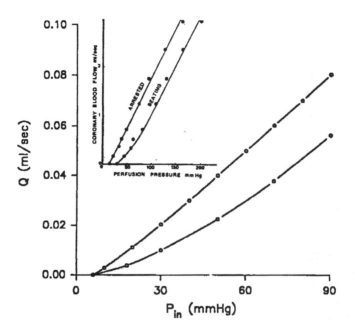

Fig. 6.8 Arrested state input pressure flow relations (*upper curve*) compared to dynamic conditions (*lower*) in Frasch's model (1993). Inlet pressure constant and equal in both cases, outlet pressures constant and equal at 6 mmHg. External pressure equal to zero in the arrested case and a function of ventricular pressure in the dynamic case. *Inset:* static and dynamic mean pressure flow relations measured on a canine heart, adapted from Downey and Kirk (1975)

Vasomotion exhibits variations of two types, namely, alteration in frequency of occurrence as well as modification of the relative distribution of constriction and dilation phases. Stimulation of vasomotion manifests itself by higher frequency and decreasing predominance of the dilator phase. Surgical trauma and anesthesia tend to abolish it. The latter observation explains why vasomotion in many areas escaped investigators' attention until techniques had been improved significantly. The conclusion seems inescapable that contraction and dilation of normal microvessels is mostly governed by prevailing local conditions, while neurogenic activity serves to modify the intrinsic tone of the muscle cells.

The consequences of combined vasomotion upstream and venomotion downstream of the capillaries were investigated by Mayrovitz et al. (1978) with the aid of a model of the bat wing's vasculature. One particular pathway was represented in detail, with lumped parallel pathways interconnected as dictated by the anatomy of the wing. The detailed pathway was composed of a segment of small artery, an arteriole, a terminal arteriole with precapillary sphincter, a capillary pathway, a muscular venule, a venous load, and included capillary filtration. This microvascular model was inherently nonlinear since the values of some of the parameters were dependent on pressures and flows (Fig. 6.9). The set of governing equations was solved with a hybrid computer.

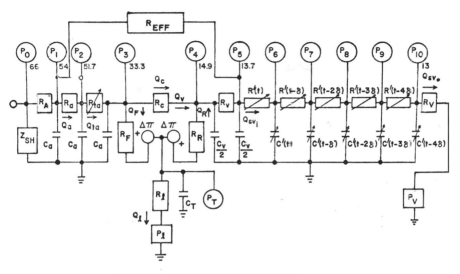

DETAILED MICROVASCULAR MODEL

Fig. 6.9 The detailed microvascular model with the bat wing as prototype, designed by Mayrovitz et al. (1978) in block format. For the relevant equations, definition of the parameters, and the numerical values applied, the reference should be consulted. Numbers adjacent to the pressure symbols (*circles*) are pressures in mm Hg

One of the clear consequences of arteriole/capillary sphincter vasomotion is the dynamic mode of capillary filtration and reabsorption. Reduction in terminal arteriole diameter produces a precipitous fall in capillary pressure and flow. Arteriolar flow is similarly reduced. When the arteriole contracts, capillary outflow is larger than terminal arteriole flow by an amount due to the increase in reabsorption, and vice versa. Superimposition of higher frequency venomotion makes the capillary component due to venomotion larger when the sphincter is open, though it is maintained at a lower level, rather than abolished, when the sphincter is contracted (Fig. 6.10). Hence, capillaries in resting tissue will induce reabsorption, lower their hematocrit, and their blood viscosity, thus facilitating flow. In exercising tissue, this dilution will be reduced or reversed. If the predictions of this model study are confirmed experimentally, they offer closure to many years of analysis of phenomena restricted to what happens within the microvasculature only, rather than in the microcirculation.

The traditional view of the peripheral resistance as a set of narrow vessels, principally arterioles, which are able to change their radii slowly, now comes across as rudimentary since a vast amount of active changes is ignored. Hence, the characterization of this peripheral vasculature by a single number, the resistance, or a pressure dependent number, should be considered as a rough approximation. Instead, as another consequence, vasomotion in conjunction with venomotion creates a local micropump. It is similar to a cardiac chamber in that a reservoir,

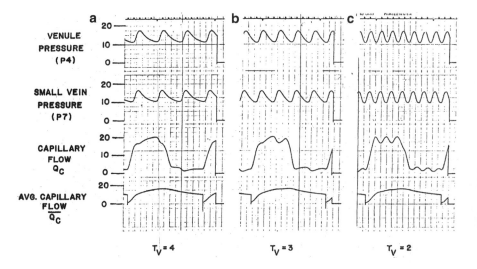

Fig. 6.10 Combined effect of vasomotion and venomotion on capillary flow. T_v denotes period of venomotion in seconds. Time marks at top are 1 s. apart. Flows are in 10^{-9} mL s^{-1} (From Mayrovitz et al. 1978)

in the form of small veins, is filled, then contracts, promoting venous return. It is different in that filling occurs from a high pressure source through a sizable impedance, the magnitude of which is subject to control effects. Thus, its contribution to venous return is subject to local and global demands and would be expected to increase with the level of exercise. The mammalian system is presumed to possess a large number of such micropumps (Sect. 8.3).

6.4   Conclusions

Discovered last, the microcirculation, not to be confused with the microvasculature, created new challenges of combining observations with an understanding of reality. Elimination of the "pore problem" in the circulation, since it had no microcirculatory system contribution to make, followed only after it continued to defy visualization.

The frame of mind underlying scientific observation may determine the conclusions reached by the observer. Analysis of the capillary as the functional unit, as opposed to the microvasculature and even more specifically, the microcirculation led to the unraveling of prior confusing observations. When the bioscientist can observe both the system as a whole and recognizes the potential limits in the orientation of his own hypothesis, new insights might appear.

6.5 Summary

This chapter forms the counterpart of Chap. 4, dealing with the multitude of microvessels in the periphery. There is reason to believe that blood flow behaves differently in glass capillaries, where blood displays anomalous viscosity, as compared to in vivo capillaries, where Poiseuille's law appears to apply. This observation (Lipowsky et al. 1978) simplified analytical studies. Examples include the comparison of different experimental approaches to evaluate the accuracy of the value of the capillary filtration coefficient and wave transmission through 28 generations of vessels from the aorta to the venule.

It could be shown mathematically that the experimentally demonstrated instability over a range of radii of strongly stimulated terminal arteries does not have to be attributed to damage of the contractile mechanism in their walls.

A detailed model of part of the pig's coronary circulation (a section through the wall containing arteries, microvessels, and veins) showed that pressures, flows, and volumes follow experimental observations without the need to invoke a vascular waterfall mechanism.

The challenge of a low hematocrit, observed for years in the microvessels, found its interpretation in reabsorption of fluid, in a sizable model of the bat wing.

References

Baxter L.T. and Jain R.K.: Transport of fluid and macromolecules in tumors. Microvasc. Res. 37: 77–104, 1989.

Burton A.C.: On the physical equilibrium of small blood vessels. Am. J. Physiol. 164: 319–329, 1951.

Chambers R. and Zweifach B.W.: Functional activity of the blood capillary bed with special reference to visceral tissues. Ann. N.Y. Acad. of Sciences 46: 683–695, 1946.

Chambers R. and Zweifach B.W.: Intercellular cement and capillary permeability. Physiol. Rev. 27: 436–463, 1947.

Chen H.I., Granger H.J. and Taylor A.E.: Interaction of capillary, interstitial, and lymphatic forces in the canine hindpaw. Circ. Res. 39: 245–254, 1976.

Downey J.M. and Kirk E.S.: Inhibition of coronary flow by a vascular waterfall mechanism. Circ. Res. 36: 753–760, 1975.

Dawson T.H.: Review. Modeling of vascular networks. J. Exp. Biol. 208: 1687–1694, 2005.

Duling B.R. and Desjardins C.: Capillary hematocrit - What does it mean? News in Physiol. Sc. 2: 66–69, 1987.

Frasch H.F.: Interpretation of Coronary Circulatory Perfusion. Ph.D. Dissertation, Univ. of Pennsylvania, Philadelphia PA, 1993.

Frasch H.F., Kresch J.Y. and Noordergraaf A.: Interpretation of Coronary Vascular Perfusion. Ch. 7 in: Analysis and Assessment of Cardiovascular Function. G.M. Drzewiecki and J. K-J. Li (eds.) Springer, New York, NY, 1998.

Fick A.: Über Diffusion. Pogggendorff's Annalen. 94: 59–86, 1855.

Fung Y.C. and Sobin S.S.: Theory of sheet flow in lung alveoli. J. Appl. Physiol. 26: 472–488, 1969.

Guntheroth W.G., Gould R., Butler J. and Kinnen E.: Pulsatile flow in pulmonary artery, capillary, and vein in the dog. Cardiovasc. Res. 8: 330–337, 1974.

Jacobsen J.:et al., 'Sausage-string' appearance of arteries and arterioles can be caused by an instability of the blood vessel wall. Am. J. Physiol. (Regulation and control) 283: R1118–R1130, 2002. [S. Kim report 2007].

Jones T.W.: Discovery that the veins of the bat's wing (which are furnished with valves) are endowed with rythmical contractility, and that the onward flow of blood is accelerated by each contraction. Phil. Trans. Royal Soc. of London, 142: 131–136, 1852.

Kassab G.S.: Morphometry of the Coronary Vasculature in the Pig. Ph.D. Dissertation, Univ. of California, San Diego CA, 1990.

Kedem O. and Katchalsky A.: Thermodynamic analysis of the permeability of biological membranes to non-electrolytes. Biochim. Biophys. Acta 27: 229–246, 1958.

Krogh A.: The Anatomy and Physiology of Capillaries. Yale Univ. Press, New Haven CT, 1922. Revised and enlarged edition, 1929.

Landis E.M.: Micro-Injection Studies of Capillary Permeability. Ph. D. Diss., Univ. of Pennsylvania, Philadelphia PA, 1927. [Also published as Am. J. Physiol. 82: 217–238, 1927.]

Leeuwenhoek van A.: Den waaragtigen omloop des bloeds, als mede dat de arterien en venae gecontinueerde bloed-vaten zijn, klaar voor oogen gestelt. Verhandelt in een brief, geschreven aan de Koninglijke Societeit tot Londen, Sept. 7, 1688. Opusc. Selecta Neerl. Arte Med. 1: 45, 1907.

Lipowsky H.H., Kovalcheck S. and Zweifach B.W.: The distribution of blood rheological parameters in the microvasculature of cat mesentery. Circ. Res. 43: 738–749, 1978.

Malpighi M.: De Pulmonibus Observatio Anatomica. Epistolae printed by G.B. Ferroni, Bologna, 1661.

Mayrovitz H.N. and Roy J.: Microvascular blood flow: evidence indicating a cubic dependence on arteriolar diameter. Am. J. Physiol. 245 (Heart Circ. Physiol. 14): H1031-H1038, 1983.

Mayrovitz H.N., Wiedeman M.P. and Noordergraaf A.: Interaction in the Microcirculation. Ch. 21 in: Cardiovascular System Dynamics, J. Baan et al. (eds.), MIT Press, Cambridge, 1978.

Michel C.C., Mason J.C., Curry F.E., Tooke J.E. and Hunter P.J.: A development of the Landis technique for measuring the filtration coefficient of individual capillaries in the frog mesentery. Q.J. Exp. Physiol. 59: 283–309, 1974.

Murray C.D.: The physiological principle of minimum work. I. The vascular system and the cost of blood volume. Proc. Nat. Acad. Sciences 12: 207–214, 1926.

Muscarella L.F.: Fluid Exchange in Distensible Capillaries. Ph. D. Dissertation, Univ. of Pennsylvania, 1990.

Muscarella L.F., Pathak A.S., Takashima S. and Noordergraaf A.: Quantitative analysis of the Landis method. Microvasc. Res. 45: 46–64, 1993.

Nicoll P.A. and Webb R.L.: Blood circulation in the subcutaneous tissue of the living bat's wing. Ann. N.Y. Acad. Sciences 46: 697–711, 1946.

Noordergraaf A.: Circulatory System Dynamics. Academic Press, New York NY, 1978.

Pappenheimer J.R., Renkin E.M. and Borrero L.M,: Filtration, diffusion and molecular sieving through peripheral capillary membranes: a contribution to the pore theory of capillary permeability. Am. J. Physiol. 167: 13–46, 1951.

Quick C.M., Baldick H.L., Safabakshs N., Lenihan T.J., Li J.K-J., Weizsäcker H.W. and Noordergraaf A.: Unstable radii in muscular blood vessels. Am. J. Physiol. 271 (Heart Circ. Physiol. 40): H2669-H2676, 1996.

Salotto A.G., Muscarella L.F., Melbin J., Li J.K-J. and Noordergraaf A.: Pressure pulse transmission into vascular beds. Microvasc. Res. 32: 152–163, 1986.

Secomb T.W., Hsu R. and Pries A.R.: Motion of red blood cells in a capillary with an endothelial surface layer: effect of flow velocity. Am. J. Physiol. Heart Circ. Physiol. 281: H629–H636, 2001.

Sobin S.S. and Tremer H.M.: Functional geometry of the microcirculation. Federation Proc. 25: 1744–1752, 1966.

Speden R.N. and Freckelton D.J.: Constriction of arteries at high transmural pressures. Circ. Res. 26/27, Suppl.: 99–112, 1970.

Starling E.H.: On the absorption of fluids from the connective tissue spaces. J. Physiol. 19: 312–326, 1895–1896.

Wayland H. and Fox J.R.: Quantitative Measurement of Macromolecular Transport in the Mesentery. Ch. 23 *in*: Cardiovascular System Dynamics, J. Baan et al. (eds.), MIT Press, Cambridge MA, 1978.

Weibel E.R.: Morphometry of the Human Lung. Academic Press, New York NY, 1963.

Wiederhielm C.A.: Physiologic Characteristics of Small Vessels. *In*: The Microcirculation, W.L. Winters and A.N. Brest (eds.), pp. 75–88, Thomas, Springfield, IL, 1969

Wiederhielm C.A.: Dynamics of capillary fluid exchange: a nonlinear computer simulation. Microv. Res. 18: 48–82, 1979.

Wiederhielm C.A., Shaw M.L., Kehl T.H. and Fox J.R.: A digital system for studying interstitial transport of dye molecules. Microvasc. Res. 5: 243–250, 1973.

Zweifach B.W. and Intaglietta M.: Mechanics of fluid movement across single capillaries in the rabbit. Microvasc. Res. 1: 83–101, 1968.

Zweifach B.W. and Lipowsky H.H.: Quantitative studies of microcirculatory structure and function. III. Microvascular hemodynamics of cat mesentery and rabbit omentum. Circ. Res. 41: 380–390, 1977.

Appendix

Questions

6.1 The Moens-Korteweg formula (Eq. 5.8a) predicts a phase velocity in vessels as narrow and as stiff as the capillaries in the range of 10 m/s. The measured velocity is, in contrast, in the cm/s range. Identify the reason for the discrepancy.

6.2 Calculate the ratio between red cell velocity and average plasma velocity in a small vessel assuming that the erythrocyte travels along the center line.

6.3 If a minuscule bolus with a high osmotic value, and containing a dissolved drug, travels through a capillary, is the drug likely to diffuse into the surrounding tissue?

6.4 Is the dimension of L_p in Eq. 6.2a that of a resistance or its inverse?

6.5 Does the diastolic pressure in the aorta qualify as the mean arterial pressure, driving peripheral perfusion?

6.6 Equation 6.3 originally assumed that the capillary was rigid. This assumption eventually had to be abandoned. At what time after micro-occlusion ($t = 0$ in Fig. 6.3) would capillary compliance most adversely affect the estimation of L_p?

6.7 Show that Eq. 6.5 does not necessarily contradict the Poiseuille relation between pressure gradient and flow.

6.8 Explain the large number of experimental observations in which capillary hematocrit is found to be less than arterial or venous hematocrit.

6.9 Argue for or against the view that unstable blood vessels act as valves to strongly augment or reduce flow by operating on vessel radius.

6.10 Much work has been done in the search for scaling laws for vascular networks, including capillary networks, in resting mammals of vastly different size. Inturn, this led to the question of whether such scaling laws should equally apply to exercising mammals (Dawson 2005). Argue the likely validity of a yes/no answer.

6.11 Discuss the applicability of the popular equation for the computation of the peripheral resistance, $R_{peripheral}$ (regional or global): $p_{arterial} - p_{venous} = R_{peripheral}Q_{through}$. Is this R necessarily a real number as distinct from a complex one?

6.12 Make a rough estimate of the total number of venular pumps using extrapolations from actual venule counts (start, e.g., with Table 6.1 in Noordergraaf A (1978)).

6.13 Can the appearance of "sausage-string" blood vessels (Jacobsen et al. 2002) be interpreted as resulting from vessel instability?

Answers

6.1 The Moens-Korteweg formula was derived taking into account the inertial properties of blood, but not its viscous properties. In narrow vessels, the viscous properties dominate the inertial ones. If c_{ph} is computed from Eq. 5.8i instead, the predicted value drops to the cm/s range.

6.2 Assuming a parabolic profile in a vessel with radius r_0 and centerline velocity v_0, the velocity v at any radial location r may be written as $v = v_0(1 - r^2/r_0^2)$. The average velocity

$$v = \frac{1}{\pi r_0^2} \int_0^{r_0} 2\pi r v \, dr = \frac{1}{2} v_0 \tag{6.9}$$

The desired ratio is therefore $v_0/v = 2$

6.3 No, the bolus will cause reabsorption of tissue fluid owing to the disturbance of pressure values, as confirmed by experimental observations.

6.4 The dimension of L_p

$$[L_p] = \frac{[J_v]}{[\text{pressure}]} = \frac{\frac{\text{flow}}{\text{area}}}{\frac{\text{force}}{\text{area}}} = \frac{\text{flow}}{\text{force}} = \frac{\text{cm}^3 \, \text{s}^{-1}}{\text{gcm} \, \text{s}^{-2}} = \frac{\text{cm}^3 \, \text{s}}{\text{g}} \tag{6.10}$$

while that of a resistance, also in the centimeter, gram, second system, equals

$$[R] = \frac{\text{pressure}}{\text{flow}} \quad \frac{\text{g}}{\text{cm}^4 \, \text{s}} \tag{6.11}$$

The dimensions are neither equal nor inverse.

6.5 It is lower than the mean pressure (Eq. 5.0), hence, no.

6.6 While the axial pressure gradient is being eliminated, promptly after occlusion; see Fig. 6.3.

6.7 If the pressure gradient is inversely proportional to the radius, Q in Eq. 6.5 becomes proportional to the radius cubed.

6.8 When the sphincter is contracted, capillary pressure is decreased and reabsorption increases, diluting the capillary blood.

6.9 It appears as a mechanism by which a modest change in pressure (e.g., from p_{max} to p_{min} along the vertical axis in Fig. 6.5A can impose a larger reduction in perfusion and vice versa.

6.10 Dawson (2005) argued for a "no" answer, primarily on the basis of the larger number of capillaries that contribute to flow during exercise.

6.11 It assumes that viscous effects of blood dominate all other properties, including micro pumping.

6.12 In the referenced table, Wiedeman reports a count of 345 venules in the vascular bed of a bat wing supplied by a single arterial branch in vivo. Earlier, Green extrapolated to the vasculature of a 13 kg dog and arrived at 80×10^6 for the sum of postcapillary venules.

6.13 Yes, promising attempts in that direction have been made, which could add a third dimension to the interpretation of instability in strongly stimulated small vessels, offered by Quick et al. (1996).

Chapter 7
The Lymphatic System

[....], non nisi istarum venarum vitio incidere,
praefertim cum medium canalem angustia,
vnde, vi perruptis valuulis, & dilatatis,
patefactisq; oscillis, in intes-ina [....]

— G. Asellius: De Lactibus, 1627, p. 78.

Digest: The network of lymphatic vessels drains the interstial tissue by returning fluid and particulates to the central veins. Under normal circumstances this is considered an active process, resulting in negative interstitial pressures. The active process is attributed primarily to contractile lymphangions, numerous tiny valved pumps, able to move fluid against a pressure gradient. The possibility that capillary lymphatics have the same ability without the benefit of valves.

The lymphatic system appears able to move fluid "uphill" from the interstitial spaces. Transmural pressure becomes a topic of study.

7.1   Introduction

The first description of the system of lymph vessels is ascribed to Asellius (1627), one year prior to the publication of Harvey's book *De Motu Cordis et Sanguinis*. In the style of his time, Asellius considered the liver the propelling source of the lymph circulation (Sect. 2.4).

From their origin to their outlet in tissue, lymph vessels are identified as lymphatic capillaries, often in the form of a plexus, frequently with blind cul de sacs and free of valves. These capillaries coalesce to form regional ducts; the ducts lead to the lymph nodes; finally, postnodal ducts come together to form the main lymphatic ducts.

Valves occur at least in the main ducts, which are also supplied with mural smooth muscle. Spontaneous rhythmic contractions have been observed for decades. Kinmonth and Sharpey-Shafer (1959) recorded oscillatory pressure in

A. Noordergraaf, *Blood in Motion*, DOI 10.1007/978-1-4614-0005-9_7,
© Springer Science+Business Media, LLC 2011

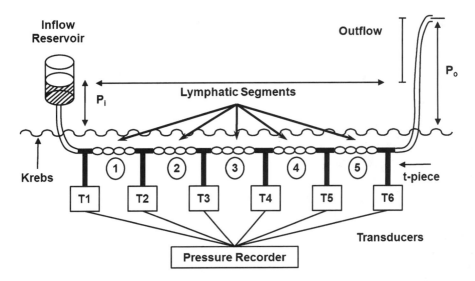

Fig. 7.1 Five bovine mesenteric, valved, lymph vessels in Krebs solution, connected in series with T-pieces are provided with pressure transducers T_i, $i = 1, 2,\ldots,6$, a fixed positive inlet pressure and a variable positive outlet pressure. Lymphangions contracted spontaneously (Adapted from Eisenhoffer et al. 1995)

the human thoracic duct with an amplitude of 10–15 mmHg and a frequency of around 0.1 Hz. Contractions were also observed in the other parts of the lymphatic system, even in isolated vessels (McHale and Roddie 1976) suggesting that it is a more general manifestation (Nicoll and Hogan 1978; Eisenhoffer et al. 1995, Figs. 7.1 and 7.2). Sympathetic innervation was noted as well.

More recently, Benoit et al. (1989) used cardiac concepts, terminology, and measurement procedures (Sect. 4.3) in their description of an in vivo lymphatic pump. This proved to have appeal (e.g., Gallagher et al. 1993; Eisenhoffer et al. 1995), though the approach needs more scrutiny.

7.2   Operation

Fluid and particulate matter, such as protein molecules and cells, enter at the capillary level of the lymphatics, propagate via the nodes, where processing takes place, and the ducts, to be returned to the venous system in a number of central areas (Threefoot 1968). This process has often been captured by the statement that the lymphatic system serves to drain the interstitial tissue, since no physical connection with blood carrying capillaries is in evidence.

The question of why fluid and particulate matter enters the lymphatic capillary has been answered in two different, rather contradictory manners. The older interpretation is based on the conviction that positive interstitial pressure provides the driving

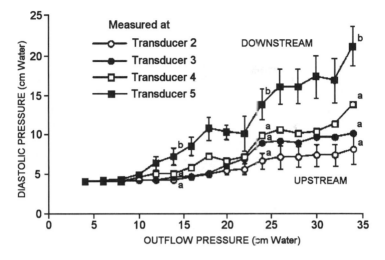

Fig. 7.2 As outflow pressure (abscissa in cm H_2O) was increased local diastolic pressures tended to increase as well, more so the closer the lymphangions were to the exit (Adapted from Eisenhoffer et al. 1995)

force. Positive pressures of several mm Hg were measured, reproducibly, by inserting the tips of fine needles into many different kinds of living tissue. Reddy et al. (1977) based an elaborate mathematical model with around 300 compartments on this concept. This model deals with the larger lymphatic vessel only. The vessels are subdivided into lymphangions, i.e., compartments bounded by valves, oriented in the central direction. The energy for propulsion is provided by active contraction of mural smooth muscle, proposed to be triggered by distension to a level exceeding a threshold, or by passive compression generated by the respiratory system, skeletal muscle activity, etc. Since, in the model, central venous pressure was set at a level below capillary blood pressures, it will be self-evident that lymph was returned to the jugular vein, the exit of this lymphatic network.

The younger interpretation was advanced by Guyton (1963), who introduced implanted perforated capsules, measuring the pressure inside the capsules by needle insertion weeks after implantation. Guyton observed negative interstitial pressure, averaging −6 mmHg outside edematous areas and positive values within such areas. He was able to demonstrate that intracapsular pressure followed the predictions of Eq. 6.2b, while those measured via needles inserted directly into the tissue did not, presumably due to tissue distortion. This appears to settle that interstitial pressure in normal tissue is negative. The capsular method has a very long response time, ruling out the detection of pressure pulsations, even if they occur at a frequency well below the respiratory rate.

Venugopal (2004) compared the performance of his mathematical model of lymphangions with in vitro measurement on bovine mesenteric lymphangions for both positive and negative axial pressure gradients among positive pressures. In this model, the lymphangion is viewed as having contractile properties, described by

Eq. 4.3b, as well as vessel properties expressed by a simplified form of Eq. 5.14. It was observed that under conditions of a positive pressure difference, the valves were always open and contraction impeded flow, while for opposite conditions, the valves were functional with flow occurring only during contraction. Lymph flow levels were significantly different in the two cases and were sensitive to timing coordination among lymphangions' contractions (Venugopal et al. 2003).

The mechanism responsible for the creation of negative interstitial pressure was attributed to suction exerted by the lymphatics, in other words to a lymphatic pump (Guyton and Barber 1980), not further specified.

The creation and maintenance of negative interstitial pressure may be interpreted in the following way. In Fig. 7.3 three Cartesian coordinate systems are shown, with lymphangion volume, V plotted along the horizontal, and lymphangion pressure, p, along the vertical axis. Since negative volumes are physically impossible, the horizontal axis does not extend into the negative range. This restriction does not apply to pressure (nor to flow). For a closed lymphangion, the pressure–volume relation is sketched in Fig. 7.3a. It is nonlinear with positive pressure for volumes exceeding a level denoted b. For $V = b$, the pressure equals to zero. For even lower (i.e., negative) pressures, the volume eventually decreases to zero (i.e., the lymphangion collapses). This means that for any volume smaller than b, internal pressure falls below external pressure (broken line). If external pressure is atmospheric, usually denoted "zero," internal lymphangion pressure will be negative. The cardiac chambers, when passive, display similar p–V relations, as do blood vessels. If the nonlinear nature of the p–V relation is quadratic, as it was measured to be for the cardiac chambers, the passive lymphangion's pressure–volume relation may be described by

$$p = \pm a(V - b)^2 \tag{7.1}$$

where the plus sign applies for volumes larger than b and the minus sign otherwise (Noordergraaf G.J et al. 2005). Hence, a nearly empty lymphangion, connected to capillaries emerging from tissue is able to accept lymph from a negative pressure environment to a magnitude determined by the lymphangion's wall properties. Subsequent contraction is assumed to occur after the volume surpasses a threshold. Equation 7.1 then gains an additional term

$$p_2 = \pm a(V - b)^2 + [cV - d]f(t) \tag{7.2}$$

which raises the pressure within the lymphangion first isovolumically (marked by a vertical arrow), then ejects its lymph into the next lymphangion, followed by relaxation of the first (Fig. 7.3b). This process may repeat itself along a string of lymphangions, probably at increasing pressure and volume levels and reduced ejection fraction. The buildup of pressure has been observed in experimental results (Fig. 7.2). This proposed sequence of events is schematized in Fig. 7.3a–c.

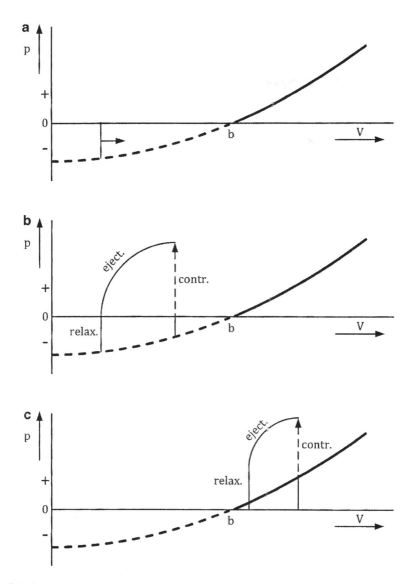

Fig. 7.3 Schematic representation of the proposed sequence of events that carries lymph from a negative pressure environment to a positive one, thereby maintaining negative tissue pressure. a) Pressure p –volume v relations of passive cavities, such as relaxed lymphangions or other biological chambers, including the cardiac ones during their diastolic phases, display a negative pressure range for low volumes enabling them to accept fluid in a negative pressure environment. b) Subsequent lymphangion contraction initiates a chain reaction, propelling the lymph to higher and higher pressure environments **b**) to **c**), until the lymph can exit into a central vein

When the pressure of the lymph is elevated enough at the exit, the lymph will mix with venous blood (Zhou 2007).

Similarity and differences with the cardiac cavities may be identified easily. Similarities include that the cardiac cavities are filled when passive, then eject upon stimulation under the influence of the first and second terms on the right in Eq. 4.7b, here on the right of Eq. 7.2. Differences are that for the cardiac cavities volumes are very much larger rendering the effect of suction (negative pressure) insignificant, while for the tinier volumes of the lymphatic capillaries, the suction effect appears dominant during their filling phase. Also, the nature of the triggering mechanisms appears to be fundamentally different.

Gibson (1974) estimated lymph flow, extrapolated to the entire human body, at around 2 L/day, representing a significant drainage flow, though probably an insignificant contribution to venous return.

The pumping performance of the lymphatics, attributed to lymphatic smooth muscle (Von der Weid and Zawieja 2004) appears to be unusually versatile. They appear to pump under circumstances of a positive or negative axial pressure gradient, and for upstream and downstream contraction sequences, both with a speed measured at several millimeters per second (Zawieja et al. 1993). Their contractile properties and their frequency of contraction can be adjusted, complexities which may be attributable to their claimed sensitivity to neural and hormonal influences and the possibility of cell to cell electrical communication.

7.3   Conclusions

The lymphatic system is a unique and fascinating component in the circulatory system, while it differs in a number of the essential characteristics of that very system. It is not, at its origin, even connected to blood vessels. The lymphatic system challenges an accepted agreement that volume cannot be recruited from a negative pressure environment, a realistic expectation since blood pressures are positive.

The movement of lymphatic fluid shows the bioscientist the value which respects and accepts biophysical laws as well as what his experimental observation may bring. Fluid dynamics defines that fluid will move from a higher to a lower pressure area, regardless of the sign involved. That nature may make a specific exception to the avoidance of the nonphysiological phenomenon of negative pressure, is stimulating for the fundamental researcher.

7.4   Summary

This chapter is focused on the lymphatic system, in particular on the effort to understand the mechanism enabling lymph vessels to fill with lymph in a negative (i.e., below atmospheric) pressure environment (as measured by Guyton).

Although presented at different pressure levels, the property is shared by all blood vessels and by the cardiac chambers. It relates to suction as well. Visualize a lymphangion, or a ventricle that contains enough fluid to exhibit a positive transmural pressure (inside pressure exceeds outside pressure). The transmural pressure will decrease with decreasing internal volume. Eventually, the transmural pressure will drop to zero, though the chamber is not empty yet. To empty the chamber, the recoil of its elastic wall has to be overcome, meaning that the inside pressure goes negative as it is emptied further. If this chamber is moved into an environment that is less negative, its inlet valve will be pushed open in response to the pressure difference across it and the chamber will accept fluid from the negative pressure environment.

References

Asellius G.: De Lactibus sive Lacteis Venis, Mediolani, 1627.

Benoit J.N., Zawieja D.C., Goodman A.H. and Granger H.J.: Characterization of intact mesenteric lymphatic pump and its responsiveness to acute edemagenic stress. Am. J. Physiol. 257 (Heart Circ. Physiol. 26): H2059-H2069, 1989.

Eisenhoffer J., Kagal A., Klein T. and Johnston M.G.: Importance of valves and lymphangion contractions in determining pressure gradients in isolated lymphatics exposed to elevations in outflow pressure. Microvasc. Res. 49: 97–110, 1995.

Gallagher H., Garewal D., Drake R.E., Gable J.C.: Estimation of lymph flow by relating lymphatic pump function to passive flow curves. Lymphology 26: 56–60, 1993.

Gibson W.H.: Dynamics of Lymph Flow, Tissue Pressure and Protein Exchange in Subcutaneous Tissue. Ph.D. Diss., Univ. Miss. Med. Ctr., Jackson MS, 1974.

Guyton A.C.: A concept of negative interstitial pressure based on pressures in implanted perforated capsules. Circul. Res. 12: 399–414, 1963.

Guyton A.C. and Barber B.J.: The energetics of lymph formation. Lymphology 13: 173–176, 1980.

Kinmonth J.B. and Sharpey-Schafer E.P.: Manometry of the human thoracic duct. J. Physiol. 145: 3P, 1959.

McHale N.G. and Roddie I.C.: The effect of transmural pressure on pumping activity in isolated bovine lymphatic vessels. J. Physiol. 261: 255–269, 1976.

Nicoll P.A. and Hogan R.D.: Pressure associated with lymphatic capillary contraction. Microvasc. Res. 15: 257–258, 1978.

Noordergraaf G.J., Tilborg van G.F.A.J.B., Schoonen J.A.P., Ottesen J., Scheffer G.J., Noordergraaf A.: Thoracic CT-scans and cardiovascular models: the effect of external force in CPR. Int. J. Cardiovascular Med. and Science. 5: 1–7, 2005.

Noordergraaf G.J., Dijkema T.J., Kortsmit W.J.P.M., Schilders W.H.A., Scheffer G.J. and Noordergraaf A.: Modeling in cardiopulmonary resuscitation: Pumping the heart. Cardiov. Eng. 5: 105–118, 2005.

Noordergraaf G.J., Schilders W.H.A., Scheffer G.J., Noordergraaf A.: Essential factors in CPR? Modeling and clinical aspects (abstract). 2nd Science day, Dutch Society for Anesthesia (Amsterdam), 2005.

Reddy N.P., Krouskop T.A. and Newell P.H.: A computer model of the lymphatic system. Comp. Biol. Med. 7: 181–197, 1977.

Threefoot S.A.: Lymphaticovenous Communications. Ch. 2 in: Lymph and the Lymphatic System, C.C. Thomas, Springfield IL, 1968.

Venugopal A.M.: A Computational Approach to Study the Effect of Multiple Lymphangion Coordination on Lymph Flow. Masters Thesis, Texas A&M Univ., 2004.

Venugopal A.M., Stewart R.H., Rajagopalan S., Zawieja D.C., Laine G.A., Quick C.M.: Applying the time-varying elastance concept to determine the optimum coordination of lymphangion contraction in a lymphatic vessel. 25th Ann. Int. Conf. IEEE, Cancun, pp. 323–327, 2003.

Weid von der P-Y., Zawieja D.C: Lymphatic smooth muscle: the motor unit of lymph drainage. Int. J. Biochem. & Cell Biol. 36: 1147–1153, 2004.

Zawieja D.C., Davis K.L., Schuster R., Hinds W.M. and Granger H.J.: Distribution, propagation, and coordination of contractile activity in lymphatics. Am. J. Physiol. 264 (Heart Circ. Physiol. 33): H1283–1291, 1993.

Zhou B.: The origin and maintenance of negative tissue pressure. Project report in a course taught by A. Noordergraaf, Univ. of Pennsylvania, 2007.

Appendix

Questions

7.1 Argue whether or not, in a single channel, the average value of the lymph flow entering the most distal lymphangion should equal the average flow entering the vein from the most proximal lymphangion.

7.2 Clarify how it is possible that the capsule (and wick) techniques yield negative interstitial pressure, while direct needle measurements, long considered the gold standard in the determination of blood pressure, show positive values, both in nonedematous tissue.

7.3 It has been found that lymphangions exhibit different contractile properties for different levels of filling. Do cardiac ventricles snare this property?

7.4 It has been claimed that lymphangions "work harder" when pumping against a higher pressure and vice versa. Does this apply to a cardiac ventricle also? And to cardiac atria?

7.5 Is it to be expected that failure of the contractile mechanism in lymphangions might result in the local formation of edematous tissue?

Answers

7.1 The valved lymphangions will not permit back flow. Yes, for an isolated channel.

7.2 The difference is attributed to tissue distortion caused by needle insertions into the interstitial space.

7.3 Yes, they do as observed by Frank (Fig. 4.21) and Starling (Fig. 4.23) and confirmed many times.

7.4 If "working harder" is interpreted as doing more mechanical work, the answer can be determined by evaluation of Eq. 4.2a. Whether or not W increases as aortic pressure goes up depends, in this case for the left ventricle, on how much ejection flow goes down. Starling found that W initially increases.

7.5 Yes, in the face of continuing filtration out of the blood capillaries and lymph outflow interrupted until exit lymph pressure reaches venous blood pressure levels, edema should develop.

Part III
Impedance Defined Flow and the Closed Loop

Chapter 8
The Closed System

Iam denique nostram de circuitu sanguinis sententiam ferre,
& omnibus proponere liceat... Necessarium est concludere
circulari quodam motu in circuito agitari in animalibus
sanguinem; & esse in perpetuo motu, & hanc esse actionem
sive functionem cordis, quam pulsu peragit, & omnino motus
& pulsus cordis causam vnam esse.

— William Harvey, 1628

Digest: Galenus' beloved theory rejected and replaced by a closed loop with a single central pump, the heart. The two ventricles pump directly into two arterial high pressure reservoirs, which are assigned responsibility for perfusion of their peripheries. Starling's observations that cardiac output is exquisitely sensitive to venous return to the heart. The validity of this conclusion becomes a battle ground. This issue resolved by the introduction of the family of cardiac function curves leading to the concepts of homeometric and heterometric autoregulation, in turn supplemented with pressure autoregulation. Effects of physical exercise, gravity, and acceleration. Efforts to model the closed loop quantitatively commence early and continue today. Three different types of basic models for the purpose of describing the closed loop, with a fourth added to accommodate control phenomena. Doubts about adequate pumping ability of the heart lead to the discovery of impedance-defined flow, generalizing Harvey's teaching from unidirectional flow to uni – and bidirectional flows. Regions of uni – and bidirectional flow.

The normal heart performs impedance transformation, the valveless heart does not.

8.1 The Normal Circulation

8.1.1 Introduction

After the renaissance movement had spread to include northern Europe, Harvey published his book *De Motu Cordis et Sanguinis*. In this book he rejected the theory by Galenus about the operation of the cardiovascular system and replaced it by

A. Noordergraaf, *Blood in Motion*, DOI 10.1007/978-1-4614-0005-9_8,
© Springer Science+Business Media, LLC 2011

the new concept of the closed circulatory circuit, in which the heart provides the sole motive force. As part of his education, Harvey had spent a few years of study in Italy, where the renaissance blossomed earlier. In Italy the same concept of the closed circulatory circuit was published, perhaps not surprisingly, 35 years earlier by Caesalpinus (1593). Although Harvey gives credit to a number of investigators preceding him, he does not mention Caesalpinus. The latter provides one example where a peripateticus, read: theoretician, developed a new concept prior to the experimenter.

Since Galenus' theory was admired for its flexibility and had become entrenched during the fourteen centuries of its life time, Harvey experienced difficulty gaining acceptance of his ideas, but eventually he prevailed. His work remains quintessential in contemporary thinking.

8.1.2   The "Closed" System and Exercise

In the preceding Chaps. 3–7, which constitute Part II of this book, major component parts of the cardiovascular system were discussed, predominantly in isolation from one another. Their interconnections create a closed loop in which blood circulates in the direction defined by cardiac and venous valves. The blood containing circuit is semi-closed owing to infusion of extracellular fluid via the lymphatics (Chap. 7) and to the facility of fluid exchange at the microcirculatory level between the circuit and its tissue environment (Sect. 6.2). The oft repeated view that the closed loop represents a closed system is manifest only when the tissue environment, a large reservoir containing around 15 l extracellularly in an adult human, as well as the lymphatics are included.

The various parts are connected differently. The ventricles and the arterial systems into which they pump are separated by valves, meaning that their connections, under normal conditions, are open or shut permitting sizable transfer of blood in a third of a heart beat. The connection between arteries and veins is provided by a multitude of narrow vessels, constituting the microcirculation, arranged individually for each organ. These microvasculatures serve core functions of their own. The veins have spacious, permanently open, connections with the atria. Finally, the atria have valvular connections with the corresponding ventricles. Valves are found in the heart, four sets of leaflets, not six generally, as well as in peripheral veins, and in the lymphatics. The central section of some parts have been studied, sometimes for centuries, because their ends seemed to invite analysis, e.g., wave transmission in arteries with a resistance at one end and a pressure/flow source at the other (Chap. 5). The different linking mechanisms employed, as well as the valves, are all functionally integrated in the operation of the system.

Studies performed during the post-Harvey period provided a more specific image of the circulatory system and its mode of operation. In a more detailed view, the heart may be considered to feature four pumps: two atria and two ventricles, of which the left ventricle is both the most powerful and the one most frequently afflicted by disease.

During each heart beat, the normal left ventricle pumps most of the blood it contains into the systemic arteries, a small high pressure reservoir, which provides perfusion with blood to most of the peripheral organs directly and the liver indirectly (Fig. 2.7). The pressure level in this reservoir is determined by its elastic properties as well as by the rate at which blood is pumped into it at the entrance of the aorta, together with the rate at which blood is allowed to escape into the peripheral organs. The latter is umbrageously determined by the total flow resistance offered by the peripheral organs, most of which are arranged in parallel. The blood that emerges from virtually all of the individual organs, as well as the fluid exiting the lymphatic ducts, collects in a large low pressure reservoir, referred to as the systemic venous reservoir, from which the right atrium and ventricle are filled.

The right ventricle provides the input to the lesser circulation by pumping directly into the pulmonary artery. Together, the lung arteries provide another high-pressure reservoir, which is smaller and maintained at a lower pressure level than its systemic counterpart. Blood flow exiting the pulmonary capillaries is collected in the pulmonary venous reservoir, from which the left atrium and ventricle are filled, again practically free of assistance by ventricular suction. Just prior to the contraction of both ventricles, the atria contract, adding a modest amount of blood (15–25%) to the already filled ventricles, despite the absence of valves at the venoatrial junctions.

Considering some of the principal properties of the major component parts, most arranged in series, some in parallel, it becomes clear that interaction must occur on an elaborate scale: According to Starling's observations, ventricular output flows depend on ventricular volumes. The latter are sensitive to venous pressures on the left and on the right. Venous pressures depend on the elastic properties of the venous systems as well as on the volumes of blood contained in these vascular systems. In addition, ventricular output is sensitive to conditions in the arterial systems into which they pump, while the difference between arterial pressures and the corresponding venous pressures are major contributors in determining flows through the peripheral organs. Although the blood carrying system constitutes a closed loop, the time averaged flow through all cross sections does not have to be precisely equal during what is thought of as steady state conditions. Although some of these conditions appear contradictory, the normal cardiovascular system is able to find a stable solution for each set of reasonable parameter values by adjustment of regional blood flows resulting in significantly different values of pressures and volumes of the component parts around the loop for these two quantities.

The flexibly of the cardiovascular system to adapt to prevailing demands on it may be illustrated by the observed fourfold to sixfold increase in cardiac output, compared to rest, in a superbly trained athlete during record physical performance. Heart rate as well as the contractile properties of the cardiac wall musculature are continuously adjusted to answer demands imposed by the current level of mental or physical exercise. The same applies to the smooth muscle in the vascular walls, which modulates their distensible properties.

Taking a broader point of view, the organization of the cardiovascular system may be seen to display two features: first, pressure–flow relations within the fluid conducting pathways, such as the arterial and venous components of the loop, are primarily linear, since the parameters they confront tend to be constant in zero order approximation (but see Sect. 5.2); second, the system relies on extensive parameter variation to exercise control, which introduces nonlinear aspects to the systems, more so in the veins under certain circumstances than in the arteries. Many of the alterations in the values of the parameters have their origin outside the cardiovascular system such as sympathetic and parasympathetic signals from the neural system, hormonal control, respiratory influences, and many others (treats this in more detail).

The validity of Starling's observations (Sect. 4.3) in the intact organism during physical exercise (bicycle ergometer) came under critical scrutiny as early as 1938, when Liljestrand et al. showed that the size of the heart never increased as much as would be expected from the associated increase in cardiac output. So much more evidence was marshaled that Hamilton (1955) felt compelled to reject the hypothesis that the heart's output is primarily governed by venous return and to deny that the heart depends mainly on changes in diastolic size to make its pumping performance fit the current need. Rushmer (1959) advanced the view that the intact animal adapts to physical exercise mainly by increasing pulse rate and only slightly by increasing stroke volume. This solution has its inherent limitations, caused by the reduced filling time imposed on the ventricle (Melbin et al. 1982).

This implied that Starling's observations incorporated another modification of the intact organism and, hence, his approach had to be generalized. The hypothesis that input–output relationships are more realistically represented by a family of curves received a strong impetus from the work of Sarnoff and Berglund (1954), who proposed that such a family of Starling curves, anabaptizedly presented as ventricular function curves, makes available a unifying concept. On the basis of this, the paradox of a smaller end diastolic volume in conjunction with a larger stroke volume can be readily explained. A move to enhanced filling is observed when the ventricle heads toward failure, but to reduced filling during the stimulation which follows, e.g., the administration of catecholamines or during exercise. Systematic investigation of neural and humoral influences by Sarnoff and coworkers (1960) and by Braunwald's group, starting in 1960, upheld the view that, within the family of curves philosophy, the ventricular function curves become applicable in mammals. This is termed "homeometric autoregulation," as distinct from "heterometric autoregulation," when output is altered in response to change in filling. Formulated differently, cardiac output then becomes a function of both preload and arterial load, as well as of the current intrinsic properties of the myocardium (Fig. 8.1). De Vroomen et al. (2000) found, in the right ventricle of newborn lambs, that augmentation of pulmonary arterial impedance can be matched by maintenance of stroke volume and heart rate through homeometric autoregulation, such that inflow remains constant.

In homeometric autoregulation, the members of the cardiac function curves were seen to be rotated counterclockwise and stretched along the ordinate

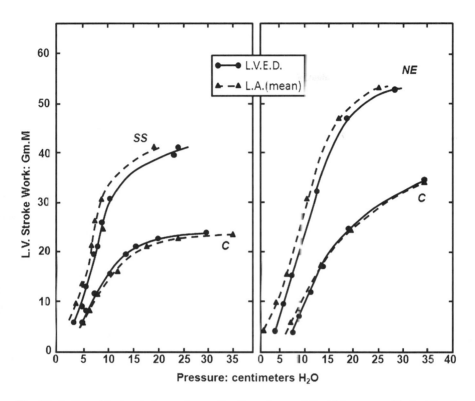

Fig. 8.1 Left ventricular stroke work as a function of mean left atrial pressure (*dashed lines*), comparing controls (*C*) with the modification induced by stellate ganglion stimulation (*left* (SS)) and by infusion of norepinephrine (*right* (NE)). The solid lines relate stroke work to left ventricular end diastolic pressure for the same conditions. Vagi were cut on both sides (By permission of Sarnoff et al. 1960)

(sometimes referred to as vertical extension), signifying modifications in ventricular work, stroke volume, cardiac output, etc. for the same end diastolic filling level.

It has recently been found (G.J. Noordergraaf et al. 2006) that still another generalization is in order: the cardiac function curves can shift along the abscissa (referred to as horizontal shift) under the influence of pressure external to the heart ($p_e(t)$) such as imposed by the respiratory system during rest and more intensively during physical exercise, or during application of cardiopulmonary resuscitation (Sect. 9.4). The generalized equation, from Eq. 4.6d, for either ventricle then takes the form

$$p_v\left(V_v, t, Q_{ej}\right) - p_e(t) = \pm a(V_v - b)^2 + (cV_v - d)F_2(t, Q_{ej}) \qquad (8.1a)$$

where

$$F_2 = f(t) - k'_1 Q_{ej}(t) + k'_2 Q_{ej}^2(t - \tau) \qquad (8.1b)$$

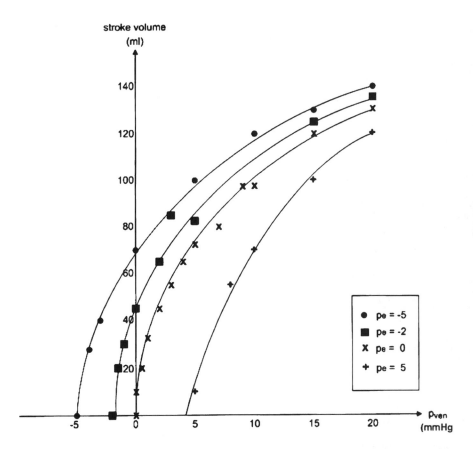

Fig. 8.2 Ventricular function curves as modified by external pressure exerted on the ventricle. Compare to Fig. 8.1, where the family of function curves exhibits shifts primarily along the ordinate, external pressure shifts the function curves primarily along the abscissa. Peripheral resistances were 0.08 and 1.2 mmHg ml^{-1}s for the pulmonary and systemic vasculatures, respectively, in this model study (Noordergraaf G.J. et al. 2006)

As depicted in Fig. 8.2, this shift may occur either to the right (for positive external pressure, as is applied in cardiopulmonary resuscitation), or to the left (for negative external pressure, as occurs during inspiration). This phenomenon might be termed "pressure autoregulation" and embodies features of homeo- and heterometric autoregulation. Pressure autoregulation allows for strong interaction between enhanced venous return and augmented cardiac output (Sects. 10.2 and 11.2). The elastic properties of the chambers' walls influence its magnitude. The effect of respiratory modulation of intrathoracic air pressure has, thus far, been largely ignored (Agostoni and Butler 1991).

8.2 Early Descriptions of the Closed Loop

The interdependence of events in the circulatory system has long intrigued investigators. To visualize the situation better, some researchers built hydraulic models of the circulation. Intentionally or unintentionally, these models were originally designed primarily for teaching purposes. Such models were published by Weber (1850) and by Marey (1863) to mention but a few of the classical ones; updated, more flexible versions were striven for, but made their debut much later (e.g., Rothe and Selkurt 1962; Osborn et al. 1967). The more complex among them modeled the left side of the heart, the aorta, the systemic peripheral resistance, and the veins, as a closed loop, with valves at a few appropriate sites. Parameters, such as peripheral resistance, arterial and venous compliances, and frequency of ventricular contraction, could be adjusted; and the resulting effects could be studied in a qualitative fashion.

Results secured in some of the mechanical analogs of this sort have been used in an attempt to judge the validity of the "forward failure" theory versus the "backward failure" theory. Starr and Rawson (1940) pointed out that these models are far too crude to serve that purpose effectively. Their hydrodynamic model contained the closed loop pathway with two pumps in series, separated by models of the vascular trees, rather than with just a single pump. Both pumps were designed so as to exhibit Starling's findings. The measurements performed on the model made it abundantly clear that the two simple theories identified above were unsatisfactory and that an improved theory must at least allow for fluid shift from one vascular system to the other, for fluid shift among the arterial part, the venous part, and the peripheral part of each vascular system, and finally for changes in the total volume of fluid that is distributed over the entire circulatory circuit. Such studies served to indicate what is required to raise model making of the closed loop to the level of quantitative studies.

The practical problems encountered in the construction of hydrodynamic models discouraged their further development. Accordingly, a search was instituted for other possibilities. An example of what the search led to may be found in Jochim's work. Starting with a hydrodynamic model, Jochim and Katz (1942) studied the effect of changes in peripheral resistance on arterial pulse pressure using heart rate and stroke volume as parameters. In later studies (Jochim 1946), the emphasis was shifted toward a mathematical approach, and still later studies utilized an electrical model (Jochim 1948). Where the effort of constructing hydraulic models has persisted it is for different reasons, like the testing of prosthetic devices, such as valves and artificial hearts (Rogers et al. 1972), as well as for the evaluation of circulatory assist devices (Chap. 9).

The wide variety of models that have subsequently been designed to aid in the study of the circulation can conveniently be divided into four classes according to key features (Noordergraaf A. 1969). The recently developed fifth class appears below.

In its simplest possible form, the circulation has been represented by a *resistive* circuit, i.e., emphasizing the viscous aspects of blood. As a consequence, the discussion is restricted to the distribution of average pressure and flow. Hill et al. (1958) designed a model of this nature to study the changes in the circulation at birth, while Vadot (1962) proposed one to predict the changes to be expected from major surgical intervention.

The next level of sophistication is exemplified by Grodins' (1959) *resistive-capacitive* model, which emphasized viscous properties of blood and compliant features of vessels, and was aimed at a description of average values of pressures, flows, and volumes. Grodins based the behavior of the heart on 's concept of 1915 in the form

$$W_s = SV_d \tag{8.2}$$

where W_s denotes the external work performed and V_d end diastolic volume, while S is a proportionality constant between the two, denoted the "strength" of a ventricle. This popularized the application of Starling's work in formulations of ventricular performance. The connection with mean arterial pressure enters the picture here, since

$$W_s \cong V_s \bar{p}_a \tag{8.3}$$

the product of stroke volume V_s and mean arterial pressure $\bar{p}_a$, resulting in a system of 23 simultaneous equations. Their solution indicated that doubling of S for the left ventricle alone increased cardiac output by some 25%.

Pulsatile phenomena were included in Warner's *resistive-inductive-capacitive* model of the closed circulatory loop (Warner 1959, Fig. 8.3), which stressed viscous and inertial properties of blood as well as the compliant properties of heart and vessels. It set the structural pattern for subsequent studies. The circuit was subdivided into a number of sections, with the condition that outflow of any section equals inflow to the next one. For each segment i a set of three equations are written. They are: (I) an equation of motion, which is commonly a version of the Navier–Stokes equation

$$p_{i-1}(t) - p_i(t) = L_{i-1}\frac{d}{dt}Q_i(t) + R_{i-1}Q_i(t) \tag{8.4}$$

in which L accounts for the inertial and R for the viscous properties of blood (Sect. 5.2); (II) an equation of continuity, which relates change in volume of blood contained by a section to inflow and outflow of that section, such that

$$V_i(t) = V_i(t=0) + \int \left[Q_i(t) - Q_{(i+1)}(t)\right]dt \tag{8.5}$$

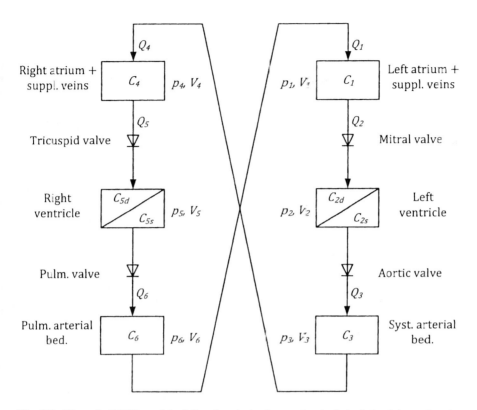

Fig. 8.3 Warner's (1959) model of the closed circulatory circuit. It includes inlet and outlet valves for both ventricles, operated by a diode function generator. Each of the six blocks in this diagram is described by three equations with p denoting pressure, Q flow, V volume and C compliance. The resulting 18 simultaneous equations were solved on an analog computer

(III) an equation of state, which relates pressure in a section to its volume through the compliant properties of the wall: (a) for vessels, with $m = 1$ for arteries, $m > 1$ for veins

$$p_i = \left(\frac{1}{C_i}\right) V_i^m \tag{8.6a}$$

(b) for ventricles, the concept of the time varying compliance was introduced, with C_{id} and C_{is} as constants for diastole and systole, respectively, such that

$$p_i = \left[\frac{1}{(C_{id} \text{ or } C_{is})}\right] V_i^n \tag{8.6b}$$

A bare-bones subdivision into six sections, such as chosen by Warner, required the solution of 18 simultaneous equations, including the conditions imposed by a multiple diode function generator for cardiac valve opening and closure. Since the principal features of this approach remain valid, they can be employed for inclusion of additional features (below and Chap. 10).

The early resistive-capacitive, as well as the resistive-inductive-capacitive model of the closed circulatory loop each exhibited some of the striking features that had been recognized in the living system, despite fundamentally different views expressed regarding the ventricles. These successes stimulated their repeated application and expansion, e.g., by Defares et al. (1963), Beneken (1965), Dick et al. (1966), and many other investigators subsequently.

The early successes also strengthened interest in the inclusion of *control phenomena*. Beneken and De Wit (1967) incorporated baroreceptor control of heart rate and of peripheral resistance. Karreman and Weygandt (1978) introduced carotid sinus control of the peripheral vascular bed resistances through a set of equations which relate carotid sinus pressure to wall deformation, wall deformation to carotid sinus nerve firing rate, sinus nerve firing rate to sympathetic nerve firing rate, and sympathetic firing rate to the elastic modulus of the carotid arterial wall and to peripheral bed resistances. To this was added a simplified description of the renal-endocrine electrolyte control loop by way of an additional set of equations, which relates renal pressure to plasma angiotensin concentration, angiotensin concentration to aldosterone secretion, aldosterone concentration to sodium content in the vascular wall, and sodium concentration to the elastic modulus of the arterial wall.

Placing the emphasis on longer-range control, Guyton et al. (1972) developed a larger set of equations (over 350). In essence, their model contains the blood conducting pathway, vascular stress relaxation, which affects circulatory pressure, membrane dynamics of the capillaries, tissue fluid volume and pressure, electrolyte shift, angiotensin and aldosterone controls, antidiuretic hormone control, kidney dynamics, control of blood flow in muscle, autoregulation, autonomic control, as well as a number of other control facets. Guyton and his coworkers concentrated their studies on the analysis of the sequence of events that lead to congestive heart failure and hypertension, the changes induced by exercise as well as the control of the volume of body fluids. Some of the conclusions to which their systems analysis led were that a decrease in the pumping capabilities of the heart was attended by decreased urinary output, increased plasma volume, increased atrial pressure and restoration of cardiac output, which had dropped initially, until a limit of cardiac impairment was reached. The modeled events were judged to be virtually identical with those observed in actual cases of progressive heart failure, including episodes of edema formation and congestion. Guyton's view that information on inadequate cardiac pumping is mediated mainly by the baroreceptors was countered by Gauer (1972) and Greenberg et al. (1973), who concluded from a long series of experiments that the main sensors of cardiac weakness are located in the atria. Guyton's systems analysis also led him to the conclusion that the peripheral resistance plays an insignificant role in the long-term regulation of arterial blood pressure.

All of these models, as well as their manifold variations, were conceived and built prior to the formulation of the concept of impedance-defined flow.

Consequently, the left and right heart, in harmony with Harvey's teaching, are the only organs assigned the responsibly to pump blood around the circuit. Impedance-defined flow adds a large number of smaller pumps as active elements to the two main ones, as discussed in several chapters, specifically in Sect. 8.3. Inclusion of any or all of these impacts directly on the systematically organized early modeling practices of the closed loop as described above.

8.3   Impedance-Defined Flow

8.3.1   The Principle, Classification, and Isolation of Its Occurrence

William Harvey held that the heart alone (solus) is responsible for steady flow around the closed circuit as well as for pulsations that occur in it. This is the key to Harvey's concept: The ventricles generate *unidirectional* flow during their ejection phases. Harvey took pains to point out that the direction in which the cardiac valves open neatly fits this picture. The rest is passive.

Ultimately, his view resulted in a multitude of studies of the cardiovascular system in which the subject, or patient, lies quietly in the horizontal position in an attempt to avoid effects of body motion and of gravity. The analysis of the arterial system, summarized in Chap. 5 (excluding Sect. 5.2) is functionally based in Harvey's view, as described in Sect. 2.4.

Research inspired by Harvey, though carried out long after his life time, made it abundantly clear that pressure–flow relations within the system are governed by impedances, originally treated as constants, i.e., as resistances, such as R_s and R_p in Eqs. 5.1. Subsequently, they were allowed to be frequency dependent and were called impedances (e.g., Z_l' and Z_t' in normalized form in Eqs. 5.13). Eventually, with the availability of the computer, they were permitted to be time-varying, such as L' in Eq. 5.34a, where the inertial property varies with cross-sectional area S, which in turn varies with time. In describing a relation between a pressure difference and flow containing time-varying impedances, differential equations may require modification for their proper description, as, e.g., in Eq. 5.32. Valves also play the role of time-varying impedances, small when open, large when closed.

Harvey's theory was criticized extensively during the nineteenth century (Sect. 2.3), though most of the criticism did not rise above the debating level. This changed in the twentieth century with the advent of the construction and operation of fluid-filled physical models by Liebau (Sect. 2.4), who demonstrated experimentally that steady flow could be generated around such closed systems by periodic, local, tube compression and release, despite the complete absence of valves. Since this appeared to conflict with Harvey's teaching, Liebau's shows at scientific conferences were, during his life time, viewed as amusing, possibly absurd.

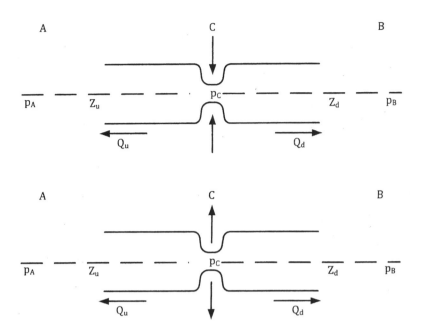

Fig. 8.4 Schematic of a local compression or contraction in an elastic vessel at location C (*upper panel*). An upstream location at a suitable site is denoted A, B similarly downstream; the pressures at these locations are p_A and p_B. The impedance between A and C is represented by Z_u, Z_d between B and C. Flows Q are marked for the upstream and downstream directions, with the *arrows* showing their positive directions. Upon release, p_C will tend to turn negative initially as a result of the recoil of the elastic vessel wall (*lower panel*). The pressure p_C in Eqs. 8.7a, b becomes the pressure in the local compliance for the relaxation or release phase

The problem was eventually isolated. Its essence is illustrated in Fig. 8.4. When a tube or vessel segment is compressed, part or all of the blood displaced can, in principle, escape in two directions. It is fundamentally *bidirectional*. When the compression subsides, refilling of the segment may occur from two directions as well. This was not envisioned in classical wave transmission theory (Chap. 5) and thus requires a more general approach.

A simplified formulation of one of Liebau's original fluid-dynamic models was described in equation form (still requiring two sets of four simultaneous equations, despite the simplification to keep the mathematics transparent). The two sets of equations were solved sequentially until steady state was achieved. Sample results are displayed in Figs. 2.11 and 2.12, showing steady flow around the circuit and exposing the reason for its appearance. The secret proved to lie in the distribution of impedances. Inasmuch as the cardiovascular system is strongly asymmetric, its distribution of impedances is far from uniform (Moser et al. 1998).

If Harvey's term "solus" is dropped, the two concepts merge, and unidirectional becomes a special case of bidirectional. It is referred to as impedance-defined flow, or Z-flow for short. The Z-flow concept, applied in this and subsequent chapters, permits quantitative analysis of systems with or without valves.

Gratifying as the solution of the Liebau problem may be, dealing with a closed circuit, free of valves, rarely applies to the mammalian cardiovascular system. There are, probably, only two exceptions, both of brief duration. The first is the human embryo, which by the end of the 3rd week has a coordinated heart beat prior to the formation of the cardiac valves about a week later (Moore 1985); the second exception can reportedly occur during total circulatory and respiratory collapse. Rudikoff et al. (1980) observed in dogs with arrested hearts, that pressures in the left ventricle, aorta, right atrium, and pulmonary artery were essentially equal during cardiopulmonary resuscitation, suggesting that the heart serves as an open conduit, until resuscitation efforts are successful (within minutes). Under these two circumstances, the systemic and pulmonary arterial pressure reservoirs (Sect. 5.1) are no longer functional.

Consequently, the contribution of impedance-defined flow in the normal must be evaluated with full awareness of the fact that the complete circuit is normally interrupted by at least one pair of closed valves at a cardiac location. In other words, the evaluation of regional effects of impedance-defined flow should concern subsystems. In retrospect and by implication, the criticism on Harvey's theory focused primarily on venous return. "The sphere of the heart's influence" (Jones 1852) was accepted to embrace all arteries constituting the arterial reservoirs.

Such subsystems may be classified in a few kinds. These were listed earlier in Sect. 2.4.3, the second, third, and seventh items. The first kind concerns those organs that display active muscle contraction and relaxation in their walls. It includes the atria and ventricles, the lymphatics, and venomotion in the peripheral organs.

The second kind deals with vessels that are passively compressed or distended, then released, by an external agent. It includes the respiratory action on the central veins, direct skeletal muscle effects on veins embedded in muscular tissue, indirect muscular effects such as on the coronary veins, the operation of the footpump, and the influence of arterial pulsation on blood flow in their companion veins.

The third kind addresses human inventions, designed for the purpose of promoting arterial flow and/or venous return (Chap. 9).

Taken together, these kinds add a new class to the four listed above. It expands the circuit drawn in Fig. 8.3 from one pump (the heart) to multiple pumps (heart and vessels) and the likelihood of more nonlinear phenomena (such as accompany significant compression, Chap. 5).

The mechanism behind impedance-defined flow, in its most basic form, may be visualized as periodic alternation between disturbing a (dynamic) equilibrium of blood in a compliant system (the active phase) and allowing the system to gain (a new) equilibrium (the passive phase), which may or may not be overtaken by the next active phase. In a scattered way, probably all of these have appeared in the literature at some point, though without any effort to arrive at a concept.

A state of equilibrium may be disturbed in several ways, such as local compression and release, contraction and relaxation, acceleration or deceleration of the system, or modification of the gravity vector (Chap. 2). The disturbance selected requires expenditure of energy on the system and results in alteration of the distribution of blood, hence in the generation of flow. Termination of the disturbance permits the system to seek a new equilibrium state, involving another redistribution of blood and generation of flow.

In a nonuniform circuit like the cardiovascular loop, compression at some point, or over some length, will tend to create two unequal exit flows. Upon release, the return flows will, in general, not match the exit flows. A pertinent consideration here is that, since the frequency contents of disturbance and recuperation are different, while most impedances are frequency dependent, impedances may have different values during the two phases, resulting in effects not expected at first sight, such as both average flows occurring in the same direction. Impedance-defined flow will display a surprising range in flexibility as will become apparent in this and subsequent chapters.

Figure 8.4 displays a conceptual scheme of selected conditions that permit computation of impedance-defined flow. A vascular system between the points A and B, is subject to compression or contraction at C, a radial effect (upper panel), which makes the pressure at C, p_C, a function of time. If the pressures at A and B are fixed, e.g., by conditions outside the sketch, the newly created upstream (u) and downstream (d) axial pressure differences are

$$\Delta p_u = p_C - p_A \qquad (8.7a)$$

and

$$\Delta p_d = p_C - p_B \qquad (8.7b)$$

and the corresponding impedances are Z_u and Z_d (used as generic symbols here; their values to be derived from the material treated in Chap. 5). The two axial flows Q_u and Q_d will be, during compression or contraction,

$$Q_u = \frac{\Delta p_u}{Z_u} \qquad (8.7c)$$

and

$$Q_d = \frac{\Delta p_d}{Z_d} \qquad (8.7d)$$

During the relaxation or release period, p_C will tend to turn negative initially, as a result of the recoil of the deformed elastic wall. Prevailing conditions have now changed in a basic fashion: the flow source at C is replaced by a (possibly nonlinear) compliance, serving as a receptacle. The pressure p_C in Eqs. 8.7a, b becomes the pressure in the local compliance during the relaxation or release phase (Sect. 6.2). Hence, the pressure differences in Eqs. 8.7a, b will change also. Other changes may impose alterations in the impedances simultaneously. Taken together, constriction or compression flows are likely to be different, both in magnitude and in direction, from relaxation or release flows.

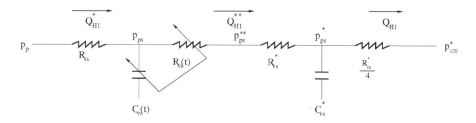

Fig. 8.5 Diagram of a small nonlinear network including the local peripheral resistance, R_{ss}, a contracting and relaxing vessel with compliance $C_{vs}(t)$ and resistance $R_{vs}(t)$, representing a number of muscular venules (venomotion). Fixed downstream small veins are identified by their resistant or compliant features as R_{vs}^*, C_{vs}^*, and $R_{vs}^*/4$. Pressures are called p and flows Q, the latter with their assigned positive directions

If no suitable points A and B are available, the contribution of impedance-defined flow can still be determined by comparing the difference between the solutions of the set of equations including and excluding possible impedance-defined flow. This may be applied for any quantity of interest in the system under scrutiny.

If one of the impedances in Eqs. 8.7c, d becomes very large (e.g., a closed valve or a vessel terminating in a blind end) the corresponding flow will be zero and the corresponding pressure difference becomes immaterial. The other flow in Eqs. 8.7c, d remains as the only unknown. The arterial reservoirs generating outflows during cardiac diastole offer prime examples: the elastic recoil of the arterial walls provide the forces.

To provide a detailed nonlinear example of the first kind on the use of Eqs. 8.7, the diagram of an analyzed network with constant terminal pressures is depicted in Fig. 8.5. The network considers contractile venules. It distinguishes the arteriolar component R_{ss}, the contractile venules with $C_{vs}(t)$ for the compliant aspect together with $R_{vs}(t)$ for the resistive aspect of these venules (marked by interconnected arrows). In addition, fixed downstream resistive and compliant features, R_{vs}^*, C_{vs}^*, and $R_{vs}^*/4$ are identified. Entrance and exit pressures (p_p and p_{100}^*) are constant. Each of these elements lumps a considerable number of vessels, owing to lack of detailed information. The emphasis here is on demonstrating that contractile venules can operate as small peripheral pumps, promoting venous return. The number of such pumps is, of course, potentially very large.

The following set of 11 equations evolved:

$$Q_{H1}^* - Q_{H1}^{**} = p_{ps}\frac{dC_{vs}}{dt} + C_{vs}\frac{dp_{ps}}{dt} \tag{8.8}$$

$$Q_{H1}^{**} - Q_{H1} = C_{vs}^* \frac{dp_{ps^*}}{dt} \tag{8.9}$$

$$p_p - p_{ps} = R_{ss}Q_{H1}^* \tag{8.10}$$

$$p_{ps} - p_{ps}^{**} = R_{vs}Q_{H1}^{**} \tag{8.11}$$

$$p_{ps}^{**} - p_{ps}^{*} = R_{vs}^{*}Q_{H1}^{**} \tag{8.12}$$

$$p_{ps}^{*} - p_{100}^{*} = \frac{R_{vs}^{*}}{4}Q_{H1} \tag{8.13}$$

$$V = \pi r^2 l \tag{8.14}$$

$$R_{vs} = \frac{8\eta l}{\pi r^4} \tag{8.15}$$

$$C_{vs} = \frac{3\pi r^3 l}{2hE} \tag{8.16}$$

$$rh = \frac{1}{30} \tag{8.17}$$

$$\frac{E(t)}{E(t=0)} = \left[\frac{r(t=0)}{r(t)}\right]^3 \tag{8.18}$$

The single contracting vessel's volume is denoted V. The modulus of elasticity E (t), which is responsible for contraction and relaxation, was taken to follow a parabolic ascent and an exponential descent, with the functions and their derivatives matched at the transition point to preserve continuity. In this example, the stronger the pumping function, the faster the relaxation. The simplicity of the model used here dictates that flows depend on the structure of the relevant channels.

This pilot model show that flow in the direction of the central veins is indeed enhanced by venomotion, with exit flow Q_{H1} rising from 16.1 to 17.0 ml/s during the single venomotion cycle reproduced in Fig. 8.6. As a consequence of contraction of venules, p_{ps} increases by 7.5 mmHg ($\Delta p_{ps} = 7.5$) at peak value (Fig. 8.6), while p_p remains fixed. At this instant, Q_u (Eq. 8.7c) should equal $\Delta p_{ps}/R_{ss}$ yielding 7.5/ 4.8 = 1.6 ml/s. Q_{H1}^{*} (Fig. 8.6b) is indeed reduced by that amount. The effect of superimposed slow vasomotion with $R_{ss} = 4.8 + 2\sin 0.63t$ is illustrated in Fig. 8.7.

Examples that do not feature A and B locations with constant pressure are available in Sects. 3.3, and in Sect. 10.2.

Attention should be drawn to a few specific features. First, tiny veins in the proximity of the capillaries invariably face a large impedance in the upstream direction, since venous pressure is significantly below arteriolar pressure. Therefore, venular contraction is in a favorable location to promote venous return. Second, where venular contraction increases flow impedance (such as by the in series $R_{vs}(t)$ in Fig. 8.5), outflow is impeded for the duration of the elevated impedance state. Hence, these effects tend to oppose each other, and the time course of the contraction-relaxation phenomenon becomes of interest.

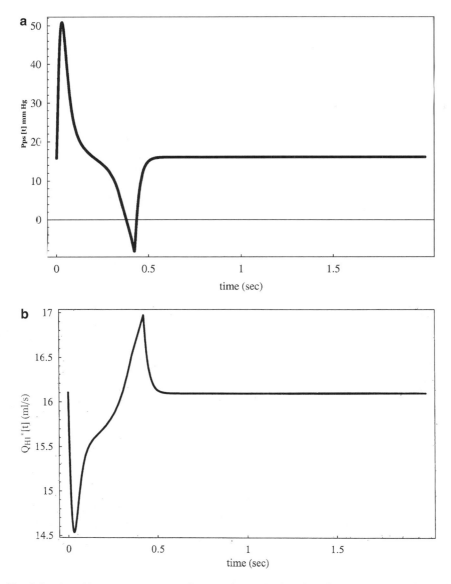

Fig. 8.6 (a) $p_{ps}(t)$ as a consequence of contraction and relaxation, (b) concurrent $Q_{H1}*(t)$ and (c) outflow $Q_{H1}(t)$ for the condition that input pressure p_p and output pressure $p_{100}*$ are constant. In all three plots the values indicated at $t = 0$ are those for a relaxed vessel. See Chap. 11 for definitions

Whether the active phase should be faster than the recovery phase depends on the structure of the circuit of interest. In the example of Fig. 2.12, the two phases concern two physically different parts of a closed loop favoring slower relaxation. In venomotion, it is the same component that contracts and relaxes. The contraction

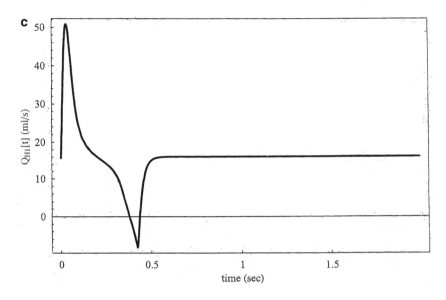

Fig. 8.6 (continued)

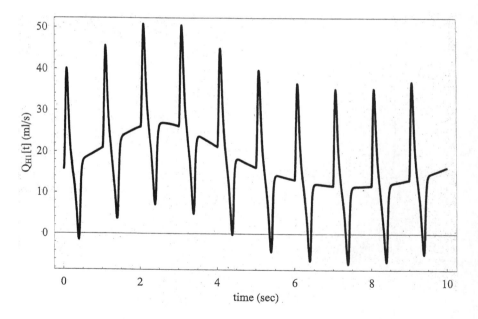

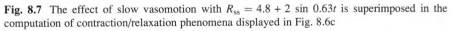

Fig. 8.7 The effect of slow vasomotion with $R_{ss} = 4.8 + 2 \sin 0.63t$ is superimposed in the computation of contraction/relaxation phenomena displayed in Fig. 8.6c

moves blood out of the venules, causing the flow impedance to increase during this phase. This would hamper continued flow from the arterial impedance after the contraction has run its course, unless the venules relax quickly. Rapid relaxation has indeed been observed in such situations, e.g., in lymphatics (McHale and Roddie 1976) and in the respiratory system, where inspiration tends to last much longer than expiration itself, despite the often quoted inspiratory to expiratory ratio of 1:2 (Fig. 11.2). Coronary veins do not fit this picture, since the duration of compression by the cardiac musculature is set by other requirements, such as the magnitude of stroke volume.

8.3.1.1   The Transformation Assigned to the Heart

When one continues to look at regional effects of (quasi) periodic compression and release, or contraction and relaxation, it will be immediately apparent that it is impossible for blood to flow continuously to regions of lower pressure and lower impedance in a closed circuit. Therefore, the simple pattern must be interrupted at some point to make room for a more complex solution. Nature accomplished this at the level of both ventricles. In a valveless system, it would be preferable for the ventricles to pump into the corresponding atria rather than into the arterial systems, disturbing continuous flow in a consistent direction. Placement of the mitral and tricuspid valves introduces high value impedances during ventricular systole, which resolves this difficulty (Noordergraaf G.J. et al. 2005). The same solution is applied to the arterial systems for which it would be more convenient to apply their potential energy to moving blood back into the ventricles: the aortic and pulmonary valves. This is referred to as impedance transformation. Four sets of leaflets are satisfactory to achieve this solution, six are not needed (Noordergraaf G.J et al. 2006).

8.3.1.2   Examples of Impedance-Defined Flow

The term impedance-defined flow will encompass unidirectional as well as bidirectional flows.

(a) *Fluid mechanical example of the first kind*

Peristalsis. Extensively studied in the gastrointestinal tract, as well as in other tubes with syncytial smooth muscle, this phenomenon is related to the movement of food. It apparently has not been demonstrated in the blood circulation, though similarities with impedance-defined flow are striking. Local electrical stimulation of such a tube generates a local contracted ring that is capable of propagating in two directions, though they tend to die out over short distances.

The common stimulation is thought to be caused by local distention, followed by contraction of the distended section and simultaneous relaxation of the distal adjacent section of tract, which can be intensified via a nerve plexus under parasympathetic control. The resulting movement of material within the tract will primarily cause a slowly propagating contraction wave in the distal direction. This has been referred to as "the law of the gut" (Guyton 1963).

(b) *Fluid mechanical examples of the second kind.*

Liebau's model. In Sect. 2.4.3, a reconstituted model, originally designed by Liebau, was tested theoretically for steady flow around the closed loop for the linearized and the nonlinear version. Both show similar steady flows.

Isolated segment of bovine aorta. Figure 8.8a shows an arrangement for a (small) subsystem that was tested experimentally and mathematically. It consists of a uniform segment of bovine aorta horizontally suspended in a water-filled tank. Alternate compression and release at the midpoint does not effect any steady flow through the aortic segment, but at other points it generates appreciable average flow visualized by dyed fluid. This example demonstrates flow without a pressure difference between the ends. The energy that moves the fluid derives from the external compression, and does not follow from the traditional pressure–flow relationship for this segment of aorta. The core of the interpretation for the compression phase is in Fig. 8.8b, displaying the absolute values of the input impedances of the long (1) and short (2) segments of the aortic specimen (Sect. 5.2). Both input impedances are strongly frequency dependent. The two are equal or unequal depending on the selected frequency of compression and release. Thus, for a frequency at which the input impedance is smaller for the long segment, ejection flow will be from left to right in Fig. 8.8a.

For the release phase, the negative transmural pressure difference assumed to be on the right of the once compressed part changes with time at a rate that depends on inflow into that part, coupling two unknown variables. In the example displayed in Fig. 8.8c most of the restoration flow enters through the short end (Buckley and Kim 2006), making both ejection and restoration flows move from left to right in Fig. 8.8a.

Fig. 8.8 (a) The *arrows* indicate an asymmetric compression site along a length of bovine thoracic aorta. Under a scenario of periodic compression and release, large steady flows can be generated in one direction or the other, depending on the selected frequency. Such passive compression at the midpoint generates pulsatile flow free of a steady component. (Described in Moser et al. 1998.) (b) The absolute values of the input impedances seen from the compression site looking into the long end Z_{in1} (*thin line*) and the short end Z_{in2}. Their frequency behavior is seen to be different, owing to the difference in lengths. Fluid inertial and viscous properties are taken into account as well as the open end reflection constants. For a frequency of 3.5 Hz, for instance, the long end has an impedance that is a small fraction of that experienced along the short end, resulting in compression flow to exit primarily through the long end for this frequency. (c). During relaxation (negative), substitution flows enter at both terminations. Flow coming in through the short end (*heavy graph*) is clearly several times larger (three times in this example) than that entering through the long end. Consequently, both main flows occur in the same direction

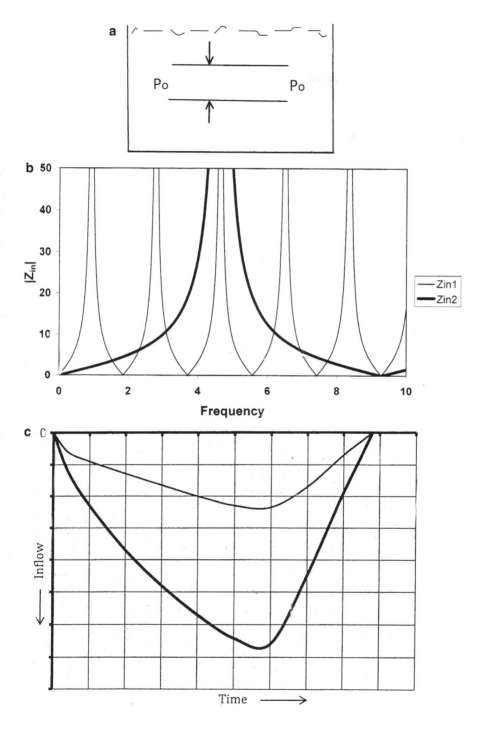

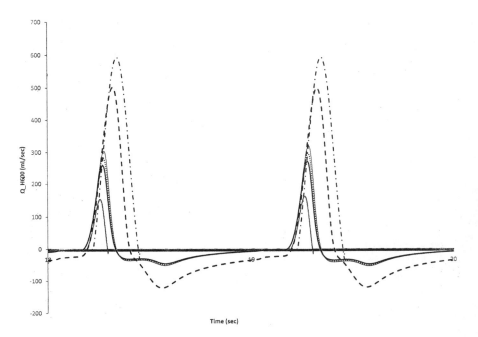

Fig. 8.9 Left ventricular ejection curves (Q_{H600}) for a number of valvular conditions: *dash-dot line*, all four valves intact ($V_s = 75$ ml); *broken line*, only the mitral valve intact ($V_s = 9.5$ ml); *fully drawn thin line*, only the pulmonary valve intact ($V_s = 4$ ml); *dotted line*, only the tricuspid valve intact ($V_s = 2.7$ ml); *fully drawn thick line*, no intact valves ($V_s = 1.4$ ml); *fully drawn line* with smaller amplitude, only the aortic valve intact ($V_s = 9$ ml) (Data assembled by Stein 2008)

(c) *Cardiovascular examples*

1. *The ventricles and the valveless heart.* With normal anatomy and normal performance, both ventricles make simple examples of impedance-defined flow of the first kind, employing two mechanisms: contraction, resulting in ejection, and relaxation, permitting filling owing to a negative Δp_u between central veins and ventricular cavities which are complemented by atrial contraction just prior to the onset of ventricular contraction. Ejection flows have no choice but to enter the receiving arteries. This condition changes when the mitral valve and/or the tricuspid valve become deficient and flow becomes bidirectional. It changes even more profoundly during cardiac collapse when the heart becomes passive (Chap. 9).

   It may be noted that when none of the cardiac valves close, the pumping ventricles generate negligible steady flow (Stein 2008, Fig.8.9), but large pulsatile flow moving back and forth, which is referred to as sloshing. [Pure sloshing may be defined as pulsatile flow, going back and forth, with an average value equal to zero.] The situation improves when either the mitral, or the tricuspid valve, or both are able to close. These results were obtained with the aid of the closed loop model described in Chap. 11 (Noordergraaf G.J. et al. 2005).

Since both ventricles normally offer the only pathways from the venous systems to the respective arterial systems, they display the power of adaptation to accommodate resting cardiac output (~5 l/min in the human) to cardiac output during exercise (~20 l/min) and heavy exercise of trained athletes (~30 l/min), based on the adaptability of the cardiac function curves, augmentation of venous return, change in heart rate together with neural plus metabolic stimuli (Chaps. 3 and 10).

2. *Systemic and pulmonary arterial outflow.* During ventricular systole, cardiac activity maintains a pressure difference across the periphery resulting in unidirectional flow downstream. During ventricular diastole, compression caused by elastic recoil of the distended arterial walls sustains this unidirectional flow without ever reaching a relaxed phase.

3. *The coronary vasculature.* The detailed model of coronary perfusion, described in Sect. 6.3, indicates that the veins are practically emptied in the atrial direction under the influence of ventricular contraction. Hence, the venous vasculature serves as a pump, expending energy supplied by the ventricular musculature. It is estimated that around 80% of the coronary blood volume is expelled to the right atrium during early systole, the entire compression period lasting about 30% of a beat. During renewed filling, though Δp_d, between the right atrium and the coronary veins, becomes negative (Eq. 8.7b), but much less significantly so than the also negative Δp_u between the coronary veins and arteries (Eq. 8.7a), while downstream impedance is less than upstream impedance, it is difficult to predict from the formulas alone without details as to numerical values whether Q_u or Q_d will dominate. However, Fig. 6.7, resulting from a model providing such details, suggests that filling of these veins comes principally from the arteries, since venous reflux at the onset of diastole appears either absent or negligible. The precise numbers depend on the imposed boundary conditions at the arterial inlet and the venous outlet. The latter was set at a constant 6 mmHg in this study (Frasch et al. 1998). In reality, atrial pressure may drop below this level at this phase in the cardiac cycle. During the remainder of the diastolic period the coronaries are essentially passive blood carrying channels, with perfusion driven by the aortic to right atrial pressure difference. This conclusion does not support Porter's contention (1898) that the emptying of intramural vessels by the contraction of the heart favors the flow of blood through the heart walls chiefly by the diminished "resistance" that the empty patulous vessels offer to the inflow of blood from the aorta when the ventricules relax. Instead, ventricular contraction inhibits blood perfusion (Figs. 6.7 and 6.8). This finding is attributed to the time-varying distribution of impedances, which becomes understandable from Eqs. 8.7 and illustrates a set of conditions where vascular compression fails to operate as an effective pump. This phenomenon may serve a different purpose, however (Sect. 10.2). Coronary venous valves, when mentioned at all in earlier texts, are commonly described as incomplete and insufficient.

4. *Peripheral perfusion and vasomotion.* Analyzed in some detail in Sect. 6.3, vasomotion adds a dynamic feature to blood flow through the peripheral resistance. At the local level, it converts steady flow into pulsatile flow with a steady component, just as it happens to ejection flow of the ventricles. As discussed in Sect. 5.2, this conversion facilitates blood flow downstream by allowing its compliant properties to participate in input impedance considerations. This participation reduces the input impedance of the downstream vasculature by making it frequency dependent. In the case of vasomotion, conditions are complicated by downstream venomotion. The details of this have not been scrutinized adequately owing to paucity of quantitative data on vessel properties.

5. *Venomotion and reflection in the venous system.* If it is valid to consider the bat wing (Sect. 6.3) as a prototype of mammalian peripheral vasculatures in general, their respective venomotion activities qualify as so many active elements. In the detailed model studies by Mayrovitz et al. (1974), (Figs. 6.9 and 6.10) there is forward flow through the capillaries at all times (Δp_u in Eq. 8.7c being always negative). On the other hand, the contracting venule (the segments from P_5 to P_{10} in Fig. 6.9) are prevented from pumping into a larger vein owing to a particular feature in the model's design (its large load resistance, R_V). If this is adapted to recognize the compliant properties of the downstream small veins, the muscular venule becomes a tiny active pump, irrespective of whether the time delay δ in Fig. 6.9 is zero or positive. In the reduced models in Eqs. 11.88 and 11.89, this is incorporated. Since the potential number of muscular venules is very large, this engenders the picture of a powerful river close to its exit, starting at its origin with a multitude of minute tributaries, with the flow subject to strong cross-sectional area reduction as the fluid moves along the river bed. (The arterial vasculature leads blood along the inverse anatomical arrangement).

   In view of the active processes in the periphery, it would seem optimistic to expect that its pressure difference to flow relation is linear or just slightly nonlinear over the entire systemic pressure range of interest, less so in the pulmonary system (Shoukas et al. 1984; Burattini 1985).

   One may speculate that reflection in the venous system enhances the flow pulse at the expense of the pressure pulse, though evidence bearing on such speculation does not appear to be available at the present time (Question 5.8). Strong reflection at some point could be misinterpreted as the presence of a valve.

6. *The lymphatics.* Lymphatics are claimed to be able to pump uphill from areas of negative interstitial pressure to positive central venous pressure. They feature lymphangions, i.e., segments demarked by centrally opening valves. At least one valve close to their outlet is necessary to prevent venous blood from irrigating the lymphatics; in reality, the valves appear to be abundant (Chap. 7).

   The mechanism of uphill pumping with the aid of impedance-defined flow may be visualized conveniently as described in Chap. 7 and illustrated in Fig. 7.3. The analogy to cardiac pumping becomes alluring.

7. *Physical exercise involving dependent body parts, the footpump, and the rocking chair.* The hand and arm veins are endowed with a spatial distribution of simple valves in many species of mammals. So are the foot and the leg veins. Some equatic mammalian species have been reported to have few or no such valves. Instead, some species have a sphincter in the vena cava close to the diaphragm. This sphincter permits control of blood flow to the heart during dives (Rommel and Lowenstine 2001).

A great deal has been written about valvular function, not all of it is enlightening. The hydro(hemo)static effect, caused by the earth's gravitational field, attracted much of the attention. When it is appreciated that the feeding arteries are subject to the same gravitational effect, it will be clear that this presents no problem in its own right (Sect. 10.2). The perceived difficulty then relates to the much more distensible properties of venous walls compared to their arterial counterparts Most of the smaller veins in the dependent parts are embedded in skeletal muscle. Hence, in the vertical position and with the skeletal muscle relaxed a significant volume of blood can be stored in these veins. The segmentation of the veins by valves does not prevent such storage over a sufficiently long time interval, since these simple valves tend to be incompetent.

Skeletal muscle contraction and relaxation, however, prevents such undesirable storage by shifting blood from (a) compressed segment(s) in the direction of the venae cavae, while (b) short-term reflux is impeded by valves.

Le Dentu (1867) postulated the venous foot pump by arguing that the nonweight-bearing foot collects a significant amount of blood in the plantar plexus, which is expelled in the direction of the central veins upon weight-bearing by that foot (roughly estimated at 20 ml from data by Gardner and Fox 1993). The plantar plexus constitutes an elaborate network of veins in the sole of the foot. The plexus may be made visible by adding a contrast medium to the blood. The contrast medium disappears promptly with loading (compression of veins in) the foot as would be expected from the proximity of the microcirculation. The plexus is heavily endowed with venous valves, so that, even in the dependent position of the leg, refilling (subsequent to relaxation) is provided by the arteries (Gardner and Fox 1993). Although the debate on the interpretation of the operation of the natural foot pump has not been closed, the experiments demonstrate clearly that ambulation promotes movement of blood out of both feet in the central direction within the venous system. A clinical application of this phenomenon is described in Sect. 9.4.

The rocking chair may well qualify as a long-term application, mostly enjoyed by seniors, to help propel venous blood out of the legs into the vena cava inferior.

8. *Pumping by influence.* Ozanam, in his book (1886), states on the basis of his own experiments that there is "circulation by influence" (Sect. 2.3). Ozanam pointed out that in the mammalian body there are many pairs formed by an

artery and its somewhat larger companion vein, with the pair wrapped in a sheath that is presumably indistensible. Ozanam lists numerous locations where this applies, though it is not true for every pair throughout the body. While observing sheathed pairs he noted that the venous system is influenced by the passing arterial pulse wave, which distends the artery briefly and compresses the vein during that interval. One example of such a sheathed pair is provided by a common carotid artery and an internal jugular vein (a vagal nerve is also enclosed in this sheath).

Analysis with the aid of a small regional, distributed model of a number of tiny veins shows that the venous flow pulse is magnified by the arterial pulse (Mawn 2002; Levine 2005). Another study, also carried out on a small network of veins of which one vein was subjected to the passing arterial pulse, showed that venous pulsations were indeed enhanced, but that for slow imposed pulsations, average flow at the exit of the network was reduced (Hu and Simone 2007, Fig. 8.10).

9. *The respiratory blood pump.* The systemic venous pathway furnishes the principal route for returning blood to the right heart. As such it determines the filling pressure to the right ventricle and therefore influences its output into the pulmonary artery. Guyton et al. (1973) quoted experiments in which an increase of central venous (i.e., filling) pressure by 1 mmHg doubled right ventricular output under certain conditions. Clearly, central venous pressure can play a key role in setting the level of cardiac output (Figs. 8.1 and 8.2).

The central veins receive their inputs through the upper and lower divisions of the systemic peripheral vasculature. In view of the highly compliant properties of the central veins, they essentially serve as a low pressure blood reservoir of large capacity.

Donders (1856) belongs to the early observers of the influence of the respiration on the circulation: "[...] with the play of inspiration and expiration, blood pressure and blood flow change very significantly. This effect can easily be demonstrated by direct observation. If the neck veins are exposed, it will be seen that they collapse during each inspiration; in contrast, during each expiration, they fill more with blood." This convinced Donders that the respiratory system assists the heart in its pumping effort by periodically increasing and decreasing the pressure around the superior and inferior thoracic veins. His view proved to be conflictive.

Fig. 8.10 A single vein in a network of 11 small veins with six input locations and a single exit is exposed to a passing arterial pulse (Ozanam 1886). The deformation is defined as causing a sinusoidal compression of 10%of its original radius at a heart rate f of 1 Hz. All six entry locations are exposed to a constant pressure of 10 mmHg, while the exit is subjected to a pressure of 4 + sin $(2\pi ft)$ (**a**). The *top curve* in (**b**) (*broken line*) shows venous exit flow without arterial exposure, while the *bottom curve* (*solid*) depicts flow under conditions of steady compression. The *dotted curve* represents exposure to the sinusoidal compression as defined above. Note that (1) the central curve is not a pure sinusoid owing to nonlinearities, (2) its amplitude is magnified, (3) its average is reduced (**b**)

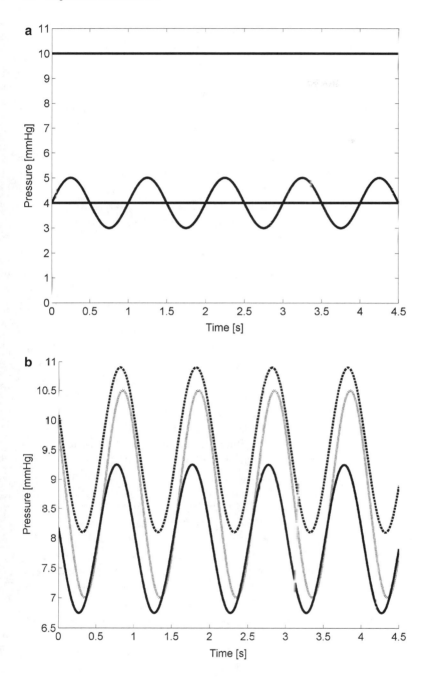

A normal intrathoracic pressure curve during activity is reproduced in Fig. 10.4. The pressure shows a minimum value at the end of inspiration. Hence, the interval of inspiration, together with the early part of expiration, favors filling of the central veins and the right atrium. When the right ventricle relaxes, it benefits directly from this filling state as well. This filling phase occurs at the expense of the neck veins, located outside the chest cavity, which may collapse as a consequence. The resulting increase in stroke volume propagates through the heart to become visible as a rise in root aortic pressure. During the remainder of the respiratory cycle, the respiratory effect wanes, completing the respiratory-induced modulation of aortic pressure.

During rest, when the demand for cardiac output is reduced, the amplitude of the respiratory signal attenuates and its support of the blood circulation reduces concurrently.

During deep sleep, in the gravitational field and in the microgravitational environment the respiratory influence may reduce further and an integer relationship between heart rate and respiratory rate (e.g., 4) may become observable (Hildebrandt et al. 1998). It has been shown that inspiration tends to shift to the middle of the cardiac phase (Moser et al. 1995; Noordergraaf A et al. 2001), thereby protecting the right heart more firmly against inspiratory filling. Under normal resting conditions, the pressure around the thoracic veins is negative compared to atmospheric at the level of a few mmHg. As a result of the peripheral sources of blood, in conjunction with the central unloading mechanism, transmural pressure in the veins is positive and the veins are wide open.

In retrospect, it is hardly surprising that Donders' idea provoked enough discord to make him redirect his interests elsewhere, in his case to ophthalmology. Respiratory's control contribution to the circulation eventually proved to be strongly versatile.

In a simplified (one segment) model of a thoracic vein, the downstream resistance was set to a real number, thereby violating one requirement of the set referred listed in Sect. 2.4. It was found that the respiration under these conditions does not promote venous return flow to the heart. But when the inertial properties of blood were taken into account (changing the downstream impedance into a complex number), the complete set of requirements was satisfied and the respiration was found to promote venous return.

10. *The atrial pumps.* The atria belong to the first kind and form a special case since Eqs. 8.7a, b require adaptation to their specific condition. They contract actively toward the end of the filling phase of the ventricles. The increased pressure ejects part of their contents into the corresponding ventricles, while another part appears as reflux into the corresponding central veins, owing to the similar upstream and downstream pressures and the similarity of the encountered impedances. This has given the atria the deserved reputation of inefficient pumps. They qualify as pumps

nevertheless owing to the prompt closure of the mitral and tricuspid valves following atrial contraction and induced by the onset of ventricular contraction. Atrial pumping remains a valuable feature in view of the fact that it assists in the transfer of blood out of the venous systems into the arterial vasculatures, lowering central venous pressures, while increasing cardiac output by 15–25% (Sect. 8.3.1.2).

11. *Body motion.* Harvey's teaching mandates that blood contained in the heart, and in the larger arteries and veins follow a strict pattern of unidirectional progression, modified only by almost periodic superimposed antegrade and retrograde waves generated by the heart. It has since become clear that reality displays a vastly more complex picture

   The phenomena involved may be subdivided into two classes. The first includes, but is not limited to, venomotion and the respiratory system's influence on the circulation, both occurring at frequencies that are basically different from the heart rate. The other class concerns effects caused by the motion of the body operating directly on the mass of blood, such as those imposed during walking, jogging, running, jumping, bicycling, etc. as well as during the performance of routine daily, or nonroutine, activities. Section 5.2.6 offers a closed form analytical solution to a physiological example, while Sect. 9.4 addresses clinical examples, which have so far received little attention of an analytical nature.

12. *Variations on the same principle.* Three main variations are in evidence. (a) Inflow is stopped entirely during compression. The cardiac ventricles serve as examples. (b) Inflow continues at a reduced level. The reduction in level of inflow may or may not be substantial. For vasomotion in the peripheral organs, this reduction will be small when the regional arterioles are constricted, larger when these arterioles are relaxed. (c) Inflow is significantly impeded. The coronary veins provide an example caused by the systolic duration of their compression. In this case perfusion is seriously hindered by the compression.

   Owing to the many forms taken by impedance-defined flow, it becomes as intricate as understanding the operation of a ventricle, even in the early phases of study of the former.

13. *Sloshing.* An example of the third kind, which is spectacular, though pathological, is provided by Fig. 8.11. It deals with nonoperational valves in a noncontractile left ventricle that is subjected to cardiopulmonary resuscitation (CPR) with a peak compression pressure of 60 mmHg. Ventricular pressure, p6, and ventricular volume V_{LV} are reproduced together with flows through the mitral valve ostium, C_{H13}, and the aortic root, Q_{H15}, all predominantly resulting from the application of CPR. Flows are seen to go negative and positive, with flow through the mitral ostium far exceeding root aortic flow in accordance with Eqs. 8.7c. d. The time averages of these two flows are slightly positive, rather than zero. This is in response to a steady venous reservoir pressure of 20 mmHg in this example (Noordergraaf G.J. et al. 2005).

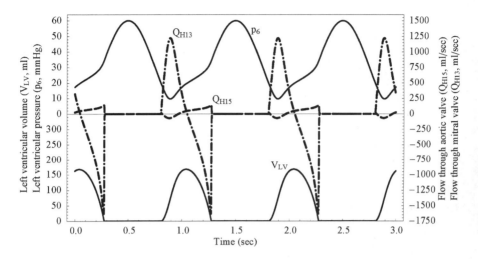

Fig. 8.11 The left ventricle in a closed model of only the systemic circulation, after removal of both left ventricular (LV) valves in an asystolic left ventricle, is subjected to a sinusoidally shaped cardiopulmonary resuscitation signal with peak values of 60/0 mmHg. The curves reproduce ventricular pressure (p_6 in this figure) and volume (V_{LV}) together with flows through the mitral valve ostium (Q_{H13}) and the aortic root (Q_{H15}). Note that flow into the aorta is negligible compared to the sloshing through the mitral ostium (Reproduced from Noordergraaf G.J. et al. 2005)

This last example permits flow from other causes, though modified, to continue in the presence of impedance-defined flow. During ventricular pumping, rather than during CPR, this is not the case; valves tend to impose alternation between various flows.

Isolation of impedance-defined flow with the aid of Eqs. 8.7 can facilitate evaluation over trying to discern it from an overall approach as in a modernized version of section 8.3 above.

8.4 Conclusions

The recognition of the circulatory system as a closed system, while a step forward, explicitly challenged the primacy of the heart as its central and only pump. Critics focused primarily on the heart's suspected inability to take care of venous return adequately. Impedance-defined flow resolved this issue by showing that the heart is not the only pump, instead that a multitude of smaller pumps can be identified as well, supporting the correct analysis of the primacy of the heart itself.

The cardiovascular system can therefore be described as a highly efficient whole: small pumps at critical locations avoid the need for an ineffective, highly demanding, central pump solution.

8.5   Summary

Chapter 8 formally introduces impedance-defined flow as a generalization on Harvey's teaching, although instances of such flow appear throughout the earlier chapters. The most basic recognition feature is the generation of bidirectional flow occurring as a result of contraction or compression of a compartment with an elastic wall, of which there is a multitude of examples. The two flows so generated tend to be unequal, owing to the difference in flow impedances faced by these two flows. Subsequent relaxation and release, leading to refilling, generally do not compensate for the difference between the original outflows. In some locations nature inserted a valve serving to enhance the difference between outflow impedances; this adjustment makes unidirectional flow a special case of bidirectional flow.

In Sect. 8.3, an initial classification among causes of impedance-defined flow is proposed. This is followed by a long, though necessarily incomplete, list of cardiovascular examples.

References

Agostoni P. and Butler J. : Cardiopulmonary Interactions in Exercise. Chapter 8 *in:* Exercise, Pulmonary Physiology and Pathophysiology. B.J. Whipp and K. Wasserman (eds.), Marcel Dekker, New York, 1991.

Beneken J.E.W.: A Mathematical Approach to Cardio-Vascular Function: The Uncontrolled Human Sytem. Ph.D. Dissertation, Univ. of Utrecht, 1965.

Beneken J.E.W., Wit de B.: A Physical Approach to Hemodyramic Aspects of the Human Cardio-vascular System. Chap 1 *in:* Physical Basis of Circulatory Transport: Regulation and Exchange. E.B. Reeve and A. Guyton (eds.) Saunders, Philadelphia PA, 1967.

Buckley E. and Kim M.: Analytical calculation of flow in a bull aorta after compression. Project report in a course taught by A. Noordergraaf, 2006.

Burattini R.: *Comments on:* Carotid sinus baroreceptor reflex control and the role of autoregulation in the systemic and pulmonary arterial pressure-flow relationships of the dog. Circ. Res. 57: 198–200, 1985.

Caesalpinus A.: Quaestionum Medicarum, Liber secundus, p. 234, Venice, 1593

De Vroomen M., Cardozo R.H., Steendijk P., Bel van F. and Baan J.: Improved contractile performance of right ventricle in response to increased RV afterload in newborn lamb. Am. J. Physiol. 278 (Heart Circ. Physiol. 47): H100-H105, 2000.

Defares J.G., Hara H.H., Osborn J.J. and McLeod J.: Theoretical Analysis and Computer Simulation of the Circulation with special Reference to the Starling Properties of the Ventricles. *In:* Circulatory Analog Computers. A. Noordergraaf, G.N. Jager, N. Westerhof (eds.). North-Holland Publ. Co., Amsterdam, 1963.

Dick D.E., Hillestad R.J. and Ridout V.C.: A computer study on the effect of circulatory system defects Proc. 19th , Ann. Conf. Eng. Med. Biol., San Francisco CA, p89, 1966.

Donders F.C.: Physiologie des Menschen, Hirzel, Leipzig, 1856.

Frasch H.F., Kresch J.Y. and Noordergraaf A.: Interpretation of Coronary Vascular Perfusion. Ch. 7 *in:* Analysis and Assessment of Cardiovascular Function. G.M. Drzewiecki and J. K-J. Li (eds.) Springer, New York, NY, 1998.

Gardner A.M.N. and Fox R.H.: The Return of Blood to the Heart. J. Libbey and Co., London, 2nd ed., 1993.

Gauer O.H.: Kreislauf des Blutes. *In:* Herz und Kreislauf. O.H. Gauer, K. Kramer, und R. Jung (eds.) Urban & Scharzenberg, München, 1972.

Greenberg T.T., Richmond W.H., Stocking R.A., Gupta P.D., Meehan J.P. and Henry J.P.: Impaired atrial receptor responses in dogs with heart failure due to tricuspid insufficiency and pulmonary artery stenosis. Circ. Res. 32: 424–433, 1973.

Guyton A.C.: A concept of negative interstitial pressure based on pressures in implanted perforated capsules. Circul. Res. 12: 399–414, 1963.

Guyton A.C., Coleman T.G. and Granger H.J.: Circulation: Overall regulation. Ann. Rev. Physiol. 34: 13–46, 1972.

Hamilton W.F.: Role of the Starling concept in regulation of the normal circulation. Physiol. Rev. 35: 161–168, 1955.

Harvey G.: Exercitatio Anatomica, De Motu Cordis et Sanguinis in Animalibus, Frankford, 1628.

Hildebrandt G., Moser M., Lehofer M.: Chronobiologie und Chronomedizin. Hippocrates Verlag, Stuttgart, 1998.

Hill W.S., Polleri J.O. and Matteo A.L.: Essay on a Hydrodynamic Analysis of the Blood Circulation. Univ. of Montevideo. ANCAP, Ministerio de Salud Pœblica, Montevideo, Uruguay, 1958.

Hu R. and Simone E.: Ozanam - Artery Pump. Project report in a course taught by A. Noordergraaf, Univ. of Pennsylvania, 2007.

Jochim K.E.: A mathematical analysis of pulse volume determinants. Fed. Proc. 5: 52–53, 1946.

Jochim K.E.: Arterial pulses simulated in electrical analogues of the circulatory system. Fed. Proc. 7: 62, 1948.

Jochim K. and Katz L.N.: Further observations on the dynamics of fluid flow in an elastic system. Fed. Proc. 1: 43–44, 1942.

Jones T.W.: Discovery that the veins of the bat's wing (which are furnished with valves) are endowed with rythmical contractility, and that the onward flow of blood is accelerated by each contraction. Phil. Trans. Royal Soc. of London, 142: 131–136, 1852.

Karreman G. and Weygandt C.N.: Theoretical Control Aspects of the Circulation. Ch. 52 in: Cardiovascular System Dynamics, J. Baan et al. (eds.), MIT Press, Cambridge MA, 1978.

Kries J von.: Studien zur Pulslehre. Akad. Verlagsbuchshandlung, Freiburg i. B., 1892.

le Dentu A.: Circulation Veineuse du Pied et de la Jambe. A. Delahaye, Paris, 1867.

Levine A.: Ozanam's idea of arterial pulsation promoting venous return. Project report in a course taught by A. Noordergraaf, Univ. of Pennsylvania, 2005.

Liljestrand G., Lysholm E. and Nylin G.: The immediate effects of muscular work on the stroke and heart volume in man. Skand. Arch. Physiol. 80: 265–282, 1938.

Marey E.J.: Physiologie Médicale de la Circulation du Sang Basée sur l'Étude Graphique des Mouvements du Coeur et du Pouls Artériel avec Application aux Maladies de l'Appareil Circulatoire. Delahaye, Paris, 1863.

Mawn T.: La circulation par influence. Project report in a course taught by A. Noordergraaf. Univ. of Pennsylvania, 2002.

Mayrovitz H.N.: The Microcirculation: Theory and Experiment. Ph.D. Dissertation, Univ. of Pennsylvania, Philadelphia PA, 1974.

McHale N.G. and Roddie I.C.: The effect of transmural pressure on pumping activity in isolated bovine lymphatic vessels. J. Physiol. 261: 255–269, 1976.

Melbin J., Detweiler D.K., Riffle R.A. and Noordergraaf A.: Coherence of cardiac output with rate changes. Am. J. Physiol. 243 (Heart Circ. Physiol. 12): H499-H504, 1982

Moore K.L.: Embryology. Schattauer, Stuttgart, 2nd ed., pp. 340–358, 1985.

Moser M., Lehofer M., Hildebrandt G., Voica M., Egner S., Kenner T.: Phase- and frequency coordination of cardiac and respiratory function. Biol. Rhythm Res. 26: 100–111, 1995.

Moser M., Huang J.W., Schwarz G.S., Kenner T., Noordergraaf A.: Impedance defined flow. Generalisation of William Harvey's concept of the circulation - 370 years later. Int. J. Cardiov. Med. and Science 1: 205–211, 1998.

Noordergraaf A.: Hemodynamics. Ch. 5 in: Biological Engineering, H.P. Schwan (ed.), McGraw-Hill, New York NY, 1969.

Noordergraaf A., Noordergraaf G..J. and Ottesen J.T.: Implications of the integer ratio between cardiac and respiratory rates. Workshop on Cardiovascular-Respiratory Control Modeling, Graz, 2001.

Noordergraaf G.J., Tilborg van G.F.A.J.B., Schoonen J.A.P., Ottesen J., Scheffer G..J., Noordergraaf A.: Thoracic CT-scans and cardiovascular models: the effect of external force in CPR. Int. J. Cardiovascular Med. and Science. 5: 1–7, 2005.

Noordergraaf G.J., Dijkema T.J., Kortsmit W.J.P.M., Schilders W.H.A., Scheffer G.J. and Noordergraaf A.: Modeling in cardiopulmonary resuscitation: Pumping the heart. Cardiov. Eng. 5: 105–118, 2005.

Noordergraaf G.J., Schilders W.H.A., Scheffer G.J., Noordergraaf A.: Essential factors in CPR? Modeling and clinical aspects (abstract). 2nd Science day, Dutch Society for Anesthesia (Amsterdam), 2005.

Noordergraaf G.J., Ottesen J.T., Scheffer G.J., Schilders W.H.A. and Noordergraaf A.: Cardiopulmonary Resuscitation: Biomedical and Biophysical Analyses. Chapter 18 in: The Biomedical Engineering Handbook, 3rd edition. Biomedical Engineering Fundamentals. J.D. Bronzino (ed.), CRC Press, Boca Raton FL 2006.

Osborn J.J., Hoehne W. and Badia W.: Ventricular Function in the Basic Regulatiuon of the Circulation: Studies with a Mechanical Analog. In: Physical Basis of Circulatory Transport: Regulation and Exchange. E.B. Reeve and A.C. Guyton, (eds) Saunders, Philadelphia PA, 1967.

Ozanam Ch.: La Circulation et le Pouls. Quatrième partie, Chapitre IV, J.B. Ballière et Fils, Paris, 1886.

Porter W.T.: The influence of the heart-beat on the flow of blood through the walls of the heart. Am. J. Physiol. 1: 145–163, 1898.

Rogers A., Morris L.B. and Williams K.R.: Artificial heart ventricular design having space and performance characteristics comparable to the heart. Int. J. Engng Sci. 10: 1037–1047, 1972.

Rommel S.A. and Lowenstine L.J.: Gross and Microscop.c Anatomy. Chapter 9 in: CRC Handbook of Marine Mammal Medicine (L.A. Dierauf and F.M.D. Gulland, eds.) CRC Press, New York, 2001.

Rothe C.F. and Selkurt E.E.: A model of the cardiovascular system for effective teaching. J. Appl. Physiol. 17: 156–158, 1962.

Rudikoff M.T., Maughan W.L., Effron M., Freund P. and Weisfeldt M.L.: Mechanism of blood flow during cardiopulmonary resuscitation. Circulation 61: 345–352, 1980.

Rushmer R.F.: Constancy of stroke volume in ventricular responses to exertion. Am. J. Physiol. 196: 745–750, 1959.

Sarncff S.J. and Berglund E.: Ventricular function. I. Starling's law of the heart studied by means of simultaneous right and left ventricular function curves in the dog. Circulation IX: 706–719, 1954.

Sarnoff S.J., Mitchell J.H., Gilmore J.P. and Remensnyder J.P.: Homeometric autoregulation in the heart. Circ. Res. 8: 1077–1091, 1960.

Shoukas A.A., Brunner M.J., Frankle A.E., Greene A.S. and Kallman C.H.: Carotid sinus baroreceptor reflex control and the role of autoregulation in the systemic and pulmonary arterial pressure-flow relationships of the dog. Circulaticn Res. 54: 674–682, 1984.

Starling E.H.: The Linacre Lecture on the Law of the Heart, Delivered at St. John's College, Cambridge, 1915. Longmans, Green, London, 1918.

Starr I. and Rawson A.J.: Role of "static blood pressure" in abnormal increments of venous pressure. I. Theoretical studies on an improved circulation schema whose pumps obey Starling's law of the heart. Am. J. Med. Sci. 199: 27–39, 1940.

Stein A.F.: Modeling valveless flow using the Donders model. Project report in a course taught by A. Noordergraaf, Univ. of Pennsylvania, 2008.

Vadot L.: Examen des problèmes d'hémodynamique au moyen d'une analogie électrique. Application particulière aux malformations cardiaques. Pathol. Biol. Semaine Hop., 10: 1499–1509, 1962.

Warner H.R.: The use of an analog computer for analysis of control mechanisms in the circulation. Proc. IRE 47:1913–1916, 1959.

Weber E.H.: Ueber die Anwendung der Wellenlehre auf die Lehre from Kreislaufe de s Blutes und ins besondere auf die Pulslehre. Ber. Verh. Kgl. Saechs. Ges. Wiss., Math. Phys. Kl., 1850.

Appendix

Questions

8.1 Hooker reported the results of his 1921 experiments on leg veins in vivo as a drop in blood pressure by 40 cm H_2O in a person switching from standing quietly erect to doing muscular exercise. Most of the flow of the displaced blood must have gone in which direction?

8.2 Give an example of a vascular bed that does not deliver its exiting blood to the central veins.

8.3 Von Kries (1892) stated in his book that root aortic pressure and ventricular ejection flow should have the same time course if there were no reflections. Correct?

8.4 Identify a clinical condition in which the requirement of equal outputs for the left and right hearts does not apply.

8.5 With the aid of a computer model of the CV loop it was found that average flow around the circuit reduced to a negligible amount after all four cardiac valve were removed, while the contractile properties of the chambers were left intact. Was this result to be expected? Argue why or why not. Does the conclusion contradict the results from the Liebau model, described in section 2.4.3.

8.6 Under the conditions described in Question 8.5, where would sloshing be most intensive?

8.7 Identify the basic reason why the coronary pump (compression and release of the embedded veins) fails to operate effectively.

8.8 A contracting cylinder (artery, vein) causes

(a) the largest volume reduction ΔV, and
(b) the smallest resistance increase ΔR,

both for the earliest change in radius Δr. Show this.

8.9 Is it possible for the compression flow and the restoration flow to be primarily in opposite directions, unlike in the example of Fig. 8.8?

8.10 In Fig. 8.8 periodic venous compression by the companion artery proved to reduce average flow. In the model that gave rise to this result, the six inlet vessels all had a radius of 1 mm. The radii of the next generation vessels were 26% larger; one of which was exposed to the arterial pulse. Can the topology of the network be changed so as to make impedance-defined flow higher than unaided flow?

8.11 The peripheral resistance, R, of (part of) a vascular bed is traditionally determined by measuring the pressures on the arterial and venous sides, and dividing the difference by the perfusing flow. Is this procedure still correct when part of the perfusing flow is caused by compression and release of small veins between the sites where pressures are measured?

8.12 In the Navier–Stokes equation (Eq. 5.11) identify the terms that deal exclusively with either inertial or viscous effects.

Answers

8.1 The direction of the central veins, with peripheral valves blocking its return.

8.2 The heart's coronary vasculature.

8.3 Yes, provided the aortic characteristic impedance, Z_0, is a real number (Eq. 3.23a). A complex number causes them to be different even without reflection.

8.4 An atrial or ventricular septal defect.

8.5 It was, in fact, predicted. When the ventricles contract, most of the ejected blood will return to the venous systems, rather than proceed through the peripheral resistances (Eq. 8.7). There is no contradiction with the results of the quoted Liebau experiment, because it lacked peripheral resistances.

8.6 Sloshing will be most intensive on the venous sides of the heart: during contraction of the ventricles most of the ejected blood will go in the direction of the veins, during relaxation it will return to fill the ventricles again.

8.7 Release of the coronary veins can only take effect after ventricular relaxation commences.

8.8 (a) $V = \pi r^2 \Delta z$, hence $\dfrac{\Delta V}{\Delta r} = 2\pi r \Delta z$, making the absolute value of ΔV maximal when r is maximal.
(b) Assuming Poiseuille flow $R = \dfrac{8\eta\Delta z}{\pi r^4}$, hence $\dfrac{\Delta R}{\Delta r} = -\dfrac{32\eta\Delta z}{\pi r^5}$, making ΔR minimal when r is maximal.

8.9 Yes, by selecting an operational frequency, where the absolute value of $Z_{in}(1)$ exceeds that of $Z_{in}(2)$.

8.10 Retrograde flow reduced antegrade flow. If the network had been chosen to be closer to the periphery, the ratio between the two flows would have been reversed.

8.11 No, flow is now determined by three pressures. As a result, part of the flow did not traverse the arterioles and the capillaries.

8.12 The inertial terms are all multiplied by the factor ρ, the viscous ones by η.

Chapter 9
Maintenance of the Circulation and Impedance-Defined Flow

*[...] und mit dem Spiele der In- und Exspiration ändert sich
auch der Blutdruck und die Elutströmung in hohem Maasse.*

— Franciscus C. Donders, 1856

Digest: Main classes of abnormality, electrical or mechanical causing heart failure. The interpretation of abnormality ascribed to mechanical causes requires more than a century for clarification. Forward and backward failure become interchangeable. Clinical treatment of slowly developing failure; space flight. Rapid failure resulting from a heart attack. Listing of types of clinical corrective measures without replacing the heart. Heart transplantation and the artificial heart. Application of impedance-defined flow based measures, including cardio-pulmonary resuscitation.

Blood flow around the circuit is fundamentally different from sloshing; flow around the circuit serves as a transport system, sloshing does not.

9.1   Failure of the Circulation

9.1.1   Basic Causes of Failure

Two cardiac systems were delineated in Chap. 2, which when operating in proper harmony, move blood out of the low pressure, low impedance veins into the corresponding high pressure, high impedance arteries. These systems are (1) electrical stimulus and conduction mechanisms, leading to (2) cardiac muscle contraction and relaxation (Chap. 3).

The condition in which the stimulus does not occur at all is referred to as asystole: no blood is expelled. At the other end of the spectrum, many stimuli may be generated resulting in irregular, uncoordinated activity of the ventricles. This condition is referred to as fibrillation. Cardiac output is reduced, typically to

A. Noordergraaf, *Blood in Motion*, DOI 10.1007/978-1-4614-0005-9_9,
© Springer Science+Business Media, LLC 2011

zero. Between these extreme cases, the stimulus can be present without following the normal sequence. The heart then manifests arrhythmias.

Asystole may be caused by strong activity of the vagus nerve which depresses the sinus node, the A-V node and impairs atrioventricular conduction. Inadequate ventilation as well as a wide range of other effects may precipitate excessive vagal stimulation.

Ventricular fibrillation may be provoked by exposure to electrical current, by myocardial ischemia, by a variety of electrolyte disturbances in the myocardium as well as by other effects.

Blood movement may, alternatively, be impaired as a consequence of anatomical defects, such as valvular malfunction (Sect. 10.2), or alteration in the mechanical properties of the musculature, though the electrical trigger mechanism functions normally.

9.1.2   Concepts in Fluid-Mechanical Failure

The cardiac patient has been a familiar figure in the clinic for a long time as witnessed by de Sénac's two-volume work on heart disease, which was published in 1749. As a cause of death, cardiac malfunction has gained, rather than lost significance since the publication of de Sénac's oeuvre. Failure of the heart to pump blood adequately may develop slowly or take an acute form.

As authors struggled to interpret the phenomena accompanying slowly manifesting insufficient cardiac performance in a convincing and comprehensive fashion, two schools of thought developed. Following Hope's (1842) lead, one school of thought ascribed the often observed venous congestion to inability of the heart to pump the blood it is offered (backward failure). The analogy with the effect of a dam in a stream, put forward at that time, was attractive to many, particularly in view of Cohnheim's (1889) experiment. Cohnheim injected fluid into the pericardium of dogs to handicap the heart and observed a venous pressure rise. Wenckebach (1934), as well as Harrison (1935), belonged to this school; it promoted the idea that venous congestion occurs upstream from the weaker side of the heart as a mechanical consequence of its weakness.

The other school of thought attributed the observed phenomena to failure of the heart to deliver enough blood to the tissues (forward failure). Mackenzie (1908) and Lewis (1933) were leaders among those who held this view. The former referred to the backward failure theory as "grievous mischief".

A major step toward the elimination of the controversy concerning forward or backward failure was taken by McMichael (1938), who introduced a new element by hypothesizing that the Starling curve would apply to the insufficient heart if its maximum possible flow is much smaller than in the normal case. He regarded a rise in venous pressure as a compensatory mechanism, rather than as a mechanical consequence. The finding of several investigators that the circulating volume in chronic congestive failure is generally enlarged was regarded by some as fitting neatly into McMichael's theory. Increased venous pressure would tend to return cardiac output to normal, provided that the heart is not "over the top of Starling's curve," whereby a vicious circle is set up. The role of the circulating blood volume, inaugurated by Weber (1850) and Starr and Rawson (1940) in the form of the notion of static pressure, led to studies of the role played by renal function (Molhuyzen 1953; Prather et al. 1969).

In McMichael's later thinking (1950), forward and backward failure are related phenomena, and it is no longer a question of either/or. In a failing heart, forward failure can frequently be diminished or eliminated by inducing backward failure, and vice versa, an observation that comes naturally with the concept of the transfer function of which McMichael's input–output relations offer specific nonlinear examples.

Since stroke volume and cardiac output are not determined solely by venous return, but also by arterial conditions, the properties of the heart itself were isolated and formulated separately in Sect. 4.3 (Eqs. 4.6b, c) and in more general forms in Sects. 8.1.2 and 9.2. The first term on the right in Eq. 8.1a describes the relaxed chamber and the second term the additional pressure caused, in time, by activation and relaxation. The parameter c carries major responsibility for the failing heart by slipping to lower values.

But the situation is even more complicated. It has been firmly established that the output of the "failing" heart may be normal or even above normal in certain clinical conditions, such as severe anemia, emphysema, and sizable arterio-venous shunts. Such observations had led to the distinction between low output failure and high output failure. The making of such a distinction by necessity raises the question of what constitutes a failing heart, when its output might be normal. McMichael (1950) proposed the following definition: "the heart is failing when its capacity to increase cardiac output is seriously impaired and when output is maintained at the expense of a raised venous filling pressure." Figure 9.1 pictures his visualization of Starling's observations as hypothesized to apply to the various cases.

Subsequent to the occurrence of a severe heart attack, the acute form of cardiac failure, the patient tends to go into a state of shock, which proves to be fatal in most instances (Scheidt et al. 1970). Hence, the symptoms of such acute attacks are entirely different from those seen in cardiac failure that develops slowly. Although there is no doubt that the cause lies in the heart-cardiac output which may be reduced to 50% or even to 25% of its normal resting, value-venous congestion commonly does not occur. Since arterial pressure tends to fall, it is apparent that a substantial volume of blood is sequestered; accordingly, expansion of the circulating volume is often used in treatment. By exclusion, the systemic venous circuit is indicated as the site where the blood is sequestered. Since this venous system normally contains more than 50% of the total blood volume, a relatively small increase in its compliance can easily harbor a significant additional volume without increase in pressure (Weil and Shubin 1970). The systems analysis appears to be much more subtle in describing the complex sequels to myocardial infarction, which cover a rather wide spectrum.

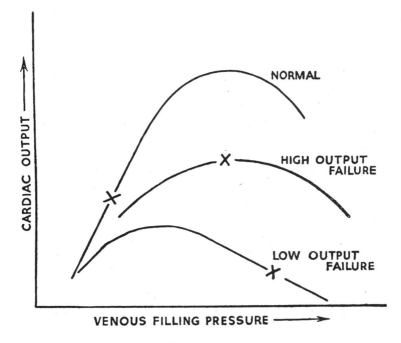

Fig. 9.1 McMichael's 1950 sketches illustrating his new ideas about the operation of the generalized Frank mechanism (Sect. 4.3) for the normal heart, the crosses marking the normal operating point during rest (*at left*), and for high and low output failure

9.2   Measures to Correct Flow

9.2.1   The Use of Drugs

Low output congestive failure is traditionally treated, and often kept under control for years, in the two ways suggested by Fig. 9.1. The first attempts to bring the cardiac function curve closer to the normal one, and in many cases this purpose can be achieved to some degree by the administration of a digitalis preparation, which improves the contractile properties of the myocardium. The second relieves the high venous pressure, by venesection in the old days, and in modern times, by the administration of diuretics, which force the kidneys to excrete more fluid. Where this measure is not taken or fails to have the desired effect, additional fluid retention by the kidneys tends to makes the patient slide down the cardiac function curve as venous pressure continues to increase and cardiac output continues to decrease, forcing the system to become unstable.

Weight loss of astronauts during early exposure to zero gravity is explained as a consequence of corrective action taken by the normal system (Pace 1977). Introduction of microgravity permits a quantity of blood, estimated at 0.5–1 l, to shift from the leg veins to the central veins. It is hypothesized that this shift results in increased filling pressure, which, in turn, tends to raise cardiac output, a situation that is corrected by diuresis.

9.2.2   The Pacemaker and the Defibrillator

In arrhythmias in which the repetition rate of ventricular contraction falls below the normal resting rate, implantation of an artificial pacemaker can have a beneficial effect.

In ventricular fibrillation, application of a defibrillator may revert the ventricle to its normal rhythm. Asystole may be terminated by use of a parasympaticolyticum such as atropine and by the application of cardiac massage.

The normal pattern of electrical stimulation, leading to contraction of the cardiac chambers, summarized in Sect. 4.1, can be disrupted by disease or deficiency and may lead to different abnormal conditions. The principal ones of interest here are asystole (the heart is quiescent), bradycardia (the ventricles beat very slowly, e.g., at a rate of around 30 beats/min, sustained by subsidiary ventricular pacemakers, Sect. 4.1), or tachycardia (the ventricles beat at a very high rate, e.g., at around 250 beats/min or even higher. This is called fibrillation if stimulation becomes chaotic). Under the first and third conditions, cardiac output is reduced to zero. In the second condition, cardiac output tends to be inadequate to meet body requirements.

The initial interest focused on bringing the heart out of its quiescent state. Steiner (1871) achieved this by invasive means in a variety of animals in which the heart was stopped by chloroform administration. He placed one electrode on the heart, the other, e.g., on the abdomen and applied an electrical signal. The noninvasive form of this followed promptly. Green (1872) placed electrodes on the neck and over the lower ribs and successfully applied an electrical signal to humans in which the heart had become quiescent after administration of chloroform, a popular anesthetic at the time.

The reason for the narrow focus was that the electrocardiogram had yet to be discovered. It was recorded in a crude form by Waller (1887), and after his development of the faster string galvanometer, more accurately by Einthoven (1895). The string galvanometer became a popular tool among physiologists and clinicians, owing to its creation of awareness of a wide variety of pathological rhythms, including total atrioventricular blockage of electrical conduction, causing ventricular bradycardia. The idea of correcting some of these abnormalities by the introduction of artificial electrical stimuli ran into a wall of technical difficulties, which were only gradually overcome. The first totally implantable, electronic, clinically successful artificial pacemaker was placed in a human in 1960 (Chardack et al. 1964). Its subsequent development has often been lauded as the greatest success, thus far, in engineering artifices. Progress is being made in making this permanently wearable device more intelligent, i.e., automatically responsive to changing demands for cardiac output (Barold and Mugica 1998; Moser et al. 2005).

9.2.3   Surgical Corrections

The arsenal of surgical techniques to correct cardiac abnormalities and related congenital vascular anomalies has grown to such an extent over the recent several decades that the study and application of these facilities became a specialty. Its presentation is the topic of a variety of textbooks addressing specialized subcategories and will not be summarized here. An exception will be made, however, for a recent revolutionary development that captivated global attention for a short period.

Batista et al. (1996, 1997) introduced ventriculectomy for the treatment of some forms of end-stage cardiomyopathy to fill the large gap left by the shortfall in the number of transplantable hearts (Sect. 9.3.1). The line of thinking is straightforward enough. Just as in the normal ventricle, the enlarged ventricle must achieve a balance of forces at the interface between blood and muscular wall. Since the dilated ventricle has a larger radius than its normal counterpart, it needs to generate a higher level of tangential wall stress, σ_t, which makes ejection more difficult. This, in turn, will promote further dilation, etc., resulting eventually in an end-stage situation. Batista's idea was to eliminate the problem of higher wall stress by dissecting a wedged-shaped segment of the ventricular wall and stitching together the remaining wall, which then had a smaller radius. Invoking a similarity principle (Dawson 1991; Li 1996), the desired radius, r, may be computed from

$$r = \frac{4\pi\rho h}{b} \tag{9.1}$$

in which ρ denotes the density of the wall musculature with thickness h, and b, experimentally determined by Batista, has a value of about 4 g/ml (Rabbany et al. 2000). Contrary to original unverified estimates, unexpectedly high mortality rates were widely experienced, which shattered the original euphoria. Nevertheless, since the need is enormous, further research and development may produce a modification that will work beneficially.

9.3   Supporting Flow by a Replacement Heart or an Assist Device

9.3.1   Cardiac Transplantation

For patients with end-stage heart disease, a possible solution may lie in replacement of the irreparably damaged organ by transplanting a healthy heart.

Beginning with the work of Nobelist Carrel and Guthrie (1905), cardiac transplantation in animals has been studied intensively. Conclusions drawn indicated that clinical cardiac transplantation was essentially a matter of finding the appropriate match between donor and recipient. A chimpanzee heart implanted in a patient in 1964 (xenograft) failed to supply adequate blood flow. The first successful transplantations of a human heart (allograft) were performed by Barnard in 1967. During the next year and a half, 136 clinical transplants were accomplished in 134 patients. They initially stimulated public enthusiasm beyond any medical event of that century, until it became clear that only a modest fraction survived for more than half a year. The clinical experience demonstrated that the surgical techniques were basically sound, but that immunological rejection was a much greater problem in cardiac transplantation than in renal transplantation instead of a lesser one as originally thought. Consequently, the rate of clinical cardiac transplantations went through a minimum in the 1970s after which new research made it possible gradually to surmount the rejection barrier (Cooper 1996a, b).

An accepted technique is to anastomose the left and right atria, the pulmonary arteries, and the aorta in this or a different order. More detailed descriptions illustrated with drawings have been published (Cooper 1996a, b; Dreyfus 1996). The sinus rhythm commonly reestablishes itself after surgery (Barnard 1968; Griepp and Shumway 1981).

From early observations in human transplants, it has been concluded that the denervated nonpaced heart is capable of altering cardiac output. This occurs predominantly through changes in stroke volume, while changes in rate are small or negligible. A 50% increase in cardiac output, brought about by rapid postural change, has been reported (Beck et al. 1969). The alteration in stroke volume corresponds with left ventricular end-diastolic pressure, as would be anticipated from the cardiac function curves. In dogs with denervated hearts, it was found that although their response to exercise comes on more slowly, they are still able to increase cardiac output to fourfold its resting value which is essentially a normal response. Although heart rate increased with the level of exercise, its augmentation appeared less than normal (Donald et al. 1964; Donald 1968).

In a preparation of this type, the pump itself is, at least initially (Dong et al. 1964, 1969; Willman et al. 1964), not subject to central nervous control; pumping frequency is often set by an indwelling pacemaker. Autotransplants, accomplished in dogs and baboons, added a new dimension to the study of the properties and control of the closed loop cardiovascular system. Furthermore, they provide the basis for separating changes in the human cardiac allotransplant due to rejection, from changes related to denervation ischemia, and other disturbances associated with the operative procedure.

9.3.2   The Enigmatic Artificial Heart

Since the heart is, in essence, a pump, it is logical that the idea of building an artificial one should evolve. Charles Lindbergh, the aviator, worked on the construction of one in the early 1930s. An apparatus to bypass both the heart and the lungs proved successful in replacing cardiorespiratory function in animals (Gibbon

1939) and, subsequently, in the treatment of the second human patient in 1953. This patient was supported by a heart-lung machine for 26 min while an atrial septal defect was closed (Gibbon 1954, 1967). By the late 1950s, the use of heart-lung machines to support patients during cardiac surgery started to gain widespread acceptance.

Efforts to improve the pump-oxygenator widened the available time interval from minutes to hours, thereby affording the thoracic surgeon the opportunity to perform intricate corrective procedures. The pump-oxygenator may be regarded as the forerunner of a wide variety of assist devices designed to improve the inadequate circulation (Sect. 9.4.3). In this role, the pump-oxygenator aided in identifying some of the problems that later proved to be disastrous to such devices.

The success of the electrical pacemaker, reinforced by the rewarding utilization of the fluid-mechanical heart-lung bypass machine buttressed the idea that the future of prosthetic devices was basically limitless. The level of enthusiasm may be gauged by the plans that were made and by the liberally funded work actually performed to realize these plans. During the period of peak activity, many researchers believed in the realizability of a four part plan consisting of the design, construction, and successful testing of: (1) emergency assist devices; (2) temporary assist devices; (3) permanent assist devices; and (4) artificial hearts. Routine recourse to the implantable artificial heart was expected to precede successful heart transplantation.

As soon as the new devices were tested in experiments on animals it became evident that there were still fundamental issues requiring solution. Most devices, though not all, proved to have catastrophic effects on the circulatory system, and animal survival time was measured in days rather than in years, as had been hoped. Eventually, under the pressure of such evidence, the difficulty of achieving the earlier goals was reassessed as no less challenging than placing a person on the moon (Harmison 1972).

The resulting analysis made it clear to surgeons and bioengineers, though it had been familiar to hematologists, that blood is too delicate a fluid to acquiesce to much mechanical manipulation. Specifically, it tends to interact with foreign material to which it is exposed, causing damage to the formed elements which may result in clotting and the generation of abnormal plasma proteins. Moving elements may further contribute unduly high shear stresses, including those caused by local turbulence.

Eventually, heart transplantation, after the immunosuppressive drug cyclosporine had been developed, gained the upper hand. Cyclosporine has since been followed by a considerable number of more advanced immunosuppressants (Renlund et al. 1993). Though research support for the artificial heart dwindled, a small number of centers continue basic research to solve the severe problems of artificial devices while new versions, such as the pneumatic total artificial heart, make their appearance. Some are used for human implantation, but as bridge devices, i.e., for temporary function, to gain time for the procurement of a suitable heart for implantation.

The shortage of hearts available for transplantation continues to provide a strong motive to sustain continued development of the artificial heart.

9.4   Impedance-Defined Flow Support (Z-Flow)

9.4.1   General Considerations

In a normal system, during conditions of rest, the external power (energy/s) delivered by the left ventricle during ejection of blood amounts to about 1.3 W; for the right ventricle this number lies around 0.3 W. The power required by the ventricles to sustain this performance is several times larger than the sum of these two, owing to the low efficiency of muscle contraction. Nearly all of this extra power is dissipated as heat. If the pulmonary artery and the aorta are briefly occluded at their roots, the external power of both ventricles drops to zero, though the power consumed by the ventricles does not, since the contractile phenomena persist, the ventricles being forced to perform isovolumetric contractions.

When the heart weakens with age, or as a result of muscle disease, its external power delivery tends to decline. It is straightforward enough to conceive the idea of adding energy to the circulation for the purpose of assisting the heart, and a variety of methods has been devised to achieve this goal. By necessity, the goal is achieved only if the added energy augments the external power delivered by the ventricles. Just enhancing blood movement in some part of the circulation may fail to achieve the purpose, since such added energy may be dissipated as heat. Lack of this insight has turned several well-intended attempts to support the heart into failures.

One way of evaluating the level of success could be to determine the augmentation in the heart's external power P attendant upon the application of the selected method of providing added energy. For a heart period T, average power delivered by the left ventricle may be computed from

$$P = \frac{1}{T} \int_0^T p_{ao}(t) Q_{ej}(t) dt \qquad (9.2)$$

and similarly for the right ventricle.

Hence, an asystolic or fibrillating ventricle that produces no flow at all ($Q_{ej} = 0$) has a P value of zero. If a cardiopulmonary resuscitation (CPR) attempt induces a stroke volume for the ventricle, P rises above zero as a consequence of added energy alone.

9.4.2   Cardiopulmonary Resuscitation

Hebrew text from Genesis 2:7, Fig. 9.2:

Texts from the peak period of the ancient Egyptian culture (prior to circa 1600 BCE, Sects. 2.1–2.3) demonstrate cognizance of air flow into the lungs and transfer of "vital spirit" into the blood of the lobes of the lungs (Bardinet 1995). In the Torah (Pentateuch), a younger Hebrew document probably initially written in

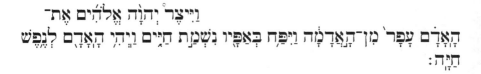

Fig. 9.2 Hebrew text referring to one of the earliest recorded modern versions of CPR (*Source*: R. Kittel, P. Kahle (eds.): *Biblia Hebraica*)

the late fifteenth century BCE, with new editions being formulated over the next several centuries, the concept is broadened to include the beginning of life (Genesis 2: 7). Vivid descriptions of revitalization appear in the subsequent historical books (1 Kings 17: 17–23; 2 Kings 4: 34–35).

In the life science world, Vesalius (1555 CE) discovered a close relation between respiration and cardiac pumping when he applied artificial respiration to animals and observed that the heart converted from its quiescent state to pumping.

Especially during the eighteenth and subsequent centuries, a wide variety of techniques was developed in efforts to improve the outcome of revitalization efforts. Early on, the primary interest was in artificial ventilation, although some of these techniques may have caused vigorous chest compression (such as in a prone victim supported crosswise over the back of a trotting horse) thereby likely administering closed chest resuscitation of the circulation as well (Weil and Tang 1999). The combination of artificial respiration and any form of cardiac massage is referred to as CPR.

It may be noted that the transition from compressing the thorax at the respiratory frequency to that at the frequency of the normal heart beat was the result of desperation, following a successful effort by Maass in 1892, to save the life of a 9-year-old boy subsequent to chloroform administration in preparation for the repair of a palatine fissure. This was a major change from twenty years earlier when it was still argued that the safety of the patient was best promoted by disregarding cardiac symptoms, such as the heart becoming quiescent, as reported by Green (1872; Sect. 9.2.2).

Closed chest resuscitation, in which the chest is compressed periodically, and open chest resuscitation, in which the chest is opened surgically and the heart itself is massaged, were introduced starting in the second half of the nineteenth century (e.g., Balassa 1858 [see Husveti and Ellis 1969], Boehm 1878, and Igelsrud 1901 [see Keen 1904], respectively). The underlying philosophy is that open chest resuscitation imitates the natural contraction and ejection of blood by the two ventricles into the pulmonary artery and the aorta, by means of hand-supplied rhythmic massage, while closed chest massage is (vaguely) viewed as imitating open chest massage by compressing the heart between the sternum and the vertebral column. Closed chest resuscitation was popularized energetically by Kouwenhoven et al. (1960) and Jude et al. (1964). These investigators initially recommended a compression depth of 3–4 cm, rather promptly raised to 1.5–2″ (3.8–5.1 cm). This approach defines the so-called cardiac pump theory, which is solidly embedded in Harveyan teaching.

The cardiac pump theory was called into question, in the 1960s, by the emergence of the thoracic pump theory (Weale 1961; Criley et al. 1976, already implied by Walters (1943)). It was noted (Rudikoff et al. 1980) that chest compression, more so than normal exhalation, increased intrathoracic pressure by up to 40 cm of H_2O with open airways, to 110, when closed (Chancra et al. 1981). Release of compression permitted intrathoracic pressure to decrease. There are two relevant aspects to consider here. First, it has been argued that increased intrathoracic pressure should dinitially promote filling of the right ventricle and therefore increase its outflow, since the right ventricle is subjected to the same increase in intrathoracic pressure. Second, however, it presupposes adequate availability of blood in the central veins. These numbers give a line to making an estimate of the attenuation factor between the pressure applied to compress the ribbed chest and the resulting increase in intrathoracic pressure. Data available clinically and in the literature, while displaying a wide scatter, support an initial estimate suggesting an order of magnitude transmission of around 10% (Noordergraaf G.J. et al. 2005).

Hence, two competing theories are envisioned as to why application of CPR should benefit the victim of cardiac and respiratory standstill. Both rely heavily on impedance-defined flow and related valve closure (mitral for the cardiac theory; tricuspid for the thoracic theory). The competition concerns two different mechanisms, though chest compression, the driving function, and the assumption of an adequate blood supply are shared. The survival rate, nonetheless, is found to lie in the rather abysmal range of 5–20% (for open chest resuscitation it was frequently reported to be well above 50%, Noordergraaf G.J 2009).

Device-oriented solutions to performing cardiac massage have been proposed as well. The Anstadt Cup (1966) was designed to offer an equivalent of open chest cardiac resuscitation. The cup consists of a rigid shell which is vacuum attached to both ventricles. The space between the shell and the pericardium contains a flexible balloon, the air pressure in which, provided by an external pump, could be made positive, causing biventricular compression and ejection, or negative, assisting the refilling of both ventricles. This compression-suction cup had no direct contact with the blood it pumped and could be operated for a longer time interval than massage by hand.

Later developments added pacemaker technology allowing compression to occur simultaneously with cardiac systole in hearts beating weakly, which elevated it to a cardiac assist device (Anstadt et al. 2002; Sect. 9.4.3).

Scrutiny of the cardiac versus the thoracic theory exposed, for the cardiac theory, conflicting findings about which valves open and close, and their reproducibility, during the CPR procedure (Rich et al. 1981; Werner et al. 1981; Kühn and Juchems 1991; Porter et al. 1992; Ma et al. 1995). Further experimental work on humans disclosed that the left ventricle may be barely compressed by reducing the distance between the sternum and the spinal column owing to its predominant location outside the line of compression. In addition, it was observed that the recommended magnitude of chest compression (4–5 cm) is often too small even if both ventricles were in the line of compression (Noordergraaf G.J et al. 2005).

With regard to the thoracic theory, there is doubt about the actual availability of venous blood, especially after the first several compressions, leading to the idea that venous return must be enhanced. In Sect. 6.3, it was found that the respiratory system increases venous return during exercise in the normal by lowering intrathoracic pressure. Taking this as a cue, it was attempted to obtain the same effect during a CPR procedure by forcing air pressure in the lungs to go strongly negative. This has not been successful since the lungs, like the atria and the veins (Sect. 6.2), are apparently unable to sustain such a load and tend to collapse instead (recognized by pulmonary clicking sounds). In the still conscious patient, sustained coughing interspersed with deep inspirations appears to be more effective (Criley et al. 1976). To imitate exercise more closely in the unconscious patient, the pressure external to the chest was made negative (negative pressure ventilation, Corrado et al. 1996). Shekerdemian et al. (1999) reported significant increases in pulmonary blood flow in response to negative pressure ventilation after tetralogy of Fallot repair in children.

Observations reported in Sect. 8.3, showed that cardiac output, in terms of flow around the circuit, becomes negligible if all cardiac valves remain open. Instead, sloshing of blood becomes the predominant feature. This tends to rule out Liebau's contention (1956) that the cardiac valves are superfluous, since this violates the requirement of impedance transformation in a circuit that embodies large peripheral resistances in series (Sect. 8.2).

Evidence has been produced to suggest that the valves may remain open during chest compression and relaxation (Rudikoff et al. 1980). This phenomenon received only cursory attention before impedance-defined flow entered upon the scene. It appears to hold one key to the reported low survival rate in CPR. A related one is the dominant attention focused on pressure, rather than on pressure and flow. This is akin to what was done in an earlier phase when attention was concentrated on the physiology of wave propagation in arteries: much attention was given to pressure phenomena. When flow became measurable and was included, a large part of the preceding discussions and of the design of models had to be revisited.

In model studies where the left ventricle was represented as a passive organ (Eq. 3.7a) offering an open circuit (both valves open), it was found that ventricular volume tended to become negative during application of CPR (Eq. 3.7d or Eq. 11.11, both with $F = 0$) (Noordergraaf G.J et al. 2005). This mathematical solution had to be ruled out in view of its physical impossibility (more details in the answers to Questions 9.11 and 9.14).

Other non-blood contacting support devices have been developed or are currently being designed. They may be classified under the headings of utilization of (trained) skeletal muscle or of artificial muscle, both wrapped around the ventricles.

9.4.3   The Ventricular Assist Device and the Intra-aortic Balloon Pump

Assist devices that operate directly on blood include (left) ventricular assist devices and the intra-aortic balloon pump.

As a consequence of the findings summarized in Sect 9.3.2, goals were redefined in two ways. First, the concept was introduced for the assist device to serve as a short-term bridge until a suitable heart for transplantation can be found (Scherr et al. 1999). Second, the scope was broadened to include assist devices suitable for small children and infants. Ongoing development and application has produced assist devices for steady as well as pulsatile flow, for either univentricular or biventricular support. Centrifugal and diaphragm pumping techniques are being applied. In some cases, the heart recovered while it was supported, postponing or eliminating the need for a replacement heart (Shum-Tim 2001).

Moulopoulos et al. (1962) introduced the balloon pump, which modifies aortic pressure in a pulsatile fashion. An elongated balloon (in some devices, more than one), mounted over one end of a catheter, is introduced into the aorta. During ventricular systole, the balloon is deflated around the catheter; it is inflated during the diastolic period, hence the term counterpulsation Initially, the R wave of the electrocardiogram was utilized for triggering purposes. This procedure was later refined by also using ultrasound (Minich et al. 1998).

Diastolic inflation of the balloon enhances aortic outflow into the peripheral vasculature; it operates as an additional pump. Hence, the ventricle must increase its output to at least maintain mean aortic perfusion pressure. If the ventricle is unable to achieve this, perfusion of the periphery may suffer, which may be viewed as a negative hemodynamic effect. The contribution by the balloon pump may be viewed as positive, if the ventricular output increases more than is required to compensate for the peripheral outflow generated by the balloon's inflation. Alteration of the peripheral resistance is likely to complicate this picture. Both positive and negative hemodynamic effects have been observed.

An example of a positive effect was reported by Weber and Janicki (1974). Under conditions of shock, attendant upon acute myocardial infarction, the balloon pump was reported to increase the cardiac index from 1.7 to 2.5 l/min m^2 on average. Subsequent studies in canines and using models, however, elicited insignificant increases in stroke volumes (Barnea et al. 1990; Platt et al. 1993; Lin 2005). The balloon pump has been the subject of a number of studies of its performance characteristics in a system of distensible vessels in which the attention was often focused on the timing of inflation and/or deflation (Fich and Welkowitz 1973; Sun 1991). Jaron and Moore (1983) observed that poor timing may have negative hemodynamic effects. Improved understanding of the balloon pump may still result from a rigorous impedance-defined flow analysis An initial model-based study along this line suggests that there is room for improvement of balloon pump performance (McLoughlin 2009).

Although the balloon pump has been effectively applied in many hundreds of patients, probably owing to balloon generated augmented coronary perfusion, the initial benefits have been easier to document than have been long-term gains. In part, less impressive long-term results may stem from the poor physical condition the patients are in, given this type of therapy, as well as from an unaltered underlying disease process (Scheidt et al. 1973).

9.4.4 The Rocking Chair

Hooker, in 1911, measured that venous pressure in a human standing erect and still, dropped by 40 cm H_2O in a leg vein upon muscular exercise performed by that leg. This observation is easily explained on the basis of impedance-defined flow of the second kind: muscular contraction and associated compression of intramuscular veins in a valved extremity (Sect. 8.3). Likewise, it might be speculated that sitting in a rocking chair and keeping it moving for hours on end by contraction and relaxation of the leg musculature, such as the quadriceps femoris, should promote propagation of blood out of the leg veins and into the central veins. There is a slowly developing body of evidence and understanding of this phenomenon, which is apparently responsible for the recent introduction of the rocking chair in some maternity hospitals (Hwang 2007).

9.4.5 The Foot Pump and Related Devices

The foot pump and its physiological features were described in the preceding chapter. This pump has found extensive clinical application for patients who cannot walk for surgical or clinical reasons. Since the physiological process cannot be called upon, a pneumatic cuff is applied to the foot, which can be inflated rapidly and imitates the action of weight bearing by flattening its arch, thus generating a flow pulse (Fig. 9.3). After a short interval, the cuff is vented to permit replacement of the blood displaced centrally, by new blood from the arteries. A computer model confirmed the production of a centrally directed flow pulse upon cuff inflation in the noncuffed popliteal vein (Hom 2006). The same approach is applicable to the hand. Clinical treatment was reported to be successful in terms of preventing the formation of deep venous thromboses, which may be interpreted as evidence in favor of physical exercise (Gardner and Fox 1993). Extremely rapid compression tends to be counterproductive, owing to the tendency of throat formation in nonsteady flow (Sect. 6.2, throat formation in steady flow).

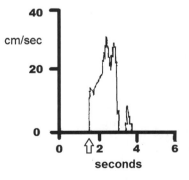

Fig. 9.3 Ultrasound recording of flow velocity in a popliteal vein of a human caused by a single compression of a foot pump on the same leg (Modified from Beckett and Wall 1988)

Other assist devices have been proposed that are based on the manipulation of blood pressure by external means. The form developed by Birtwell et al. (1969) is, in many ways, a noninvasive counterpart of the balloon pump. The instrument consists of a metal cylindrical housing constructed of two equal halves hinged on one side, while the tangential separation on the other side is varied by means of a hydraulic drive. The space between this housing and the body part enclosed by the cylinder is taken up by a fluid-filled, form-fitted bag. When the drive is triggered, in experiments on the hind limbs of dogs, average flow through the abdominal aorta was found to increase by approximately 40%. Cylinders of this type may be used to apply pressure to the thorax, to the limbs, or to both. Birtwell et al. (1969) used both simultaneously and chose a phase relationship between the external actuators and ventricular activity such that the unit surrounding the thorax produced a high pressure during ventricular systole, while the unit around the extremities produced a high pressure during ventricular diastole.

A variation of this approach sequences external pulsation. In this technique, the experimental animal is placed in a suit of which portions covering the extremities are subdivided into several segments, to allow independent pressurization. As proposed by Cohen et al. (1969), the limb segments are pressurized sequentially, commencing with the most distal segments at the onset of diastole and releasing all pressures at the beginning of the next ventricular systole. In a small number of experiments on baboons, an average rise in cardiac output of 25% was reported. The equipment misses the finesse of the intra-aortic balloon pump. Although the focus was on arterial response to external compression, venous effects must have played a large role in the augmentation of cardiac output.

9.4.6   Shaking the Entire System, BASH and EASE

It occurred to Arntzenius et al. (1970) that the inverse of ballistocardiography (Starr and Noordergraaf A 1967) might be effective as a circulatory assist device. In ballistocardiography, the patient is supported in the supine position and the motion of the support is recorded; in the inverse, the support is forced to move by an external power source. The nature of the movement initially was chosen such that the table is accelerated abruptly (at around 1 g) and returned gradually to its original position. Initial success, in terms of significant augmentation of cardiac output, was reported in a hydraulic model, in pigs, and in patients in cardiogenic shock (Arntzenius et al. 1972), when a footward acceleration was applied early in systole. This type of equipment was recommended for installation in ambulances (Ware et al. 1971).

However, a more systematic study of body acceleration in synchrony with the heart beat (BASH) did not support the initial expectations; neither the timing of the initial rapid acceleration, nor the direction in which it was applied produced consistent results. Although there is no doubt about the validity of the concept regarding inertial effects on blood flow (Sect. 4.2; Sud et al. 1985; Fig. 9.4), at least

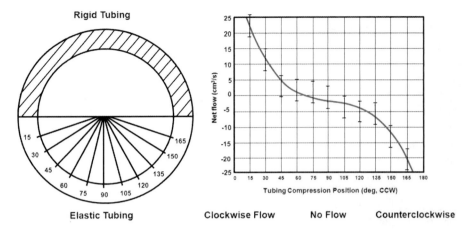

Fig. 9.4 Representation of Liebau's circular tubing, referred to in Sect. 1.1, with flow direction and the net forward flow generated in relationship to the point of compression on the elastic tubing part of the experimental apparatus (Modified from Bovard et al. 2004)

part of the explanation of the inconsistency in results of whole body experiments may reside in the poor transmission to the body of forces imparted to the support, as a result of which the patient accelerates slowly, then goes into vibrations in its own resonance frequency (Verdouw et al. 1973).

If forcing is carried out in a sinusoidal fashion, with a frequency close to the body's resonance frequency, the effect on aortic pressure and flow becomes large and variable, apparently depending on the phase relationship between the heart cycle and the forcing function (around 4 Hz in the dog, Edwards et al. 1972). When the forcing frequency equals the heart frequency (EASE), the sensitivity to the phase relationship emerges distinctly (Bhattacharya et al. 1976).

More recently, Adams et al. (2000, 2001) reintroduced whole body motion, initially to support ventilation, subsequently expanded to include CPR, applying sinusoidal forcing with adjustable frequency and amplitude. These investigators achieved about 20% of the resting control cardiac output in arrested hearts of pigs, with maintenance of normal gas parameter values in arterial blood.

9.4.7 Massage

During the late 1800s and well into the 1900s, it was widely believed that massage of a passive arm or leg increases venous return to the heart and consequently arterial inflow. Recent attempts to verify this opinion showed, however, that neither effleurage, petrissage, nor tapotement, as different modes of massage, could produce a measurable increase in either flow velocity or flow, based on observations utilizing ultrasound technology, although light exercise produced a threefold increase in the extremity of interest (e.g., Shoemaker et al. 1997).

9.5 Conclusions

Increasing understanding of the circulatory system enticed bioscientists toward the thinking that support, replacement, or modulation of sections of the cardiovascular system should be possible and even relatively simple. This implied their assumption of a low complexity in the whole system, ignoring or subverting aspects such as biofeedback. Their work illuminated features in the system previously unrecognized, such as beat to beat volume differences, rapid torus changes, and the difficult characteristics of blood itself.

Interactive support and communication between parts of the circulatory system as a whole or even local feedback, is rapid, complex, and permeated with checks and balances that external modulation can only approach it, while relying on the rest of the circulatory system to allow for the introduced inadequacies.

9.6 Summary

This chapter looks at clinical measures to sustain blood flow in the closed circulatory system. After a succinct review of what have become accepted procedures, attention is turned to impedance-defined flow support, especially cardiopulmonary resuscitation (CPR).

Two competing theories, denoted cardiac and thoracic, developed over the last half century. They arose from a common ancestor called open chest cardiac resuscitation (OCCR) in which the chest is opened surgically and the heart itself is massaged in an effort to duplicate the natural process. Kouwenhoven and associates popularized closed chest resuscitation (CCCR) as a noninvasive duplicate of the invasive procedure. The two original theories compete only fractionally, since they share the assumption of an adequate blood supply in the chest and chest compression as their methodology to move that blood. Patient survival rate dropped precipitously in the transition to the noninvasive procedure.

References

Adams J.A., Mangino M.J., Bassuk J., Inman D.M. and. Sackner M.A. (2000) Noninvasive motion ventilation (NIMV): a novel approach to ventilatory support. J. Appl. Physiol. 89: 2438–2446

Adams J.A., Mangino M.J., Bassuk J., Kurlansky P. and Sackner M.A.: Novel CPR with periodic Gz acceleration. Resuscitation 51: 55–62, 2001.

Anstadt G.L., Schiff P. and Baue A.E.: Prolonged circulatory support by direct mechanical ventricular assistance. Trans. Amer. Soc. Artif. Intern. Organs 12: 72–76, 1966.

Anstadt M.P., Schutte-Eistrup S.A., Motomura T., Soltero E.R., Takano T., Mikati I.A., Nonaka K., Joglar F. and Nosé Y.: Non-blood contacting biventricular support for severe heart failure. Ann. Thorac. Surgery 73: 556–562, 2002.

Arntzenius A.C., Koops J., Rodrigo F.A., Elsbach H. and Brummelen van A.G.W.: Circulatory Effects of Body Acceleration Given Synchronously with the Heart Beat (BASH). Bibl. Cardiol. 26: 180–187, 1970.

Arntzenius A.C., Laird J.D., Noordergraaf A., Verdouw P.D. and Huisman P.H.: Body Acceleration Synchronous with the Heartbeat (BASH); a Progress Report. Bibl. Cardiol. 29: 1–5, 1972.

Bardinet T.: Les Papyrus Médicaux de l'Égypte Pharaonique. Fayard, Paris, 1995.

Barnard C.N.: What have we learned about heart transplants? J. Thorac. Cardiov. Surg. 56: 457–468, 1968.

Barnea O., Moore T.W., Dubin S.E., Jaron D.: Cardiac energy considerations during intraaortic balloon pumping. IEEE Trans. Biomed. Eng. 37: 170–181, 1990.

Barold S.S. and Mugica J. (eds.): Recent Advances in Cardiac Pacing; Goals for the 21st Century. Futura Publ. Co., Armonk NY, 1998.

Batista R.J.V., Santos J.L.V., Takeshita N., Bocchino L., Lima P.N., Cunha M.A.: Partial left ventriculectomy to improve left ventricular function in end-stage heart disease. J. Card. Surg. 11:96–97, 1996.

Batista R.J.V., Verde J., Nery P., Bocchino L., Takeshita N., Bhayana J.N., Bergsland J., Graham S., Houck J.P. and Salerno T.A.: Partial left ventriculectomy to treat end-state heart disease. Ann. Thorac. Surg. 64: 634–638, 1997.

Beck W., Barnard C.N. and Schrire V.: Heart rate after cardiac transplantation. Circulation 40: 437–445, 1969.

Beckett C. and Wall M.: The venous pump of the foot. Nursing Times 84: 45–47, 1988.

Birtwell W., Giron F. and Soroff H.: Combined Peripheral and Thoracic Modalities of Synchronous External Pressure Assist. Chapter 42 in: Proc. Artif. Heart Program Conf., HEW, 1969.

Boehm R.: Arbeiten aus dem pharmakologischen Institut der Universität Dorpat. XIII. Über Wiederbelebung nach Vergiftungen und Asphyxie. Arch. Exp. Pathol. Pharmacol. 8: 68–101, 1878.

Bovard M.S., Connell W.R., Moore S.E., Palladino J.L.: Quantifying impedance defined flow. Proc. 30th IEEE Northeast Bioeng. Conf., Springfield MA, pp. 192–193, 2004.

Carrel A., Guthrie C.C.: The transplantation of veins and organs. Am Med. 10: 1101–1102, 1905.

Chandra N.C., Weisfeldt M.L., Tsitlik J., Vaghaiwalla F., Snyder L.D., Hoffecker M., Rudikoff M.T.: Augmentation of carotid flow during CPR in dogs by ventilation at high airway pressure simultaneous with chest compression. Am. J. Cardiol. : 48: 1053–1063, 1981

Chardack W.M., Gage A.A., Frederico A.J., Schimert G. and Greatbatch W.: Clinical experience with an implantable pacemaker. Ann. NY Acad. Sci. 111: 1075–1092, 1964.

Cohen L., Portersfield D., Mitchell J., Mullins C.: Sequenced External Pulsation in the Therapy of Cardiogenic Shock. Chapter 43 in: Proc. Artif. Heart Program Conf., HEW, 1969.

Cohnheim J.: Lectures on General Pathology. New Sydenham Soc., London, 1889.

Cooper D.K.C.: Experimental Development and Early Clinical Experience. Chapter 18 in: The Transplantation and Replacement of Thoracic Organs. D.K.C. Cooper et al., (eds.). 2nd. ed., Kluwer Acad. Publ., Boston MA, 1996a.

Cooper D.C.K.: Surgical Technique of Orthotopic Heart Transplantation. I: Standard Approach. Chapter 24 in: The Transplantation and Replacement of Thoracic Organs. D.K.C. Cooper et al., (eds.). 2nd. ed., Kluwer Acad. Publ., Boston MA, 1996b.

Corrado A., Gorini M., Villella G., Paola De E.: Negative pressure ventilation in the treatment of acute respiratory failure: an old noninvasive technique reconsidered. Eur. Respir. J. 9: 1531–1544, 1996.

Criley J.M., Blaufuss A.H. and Kissel G.L.: Cough-induced cardiac compression: self administrated form of cardiopulmonary resuscitation. JAMA 236: 1246–1250, 1976.

Dawson T.H.: Engineering Design of the Cardiovascular System of Mammals. Prentice Hall, Englewood Cliffs NJ, 1991.

Donald D.E.: Capacity for exercise after denervation of the heart. Circulation 38: 225–226, 1968.

Donald D.E., Milburn S.E. and Shepherd J.T.: Effect of cardiac denervation on the maximal capacity for exercise in the racing greyhound. J. Appl. Physiol. 19:849–852, 1964.

Dong E. Jr., Fowkes W.C., Hurley E.J., Hancock E.W. and Pillsbury R.C.: Hemodynamic effect of cardiac autotransplantation. Circulation 29, Suppl. 1:77, 1964

Dong E. Jr., Gkaze H., Stinson E. and Weaver C.: Cardiac control: Heart rate open loop response. Proc. Artif. Heart Program Conf. HEW p.327, 1969.

Dreyfus G.: Surgical Technique of Orthotopic Heart Transplantation. 2. Bicaval 'Total' Approach. Chapter 25 in: The Transplantation and Replacement of Thoracic Organs. D.K.C. Cooper et al., (eds.). 2nd. ed., Kluwer Acad. Publ., Boston MA, 1996.

Edwards R.G., McCutcheon E.P. and Knapp C.F.: Cardiovascular changes produced by brief whole-body vibrations in animals. J. Appl. Physiol. 32: 386–390, 1972.

Einthoven W.: Über die Form des menschlichen Electrocardiogramms. Pflügers Arch. 60: 101–123, 1895.

Fich S. and Welkowitz W.: Perspectives in cardiovascular analysis and assistance. In: Perspectives in Biomedical Engineering, R.M. Kenedi (ed.) Univ. Park Press, Baltimore MD, 1973.

Gardner A.M.N. and Fox R.H.: The Return of Blood to the Heart. J. Libbey and Co.. London, 2nd ed., 1993.

Gibbon J.H. Jr.: The maintenance of life during experimental occlusion of the pulmonary artery followed by survival. Surg. Gynec. Obstet. 69: 602–614, 1939

Gibbon J.H. Jr.: The application of a mechanical heart and lung apparatus to cardiac surgery. Minn. Med. 37: 171–180, with references on p. 185, 1954

Gibbon J.H. Jr.: The early development of an extracorporeal circulation with an artificial heart and lung. Trans. Am. Soc. Artif. Organs 13: 77–79, 1967

Green T.: On death from chloroform: Its prevention by galvanism. Br. Med. J. 1: 551–553, 1872.

Griepp R.B. and Shumway N.E.: Cardiac Homotransplants. Ch. 9 in: Davis-Christopher Textbook of Surgery, 12th ed., D.C. Sabiston Jr., (ed.), Saunders, Philadelphia PA, 1981.

Harmison L.T.: Totally implantable nuclear heart assist and artificial heart. Report, National Heart Lung Inst., Bethesda MD, 1972.

Harrison T.: Failure of the Circulation. Williams & Wilkins, Baltimore MD, 1935.

Hom D.: Computer model of a footpump. Project report in a course taught by A. Noordergraaf, Univ. of Pennsylvania, 2006.

Hope J.: A Treatise on Diseases of the Heart. Lea & Blanchard, Philadelphia, PA, 1842.

Husveti S. and Ellis H.: Janos Balassa: Pioneer of cardiac resuscitation. Anaesthesia 24: 113–115, 1969.

Hwang D.: Rocking chair and venous return. Project report in a course taught by A. Noordergraaf, Univ. of Pennsylvania, 2007.

Jaron D. and Moore T.H.W.: Theoretical considerations regarding the optimization of cardiac assistance by intraaortic balloon pumping. IEEE Trans. on Biomed. Eng. BME-30: 177–186, 1983.

Jude J.R., Kouwenhoven W.B. and Knickerbocker G.G.: External Cardiac Resuscitation. Monographs in the Surgical Sciences vol. 1, 59–117, 1964.

Keen W.W.: Case of total laryngotomy (unsuccessful) and a case of abdominal hysterectomy (successful), in both of which massage of the heart for chloroform collapse was employed, with notes on 25 other cases of cardiac massage. Ther. Gaz. 28: 217–230, 1904. Includes a report on Igelsrud's earlier successful open heart massage (1901).

Kouwenhoven W.B., Jude J.R. and Knickerbocker G.G.: Closed chest cardiac massage. JAMA 173: 1064–1067, 1960.

Kühn C. und Juchems R.: Öffnungs- und Schließbewegungen der Herzklappen bei kardiopulmonaler Reanimation. Beweis für die Richtigkeit der „cardiac pump theory". Dtsch. med. Wschr. 116: 734–738, 1991.

Lewis T.: Diseases of the Heart. Macmillan, London, 1933.

Li J.K-J.: Comparative Cardiovascular Dynamics of Mammals. CRC Press, New York, 1996.

Liebau G.: Möglichkeit der Förderung des Blutes im Herz- und Gefäszsystem ohne Herz- und Venenklappenfunktion. Verh. deutschen ges. Kreislauff, 22. Tagung. Seite 354–359, 1956.

Lin F.: Intra-aortic balloon pump. Stroke volume optimization. Project report in a course taught by A. Noordergraaf, Univ. of Pennsylvania, 2005.

Ma M.H-M., Hwang J-J., Lai L-P. et al.: Transesophageal echocardiographic assessment of mitral valve position and pulmonary venous flow during cardiopulmonary resuscitation in humans. Circulation 92: 854–861, 1995.

Mackenzie J.: Diseases of the Heart, Oxford Univ. Press, London, 1908.

Marinelli R., Färst B., Zee van der H., McGinn A. and Marinelli W.: The heart is not a pump: A refutation of the pressure propulsion premise of heart function. Frontier Persp. 5:15–24, 1995.

Maass F.: Die Methode der Wiederbelebung bei Herztod nach Chloroformeinathmung. Berliner klin. Wochenschrift 29: 265–268, 1892.

McMichael J.: The output of the heart in congestive failure. Q. J. Med. 7: 331–353, 1938

McMichael J.: Pharmacology of the Failing Human Heart. Thomas, Springfield IL, 1950.

Minich L.L., Tani L.Y., Pantalos G.M., Bolland B.L., Knorr B.K., Hawkins J.A.: Neonatal piglet model of intraaortic balloon pumping: improved efficacy using echocardiographic timing. Ann. Thorac. Surg. 66: 1527–1532, 1998.

Molhuyzen J.A.: De Centrale Veneuze Druk. Scheltema & Holkema, Amsterdam, 1953.

Moulopoulos S.D., Topaz S., Kolff W.J.: Diastolic balloon pumping (with carbon dioxide) in the aorta: A mechanical assistance to the failing circulation. Am. Heart J. 63: 669–675, 1962.

Noordergraaf G.J.: Cardiopulmonary Resuscitation: Are Two Hands (Really) Enough? A modeling approach to CPR. Ph.D. Dissertation. Radboud Univ. Nijmegen, Nijmegen NL, 2009.

Noordergraaf G.J., Dijkema T.J., Kortsmit W.J.P.M., Schilders W.H.A., Scheffer G.J. and Noordergraaf A.: Modeling in cardiopulmonary resuscitation: Pumping the heart. Cardiov. Eng. 5: 105–118, 2005.

Noordergraaf G.J., Schilders W.H.A., Scheffer G.J., Noordergraaf A.: Essential factors in CPR? Modeling and clinical aspects (abstract). 2nd Science day, Dutch Society for Anesthesia (Amsterdam), 2005.

Noordergraaf G.J., Tilborg van G.F.A.J.B., Schoonen J.A.P., Ottesen J., Scheffer G..J., Noordergraaf A.: Thoracic CT-scans and cardiovascular models: the effect of external force in CPR. Int. J. Cardiovascular Med. and Science. 5: 1–7, 2005.

Pace N.: Weightlessness: a matter of gravity. N. Engl. J. Med. 297: 32–37, 1977.

Platt K.l., Moore T.W., Barnea O., Dubin S.E., Jaron D.: Performance optimization of left ventricular assistance. A computer model study. ASAIO J. 39: 29–38, 1993.

Porter T.R., Ornato J.P., Guard C.S., Roy V.G., Burns C.A. and Nixon J.V.: Transesophageal echocardiography to assess mitral valve function and flow during cardiopulmonary resuscitation. Am. J. Cardiol. 70: 1056–1060, 1992.

Prather J.W., Taylor A.E. and Guyton A.C.: Effect of blood volume, mean circulatory pressure, and stress relaxation on cardiac output. Am. J. Physiol. 216: 467–412, 1969.

Rabbany S.Y., Kresh J.Y., Noordergraaf A.: Myocardial wall stress: evaluation and management. Cardiovasc. Engineering 5: 3–10, 2000.

Renlund D.G., Ensley R.D., Olsen S.L., Bristow M.R.: Future Improvements in Immunosuppression Following Cardiac Transplantation. Chapter 12 in: Heart and Lung Transplantation 2000. (M.P. Kaye and J.B. O'Connell eds.) Landes Co., Austin TX, 1993

Rich S., Wix H.L. and Shapiro S.P.: Clinical assessment of heart chamber size and valve motion during cardiopulmonary resuscitation by two-dimensional echocardiography. Am. Heart J. 102: 368–373, 1981.

Rudikoff M.T., Maughan W.L., Effron M., Freund P. and Weisfeldt M.L.: Mechanism of blood flow during cardiopulmonary resuscitation. Circulation 61: 345–352, 1980.

Scheidt S., Ascheim A. and Killip T. III: Shock after acute myocardial infarction. Am. J. Cardiol. 26: 556564, 1970.

Scherr K., Jensen L. and Koshal A.: Mechanical circulatory support as a bridge to cardiac transplantation: Toward the 21st century. Am. J. Critical Care 8: 324–337, 1999

Sénac de J.-B.: Traité de la Structure du Coeur, de son Action, et de ses Maladies. J. Vincent, Paris, 1749.

Shekerdemian L.S., Bush A., Shore D.F., Lincoln C., Redington A N.: Cardiorespiratory responses to negative pressure ventilation after tetralogy of Fallot repair: a hemodynamic tool for patients with a low-output state. J. Am. Coll. Cardiol. 33: 549–555, 1999.

Shum-Tim D.: Experimental Development of the Medos-HIV Ventricular Assist Device in Children. Chapter 18 in: Mechanical Support for Cardiac and Respiratory Failure in Pediatric Patients. B.W. Duncan, (ed.), Marcel Dekker, New York NY 2001.

Shoemaker J.K., Tiidus P.M. and Mader R.: Failure of manual massage to alter limb blood flow: measures by Doppler ultrasound. Medicine and Science in Sports and Exercise. 29: 610–614, 1997.

Starr I. and Noordergraaf A.: Ballistocardiography in Cardiovascular Research. Lippincott Co., Philadelphia PA, 1967.

Starr I. and Rawson A.J.: Role of "static blood pressure" in abnormal increments of venous pressure. I. Theoretical studies on an improved circulation schema whose pumps obey Starling's law of the heart. Am. J. Med. Sci. 199: 27–39, 1940.

Steiner F.: Über die Electropunctur des Herzens als Wiederbelebungsmittel in der Chloroformsyncope, zugleich eine Studie über Stichwunden des Herzens. Archiv f. klin. Chir. 12: 741–790, 1871.

Sun Y.: Modeling the dynamic interaction between the left ventricle and intra-aortic balloon pump. Am. J. Physiol. 261 (Heart Circ. Physiol 30): H1300–H1311, 1991.

Timerman S., Cardoso L.F., Ramires J.A.F., Halperin H.: Improved hemodynamic performance with a novel chest compression device during treatment of in-hospital cardiac arrest. Resuscitation 61: 273–280, 2004.

Verdouw P.D., Noordergraaf A., Arntzenius A., Huisman P.H.: Relative Movement Between Subject and Support in Body Acceleration Applied Synchronously with the Heart Beat (BASH). In: G. Juznic (ed.), Biomedical Sciences and Cardiovascular Dynamics, S. Karger Publ. Co., Basel, pp. 57–63, 1973. Also appeared as Bibl. Cardiol. 31: 57–62, 1973.

Waller A.D.: A demonstration on man of electromotive changes accompanying a heart's beat. J. Physiol. 8: 229–234, 1887.

Walters R.M.: Simple methods for performing artificial respiration J. 123: 559–561, 1943.

Ware R.W., Hall C.W., Fogwell J.W., Gerlach C.R., Schuhmann R.E., Ross J.R. and DeBakey M.E.: Inertial cardiac assistance. Trans. Am. Soc. Artif. Int. Organs 17: 211–212, 1971.

Weale F.E.: External cardiac massage. Lancet 1: 172, 1961.

Weber E.H.: Ueber die Anwendung der Wellenlehre auf die Lehre from Kreislaufe de s Blutes und ins besondere auf die Pulslehre. Ber. Verh. Kgl. Saechs. Ges. Wiss., Math. Phys. Kl., 1850.

Weber K.T. and Janicki J.S., 1974 Intraaortic Balloon Counterpulsation. A review of physiological principles, clinical results, and device safety. Ann. Thoracic Surg. 17:602–636, 1974

Weil M.H., Shubin H.: Changes in venous capacitance during cardiogenic shock – A search for the third dimension. An Editorial. Am. J. Cardiol. 26: 613–614, 1970.

Weil M.H. and Tang W.: CPR: Resuscitation of the Arrested Heart. Chapter 1, W.B. Saunders Co., Philadelphia PA, 1999.

Wenckebach K.F.: Herz- und Kreislaufinsufficienz. Steinkopff, Dresden & Leipzig, 1934

Werner J.A., Greene H.L., Janko C.L. and Cobb L.A.: Visualization of cardiac valve motion in man during external chest compression using two-dimensional echocardiography. Circulation 63: 1417–1421, 1981.

Willman V.L., Cooper T. and Hanlon C.R.: Return of neural responses after autotransplantation of the heart. Am. J. Physiol. 207: 187–189, 1964.

Appendix

Questions

9.1 Explain the fallacy of the "dam in stream" analogy

9.2 Cardiac output during CPR is likely to be what percentage of normal?

9.3 Does unconsciousness due to circulatory standstill, or due to asphyxia occur after different intervals?

9.4 The largest fraction of blood volume is found in which part of the CV system?

9.5 Is there a systematic difference between intrathoracic pressure under normal conditions and during CPR?

9.6 What is the effective heart rate under a CPR protocol of 15:2 (15 chest compressions at 100/min, interrupted by 2 artificial respiratory cycles of 4 s each)?

9.7 The arterial and venous changes in pressure subsequent to circulatory stand-still (negative and positive, respectively), permit estimation of the ratio between venous and arterial compliances, averaged over the ranges of the pressure shifts. Derive this mathematically.

9.8 Compare the rise in internal pressure in (α) a glass tube filled with blood and closed at both ends with (β) a thin-walled rubber tube similarly filled and closed, when external air or fluid pressure is increased by 20 mmHg.

9.9 Does Sect. 9.4.2 carry implications for the behavior of the mitral and tricuspid valves?

9.10 Over the centuries, investigators have proposed mechanisms for (partial) emptying a ventricle entirely at variance with Harvey's concept of cardiac muscle shortening. Past examples include pulsatile properties of the arteries, generation of heat, and kinetic energy inherent to blood (Marinelli et al. 1995). There is little doubt that others will be proposed in the future. Is Harvey's concept sufficiently robust to outlive all of them?

9.11 A simple equation to define a passive ventricular pressure–volume relation is given by

$$p_v(t) - p_e(t) = \pm a[V_v(t) - b]^2$$

where F_1 or $F_2 = 0$ (Eqs. 4.6), a and b are positive constants, p_v and p_e denote fluid pressure within and air pressure without this ventricle, respectively, and V_v is the volume contained by the ventricle. Experimental evidence dictates that the minus sign in front of the parameter a applies only when $V_v < b$. Show that for $p_e > p_v$, there is, in general, no physically realizable solution for V_v, i.e., ventricular volume becomes negative.

9.12 From a point in time well before Harvey, cardiovascular teaching maintained that blood flow transports the materials on which life depends. Yet, the measurement of blood pressure was far more popular during much of this time. Why?

9.13 Are the cardiac and the thoracic theories in CPR clearly separable?

9.14 Computer solutions have, on occasion, shown negative ventricular volumes. What does this mean? How can the appearance of such a flaw be prevented? Hint: consult the "remedy" (Noordergraaf G.J et al. 2005) when using Mathematica, or prevent $p_e - p_v(t)$ directly from rising above ab^2 by setting inflow and outflow of the chamber of interest equal to 0 when this inequality is violated in Matlab.

9.15 Could it be helpful for the caregiver to measure the force exerted on the sternum during CPR?

9.16 Discuss the possibility of fluid-filled catheter resonance to interpret the high peak pressures recorded in the aorta and right atrium in Fig. 2 (left) of Timerman et al. 2004.

Answers

9.1 The image of a dam, more than likely inspired by the constructions built by hydraulic engineers, implies something static and permanent, placed to prevent undesirable augmentation of river flow. For the ventricle, undesirable reduction of blood flow is (a) not static, while (b) increased venous pressure tends to augment cardiac output as McMichael pointed out.

9.2 Fifty percent or less (OCCR), 10% or less (CCCR).

9.3 Yes, less than 1 min and about 3 min, respectively.

9.4 The venous system.

9.5 During quiet inspiration it is negative throughout, during forced expiration it tends to become positive briefly; during the compression phase in CPR it is significantly positive, during its relaxed phase tending to be slightly negative.

9.6 Fifteen chest compressions take 9 s, followed by 8 s for ventilation, making a total of 17 s. Effectively imposed heart rate equals $\left[\frac{9}{17}\right]100 = 53$ per min.

9.7

$$\bar{C}_{art}\Delta p_{art} = -\bar{C}_{ven}\Delta p_{ven} \rightarrow \frac{\bar{C}_{ven}}{\bar{C}_{art}} = -\frac{\Delta p_{art}}{\Delta p_{ven}} \tag{9.3}$$

9.8 In (α) the rise will be zero; in (β) the rise will be 20 mmHg, if the stiffness of the wall is negligible, less if this is not the case.

9.9 Yes, for the cardiac theory the mitral valve should open and close, for the thoracic theory the tricuspid valve should open and close.

9.10 Consideration of the length of survival of Harvey's ideas regarding ventricular pumping since 1628 inspires confidence.

9.11 For the equation given in the question, its left-hand side goes negative, if $p_e > p_v$. This requires the right-hand side to become negative as well. This, in turn, requires the minus sign in front of the parameter a to apply. This minus sign demands that $V_v < b$. Taking both into account in solving the equation for V_v yields

$$V_v = b - \left[\frac{p_e - p_v}{a}\right]^{\frac{1}{2}}, \tag{9.4}$$

Or V_v will go negative for

$$p_e - p_v > ab^2 \tag{9.5}$$

Substitution of parameter values, listed in Table 11.1, shows this pressure difference to be very small.

9.12 The measurement of flow proved to be much more difficult for technical reasons.

9.13 Both theories rely on chest compression. The cardiac theory holds that the heart is mechanically compressed between bony structures as a result, causing ventricular ejection. The thoracic theory believes in an overall increase in pressure in the chest operating on all structures situated within the chest cavity leading to improved ventricular filling as well as augmentation of stroke volume. Since chest compression is the common denominator, the theories are difficult to separate clearly.

9.14 Negative volumes in the body, a physical impossibility, should be attributed to an oversight in a governing equation, or to an error in the corresponding computer code, or both.

9.15 Yes, indeed. Caregivers tend to tire quickly and become inclined to reduce the compression force.

9.16 The recurring damped oscillation, close to 5 Hz, suggests resonance of the catheter-manometer system. In the publication, this effect is much smaller, however, than the difference between autopulse and manual chest compression.

Chapter 10
Circulatory Control

La fixité du milieu intérieur est la condition de la vie libre, indépendante.

— Claude Bernard, 1878

Digest: The path leading up to the concept of homeostasis. Cardiac controls. Baroreceptor control with and without set-point. Impedance-defined flow phenomena. Cooperation among controls. The influence of the respiratory system on the performance of the cardiovascular system during rest and exercise. Vaso- and venomotion.

The well over a century old concerns that the heart is too weak solely to be responsible for venous return (Sect. 2.4) are resolved by the introduction of the concept of impedance-defined flow together with the appreciation of extra cardiovascular systems influencing blood flow within the cardiovascular system. This applies more firmly the higher the levels of exercise and training.

10.1 Introduction

10.1.1 Concept Development

"The constancy of the milieu interieur" was postulated by Bernard in 1878 to summarize his observations in warm-blooded animals. He claimed that for any variations that may occur, such organisms compensate continuously. Fredericq (1885) formulated Bernard's postulate more causally, viz., "The living being is an agency of such sort that each disturbing influence induces by itself the setting into motion of compensatory apparatus to neutralize and repair the disturbance". Later, Cannon (1929, 1932) elaborated on this theme, formulating the challenge fundamental to biomedical interest: The coordinated physiological reactions which maintain most of the steady states in the body are so complex, and are so peculiar to the living organisms, that it has been suggested [by himself as part of a lecture given

A. Noordergraaf, *Blood in Motion*, DOI 10.1007/978-1-4614-0005-9_10,
© Springer Science+Business Media, LLC 2011

in honor of Charles Richet in 1925] that a specific designation for these states be employed – "homeostasis."

Homeostasis implies physiological adjustment such that the organism remains in an overall consistent state. To achieve a new state, considerable adjustments may be required in the properties of the system's components, traditionally referred to as parameter changes. Depending on the state and requirements of the mammal, e.g., during exercise vs. during rest, or alteration in its environment, e.g., of temperature or gas composition, specific physiological variables (blood flow, respiratory depth, etc.) will alter as a result. Homeostasis may not be achievable under a number of circumstances.

In this chapter, two examples will be studied. One, where homeostasis works successfully during different levels of exercise, in the other where homeostasis fails as a result of cardiopulmonary function collapse, usually even despite efforts to revitalize cardiac function. [For a more general exposure to classification and terminology, reference is made to Chap. 9 in "Circulatory System Dynamics" (Noordergraaf A. 1978).]

10.1.2   Stimuli and Related Parameters Operating from Within and Without the Cardiovascular System

The listing presented here is percieved as partial, since additional mechanisms continue to be discovered. In the analyses reported here, a selection of the cardiovascular controls listed below will be called upon.

- Sympathetic, metabolic, and hormonal stimulation of the heart's contractile properties: the quantities c and d in Eq. 4.6d assume the role of parameters for the individual cardiac chambers.
- Similar stimulation of heart rate with f_h as the responsible parameter.
- Depth of respiration: intrathoracic pressure imposed by the respiratory system, p_{er} or by chest compression during CPR, p_e, can shift the cardiac function curve along the filling axis (Fig. 8.2) influencing stroke volume (Eq. 8.1a showing p_e on the left-hand side). Both pressures, represented by p_e, serve as variables in their home systems as well as time-varying parameters in the circulation.
- Frequency of respiration, a control of the type as under (the first item), with particular sensitivity to blood p_H; f_r as the designated parameter.
- The baroreceptor control, a neural control operating primarily on the basis of arterial blood pressure as reported by the baroreceptors, acting on the peripheral resistances R_s and R_p as parameters, as well as on the heart (first item, above).
- Active venomotion, operating on the vessel's luminal size as parameter, by way of its mural musculature.
- Passive venomotion, where veins are embedded in skeletal muscle that may contract and relax depending on the type of exercise.
- Circulatory filling pressure, primarily determined by the volume of circulating blood available.
- Elastic properties of blood vessels, a nonlinear property that influences the pressure–volume relation, especially in veins.

A number of these controls have been studied, primarily by experimental means, fewer have been the subject of mathematical modeling, while the remainder has hardly been scrutinized at all. Those that were analyzed in some detail, generally, were studied in isolation from other controls. Examples include a study by Guyton (1963b) to analyze the matching of cardiac output and venous return by selecting right atrial pressure as the independent variable while evaluating the dependence of these two quantities on the level of sympathetic stimulation and the value of the mean circulatory filling pressure, restricting himself to average values. Beneken and De Wit (1967) modeled baroreceptor control of heart rate and the systemic peripheral resistance, while Karreman and Weygandt (1978) expanded carotid sinus control of the peripheral resistances by modeling the physiological feedback mechanisms. Shifting emphasis to longer range control, Guyton et al. (1972) developed a larger set of equations (over 350) (Sect. 8.2). Ha et al. (2005) performed experimental studies on sheep, taking into account body position.

After a period of introspection, attention turned to focus on refining the quality of models (Cole et al. 2005) especially regarding the cardiac chambers (Palladino et al. 2000a, b) and on rethinking the strategy of model making in physiology, in particular with respect to predicting function from structure and structure from function (Palladino et al. 2006).

These models, as well as their manifold variations, were conceived and built prior to the conception of impedance-defined flow. In the following sections, impedance-defined flow will be incorporated in two examples, one for the normal loop (Sect. 2 below) and the other for the case of heart and respiratory failure (Sect. 3 below).

10.2   Control of Cardiac Output and Venous Return

10.2.1   Control by the Heart

The two ventricles probably display the most conspicuous examples of impedance-defined flow in the cardiovascular system. The quasi periodic contraction of the ventricular walls leads to closure of the mitral and tricuspid valves, interposing high impedances between the ventricles and the atria, even if closure is imperfect. The paths of lesser impedance (Eqs. 8.7c, d) lead flow into the arterial reservoirs (Eqs. 8.1 and, with more detail, in Chap. 11), despite the fact that their input impedances contain significant peripheral resistances for the steady flow components (Fig. 5.5).

When the ventricles relax, the aortic and pulmonary valves close owing to brief retrograde flow. The atrial pressures open the mitral and tricuspid valves and passive ventricular filling commences, allowing the ventricles to become part of the central venous systems, as are the atria. Just prior to the next ventricular contraction, the atria themselves contract. Owing to the small pressure and impedance differences, the atria move blood into the ventricles as well as returning some back into the venous reservoirs (Fig. 3.13). As a consequence of such sloshing, atrial contraction contributes only modestly to ventricular filling, estimated at less than 25%.

The coronary circulation, analyzed in Sect. 6.3, was concluded to exhibit compression of its veins during ventricular ejection, resulting in forward flow (Fig. 6.7). This implies, primarily for the coronary veins, that they serve as a pump themselves [propelling blood into the then relaxed right atrium]. For the coronaries, however, their compression during systole lasts long enough to diminish average coronary perfusion when compared to the relaxed ventricle. Starving the coronary vasculature for blood carrying metabolites may play a role in insuring that the crossbridges become unstable, forcing the ventricles to relax (Sect. 4.2).

10.2.2 Control of the Heart

The pumping function of the heart itself is affected by control mechanisms which have been distinguished as internal and external. The internal mechanisms that relate to alterations of the contractile behavior of the myocardium are further subdivided into: (1) heterometric, in which changes in fiber length, caused by altered venous return and/or arterial outflow (Sect. 4.3) modify the degree of interdigitation of actin and myosin filaments at the onset of contraction, resulting in a different contractile force; (2) homeometric, which is thought of as modifications in the biochemistry of the contractile machinery, resulting in changes in the generated force of contraction, in the absence of changes in the degree in overlap length between actin and myosin filaments; and (3) frequency of contraction, which has been ascribed to changes in the permeability of the cardiac pacemaker (SA node).

The external mechanisms consist essentially of effects induced by neural, humoral (Sect. 4.3), and respiratory (Sect. 4, below) influences. The first is distinguished in two antagonistic controls: (1) parasympathetic, a nervous influence which is conceived of as decreasing cardiac output and lowering the frequency of contraction under otherwise the same circumstances; and (2) sympathetic, the opposite of the parasympathetic effect. Levy (1978) demonstrated interaction between these components, which makes the total system more difficult to analyze.

10.2.3 Heart Rate

Changes in heart rate have been held responsible for increasing cardiac output, decreasing output, or leaving it unchanged, often for the same directional change in rate. A number of these apparent contradictions could be resolved by the

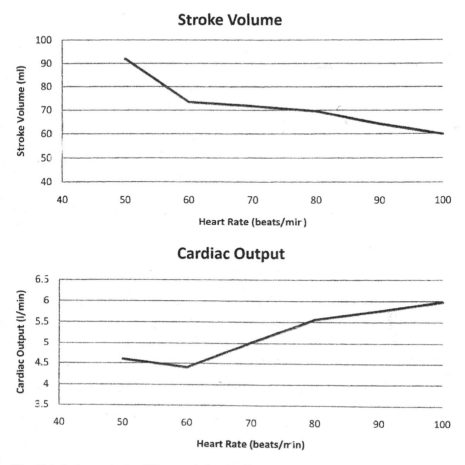

Fig. 10.1 Left ventricular filling restriction by increased heart rate under otherwise normal conditions (Donders model 2007). As heart rate increases, stroke volume decreases steadily, rapidly at first, then more slowly. In this sample, cardiac output decreases slightly at first, then increases (Melbin et al. 1982)

introduction of a single quadratic regression function relating changes in cardiac output to changes in heart rate for a sequence of experiments on dogs. Depending on the value of stroke volume at a particular heart rate, changes in rate could increase, decrease, or leave unchanged the value of cardiac output (Melbin et al. 1982). Figure 10.1 offers a computed example of left ventricular inflow restriction on cardiac output as it depends on heart rate.

Neural control experiments, which could not be represented by the same quadratic relationship, offer an example of competing control. Heart rate increase in response to sympathetic stimulation has been the subject of quite detailed investigations, e.g., by Warner (1965). The same applies to vagal stimulation and the ensuing decrease in rate (Warner and Cox 1962; Katona et al. 1970). In 1969, Warner and Russell proposed the following mathematical model for the combined effect of sympathetic and parasympathetic stimulation in setting the heart rate f:

$$f_{sv} = f_v + \frac{(f_s - f_o)(f_v - f_{min})}{(f_o - f_{min})} \tag{10.1}$$

where f_v and f_s denote heart rates resulting from vagal and sympathetic stimulation separately, f_o, the rate with all efferent nerves cut, and f_{min}, the lowest possible heart rate.

10.2.4 Respiratory Control

The elastic recoil of the lungs, causing intrapleural pressure to be below the atmospheric level, was held responsible for venous return by the nineteenth century investigators of elastic properties of the lung, the argument being that permanent traction kept the veins from collapsing. Subsequently, attention shifted from this steady component to focus almost exclusively on the more conspicuous oscillatory components induced by the respiration, already observed by Valsalva according to Morgagni (1761), with Harvey (published in 1952) as preluder.

Donders' message regarding the influence of the respiration on the circulation of blood may be reflected as "...with the play of inspiration and expiration, also blood pressure and blood flow change very significantly. This effect can also be demonstrated easily by direct observation. If the neck veins are exposed, it will be seen that they collapse during each inspiration; in contrast, during each expiration, they fill more with blood." In analyzing this statement, it is well to remember that the neck veins are extrathoracic.

Since Donders felt that the residual driving pressures from the arterial pressure reservoirs were too small to be responsible for adequate venous return, he proposed the respiratory pump as a substantial aid in promoting the return of blood to the heart. His proposal was extensively criticized by investigators who claimed that the augmentation in venous return, occurring during inspiration, was balanced by its reduction during expiration. Others held that collapse of a central vein alters flow resistance such as to nullify any net effect between inspiration and expiration. Still others simply denied that the respiration has any effect on the circulation. Both animal experiments and theoretical arguments were internally inconsistent. For example, Morgagni writes in one of his many letters (1761) that his own experiments showed the opposite of Valsalva's. Brecher (1956) presented a detailed review of these conflicts, while taking Donders' side himself primarily on the basis of his own measurements of flow in central veins. Nature appears to play a far more refined game that leaves room for just about all published conclusions. Under conditions of a fixed ratio between heart and respiratory frequencies accompanied by shallow breathing, the respiratory system's contribution to venous return may be hard to detect (Sect. 8.3). On the other hand, during physical activity, when the ratio of frequencies is variable and breathing is deeper or deep, the negative excursion of intrathoracic pressure $p_e(t)$ is more profound (Fig. 10.4). Any heart beat that is exposed to such a strongly negative respiratory pressures will experience enhanced filling and generate higher stroke volumes (Noordergraaf G.J. et al. 2006).

Other researchers, both prior to and subsequent to Donders contributed additional ideas about mechanisms serving promotion of venous return in valveless parts of the circulation (Sect. 2.3; Moser et al. 1998). In recent decades, interest has been predominantly one sided, focusing, as it did, on ventricular ejection while presuming a desirable level of filling.

Wiggers, as early as 1934, offered a more quantitative picture. Intrapleural pressure during expiration amounts to -3 to -6 mmHg. During quiet inspiration, it goes down to -4.5 to -9 mmHg, during deep inspiration, it may perhaps be reduced to -30 or -40 mmHg with respect to atmospheric pressure, which was supported by Versprille's experiments (1995) on healthy human subjects.

In some ten human subjects, Rahn et al. (1946) showed that muscular effort may change pressure during exhalation with the airways open. Hence, passive and forced exhalation should be distinguished.

In Starling's experiments, the pressure external to the heart was atmospheric (isolated heart-lung preparations). In the intact system, the respiratory system contributes an external pressure, $p_e(t)$, which oscillates at a frequency below the heart frequency.

Only vaguely referred to in the literature dealing with effects of exercise, $p_e(t)$ is able to exert a powerful influence on the ventricular function curve by shifting it along the preload axis. The shift is to the left for negative p_e and to the right for positive values, both in reference to Starling's experimental procedures $(p_e = 0)$. In as much as p_e varies with time, the ventricular curve is shifting continually with a small amplitude during quiet breathing to a large one during intensive physical exercise (Sect. 8.1).

Inclusion of the effect of pressure external to the heart, brought about by respiration (p_{er}), or by cardiac massage $(p_{ec}, \text{Sect. } 9.4.7)$, both captured by the symbol $p_e(t)$, further generalizes the description of the cardiac function curves in Eqs. 4.6 and 8.1. In time, $p_{er}(t)$ tends to assume negative values, e.g., during inspiration, while p_{ec} tends to positive values, e.g., during chest compression.

Returning to the Donders' claim that respiration enhances venous return now becomes more accessible to evaluation. There is little doubt that inspiration lowers p_e. If this effect indeed promotes venous return, it should be expected that venous filling and venous pressure would tend to rise toward the end of inspiration. This kind of reasoning may, however, be overly simplified, since p_e also plays a role in the ventricle's preload. As p_e becomes more negative, preload simultaneously grows more positive, enhancing ventricular filling. Therefore, two opposite changes will occur: more blood is returned to the central veins and the right ventricle is induced to accept more blood in its filling process, resulting in an, offhand, unpredictable change in central venous pressure. Following central venous blood pressure alone does not seem the advisable method to evaluate Donders' claim.

There is, nevertheless, an alternative: If inspiration marshalls more blood to the venous reservoir, then more blood is available for cardiac output. Taking CO as a measure of the resulting effect includes both alterations in the oscillatory aspect $(p_e(t))$ and its average value $(\bar{p}_e)$. Noordergraaf G.J. et al. (2006) demonstrated a positive relation between the latter and CO in a study utilizing the Donders model.

10.2.5   Control of Pressure; Gravitational and Inertial Effects

The overwhelming majority of laboratory studies, performed in the gravitational field, have been conducted in the horizontal plane with the idea that gravitational effects would be negligible. This concept was not fully supported by investigators interested in conditions where microgravity prevailed, since they found that space conditions could best be simulated in the circulatory system on earth by supporting the subject on a flat surface with a head down tilt of around 10° rather than 0°. The effect of the difference has attracted little attention.

In measurements on baboons in an aircraft flying, in rapid succession, Keplerian trajectories (parabolas) to achieve microgravitational conditions, then changing direction for the aircraft to recover its altitude under high g conditions, the vector sum of $\vec{g}$ and of $\vec{a}$, the imposed acceleration changes with time both in magnitude and in direction. Latham et al. (1994) observed unpredictable responses in right atrial pressures, even in the same animal, on different days. The responses were found to be sensitive to circulatory filling pressure as well as to animal posture (Latham et al. 1993).

In the larger arteries and veins, blood can be made to move easily along the axial direction of the vessel, though not perpendicular to it. This is discussed in Sect. 9.4.6 for the application of a sinusoidal acceleration/deceleration. By implication, Essler et al. (1999) raised the issue whether or not alteration in pressure and flow, resulting from variant gravitational conditions, should be related to fast changes in values of system parameters.

In a blood vessel aligned with the gravitational field, pressure differences Δp are introduced at a magnitude of

$$\Delta p = \rho g h \tag{10.2a}$$

The density of blood is denoted by ρ, the acceleration of gravity by g. Converted into historic units, this means $\Delta p = 0.76$ mmHg for each cm of height h, in a continuous blood column, independent of cross-sectional area. In long vessels, the effect of gravity may play a commanding role.

The giraffe provides an extreme example. Taking a value of 250 cm for the vertical component

$$h = L_g \cos \alpha \qquad (10.2b)$$

of the anatomical distance L_g between the giraffe's cerebral circulation and the left ventricle, with α the angle between the direction of L_g and that of the acceleration of gravity, the hemostatic pressure difference Δp between these two sites would amount to $250 \times 0.76 = 191$ mmHg. In the head up position, cerebral arterial pressure would be below root aortic pressure by this amount, in the head down position augmented by the same amount. In both situations, blood flow could be seriously compromised unless other mechanisms provide compensation. Under dynamic (wild life) conditions, α will be time dependent.

Further analysis clarifies some of these disturbing points. If the carotid arteries are occluded near their points of origin, carotid artery pressure (p_c) becomes an independent variable to be chosen by the investigator, while aortic pressure (p_a) is measured. For a range of steady values of p_c, the illustrated curve (a) in Fig. 10.2a, is obtained. It indicates that aortic pressure tends to drop as carotid pressure increases with threshold and saturation effects at the ends (Taher et al. 1988). The relationship is generally nonlinear. (Frequently, the assumption of linearity is introduced to make applicable a body of methods and criteria, the validity of which is restricted to linear systems, Fig. 10.2.)

The adjustment of systemic arterial blood pressure furnishes an example of closed loop control. If systemic arterial blood pressure drops, this change is detected by the baroreceptors. The baroreceptor output is transmitted to the central nervous system, where the information is processed. The output of the central nervous system is transmitted to the heart, which will be induced to augment cardiac output (first effector site) and to the peripheral resistance, which will be induced to increase (second, presumably stronger, effector site). The effect will thus be an increase in systemic arterial blood pressure. The inverse procedure, as occurs in exercise, will counteract arterial pressure augmentation. It should be noted that baroreceptors do not regulate (i.e., keep constant) arterial pressure, though they offer adjustments. The sensitivity of stroke volume to downstream pressure conditions is a complicating feature.

Evaluation of the operating point O for arterial pressure may be achieved, by approximation, by selecting a point (p_c^0, p_a^0) on curve a and drawing the tangent at that point. The equation for this tangent is

$$p_a = (p_c - p_c^0) \tan \theta + p_a^0 \qquad (10.3a)$$

which may be written as

$$p_a = g(p_c(t)) \qquad (10.3b)$$

This defines the neural effect. The fluid-dynamic effect (graph b in Fig. 10.2a) may be written as

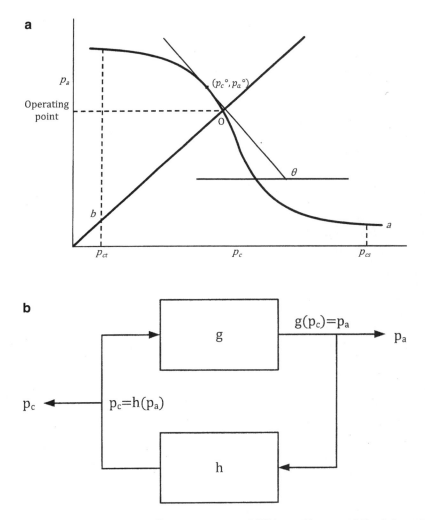

Fig. 10.2 (**a**) The two components of baroreceptor control. With carotid pressure (p_c) as independent variable, graph a depicts the resulting arterial pressure p_a. The influence of p_c on p_a shows a threshold around $p_c = p_{ct}$ and saturation at about $p_c = p_{cs}$. Graph b relates the same pressures by fluid-dynamic means. The intercept of the two graphs defines the operating point O. (**b**) Block diagram without an external set-point, yielding the same solution for the operating point

$$p_c = h(p_a(t)) \tag{10.3c}$$

If the functions g and h are known, Eqs. 10.3b, c can be solved for the intercept of the tangent to a with graph b. Iteration will yield accurate coordinates of O. The corresponding block diagram (Fig. 10.2b) is free of an externally imposed so-called set point (Cecchini et al. 1981).

Preference is often given to the use of a set point as an arbitrary convenience in a zero order model. Linearizing a segment of graph a (Fig. 10.3a) and giving names to the intercepts of its extensions with the coordinate axes, Eq. 10.3b is replaced by

$$p_a = -Gp_c + Gp_0 \tag{10.4a}$$

and Eq. 10.3c by

$$p_a = \left(\frac{1}{H}\right)p_c \tag{10.4b}$$

in which G and H are constants. The solution for the location of the operating point reads

$$p_a = \frac{Gp_0}{1 + GH} \tag{10.5a}$$

and

$$p_c = \frac{GHp_0}{1 + GH} \tag{10.5b}$$

in which p_0 assumes the role of set point, as also indicated in Fig. 10.3b. Its lack of uniqueness is suggested by Fig. 10.3c where a different set point leads to the identical solution for the operating point.

This linearized approach may be adapted easily to systemic arterial pressures in the giraffe as an extreme example. For this purpose, it will be assumed here that the giraffe possesses baroreceptors close to its brain. This assumption is still subject to debate. The hemostatic pressure difference between the heart and the brain, without control, for a vertical distance h of 250 cm in the upright position should amount to 191 mmHg, which might mean absence of brain perfusion. Assuming that Eq. 10.4a retains its validity and replacing Eq. 10.4b by

$$p_a = p_c + \rho gh \tag{10.6}$$

where h is vertical height, ρ the density of blood, and g the acceleration of gravity. p_a and p_c can then be solved from Eqs. 10.4a and 10.6 yields

$$p_a = \frac{G}{1 + G}p_0 + \frac{G}{1 + G}\rho gh \tag{10.7a}$$

and

$$p_c = \frac{G}{1 + G}p_0 - \frac{1}{1 + G}\rho gh \tag{10.7b}$$

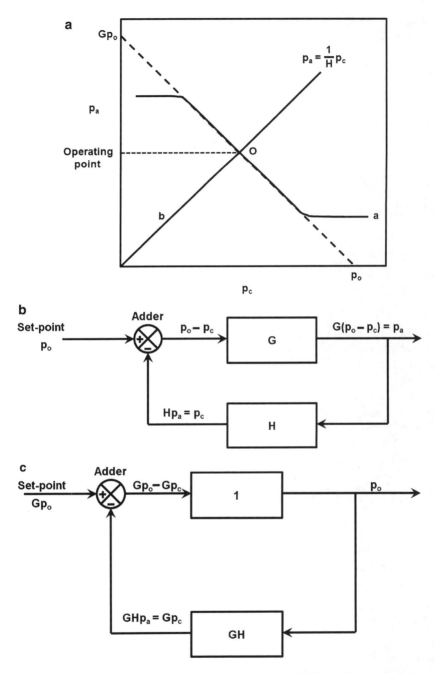

Fig. 10.3 (**a**) As Fig. 10.2 with a segment of graph *a* linearized. (**b**) Block diagram displaying set point p_0. This set point is not unique: (**c**) provides the identical solution for the coordinates of the operating point, though employing a different set point. *G* and *H* define individual steady state input-output relations of the two blocks in (**b**); 1 and *GH* in (**c**).

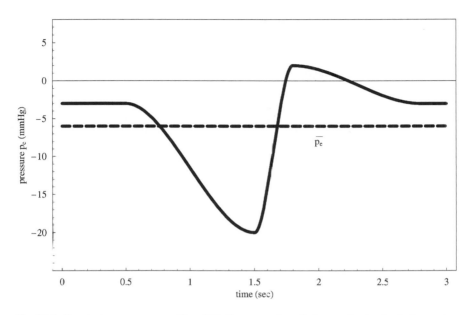

Fig. 10.4 Respiratory pressures $p_e(t)$ and $\overline{p_e}$, its mean value, during moderate physical exercise. Equations 11.121 and 11.122 in Chap. 11 offer a mathematical description of the former

which shows that p_a is raised by $G\rho gh/(1+G)$, while p_c is lowered by $\rho gh/(1+G)$ compared to the supine position ($h=0$). For illustrative purposes, if p_0, the set point, is set at 250 mmHg, $p_a = p_c = 125$ in the supine position. In the upright position, with $G = 1$, $p_a = 125+95 = 220$ and $p_c = 125-95 = 30$ mmHg. Though this change makes the left ventricle do more work to generate the same flow (Eqs. 4.2, Fig. 10.5), sustaining brain perfusion should not present any difficulty (Fig. 10.6), despite the fact that the difference between p_a and p_c remains unaltered. The experiments carried out by Goetz et al. (1960) and Warren (1974) on giraffes support the main point of this analysis.

Replacing h by $-h$ in Eqs. 10.7a, b applies the same reasoning to the head down (drinking) situation: p_a is now lowered, which reduces the hemostatic effect on arterial p_c.

Much confusion continues to reign in considering venous return. Amoroso et al. (1947) observed five tricuspid valves in the jugular vein of a giraffe and noted that this vein had a "very thick" wall, presumably counteracting collapse. It would appear that the role of the valves is critical in preventing the full hydrostatic effect to operate on venous pressure close to the brain of the giraffe while drinking from a pool. Without such valves, in the absence of a venous baroreceptor mechanism, venous pressure, close to the brain, could exceed arterial pressure in the same vicinity.

The saphenous vein was also found to be thick walled and in possession of numerous tricuspid and bicuspid valves.

Much work has been done to gain deeper insight into the detailed operation of the baroreceptor mechanism, both experimentally and theoretically (Taher et al. 1988), especially regarding the relation between blood pressure in the carotid sinus,

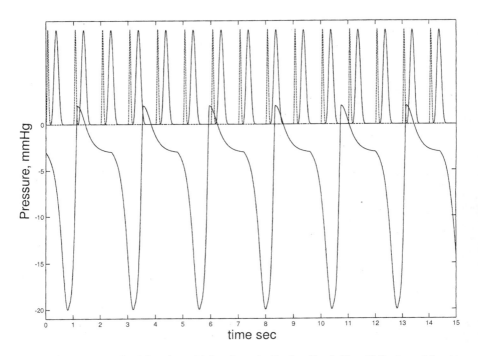

Fig. 10.5 The normalized functions $f(t)$ for the atria (*broken lines*), Eqs. 11.9a, b, and for the ventricles (*solid*) for a succession of heart beats at 60 beats/min (*top*). Intrathoracic pressure–time relationship at a frequency 2.5 times lower. The two frequencies do not display an integer ratio under most conditions

$p_c(t)$, and the rate of discharge, n, of the baroreceptors. Warner (1958) developed what became its most popular mathematical formulation:

$$n = k_1 (p_c - p_0{}^*) + k_2 \frac{dp_c}{dt} \tag{10.8}$$

where $p_0{}^*$ denotes (a constant) threshold pressure, t is time, while k_1 and k_2 are constant weighting factors. This expression incorporates both threshold and sensitivity to rate of change in pressure; it does not incorporate nonlinearity, adaptation, saturation, or asymmetry. It took a few decades before all well-established baroreceptor properties found their place in a single equation (Taher et al. 1988):

$$\Delta n = \Delta p_c \left[a_1 e^{-\frac{t}{\tau_1}} + a_2 e^{-\frac{t}{\tau_2}} + a_3 e^{-\frac{t}{\tau_3}} \right] \left[\sin \frac{n}{n_{max}} \pi \right]^{\frac{1}{2}} \tag{10.9}$$

The change in discharge rate, Δn, in response to a small step increase in pressure, Δp_c, is given by the magnitude of the increment multiplied by the sum of three exponential functions each with its own weighting factor a_i and time constant

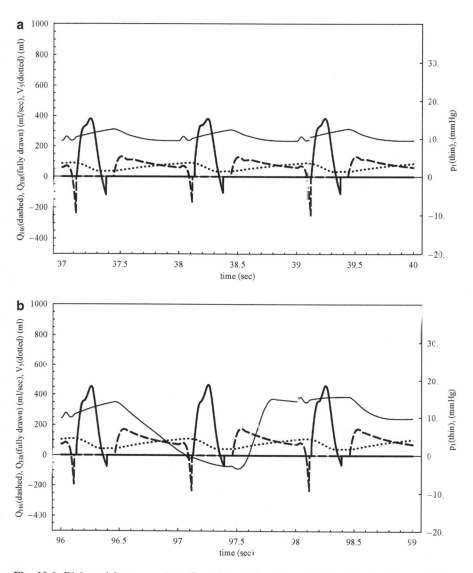

Fig. 10.6 Right atrial pressure (p_1), flow through the tricuspid valve (Q_{H6}), right ventricular ejection flow (Q_{H8}), and right ventricular volume (V_5), without respiration (**a**, $p_e = 0$) and with moderate respiration (**b**, $p_e(t)$. Cardiac output in (**b**) is 28% higher than in (**a**) (Adapted from Noordergraaf G.J. et al. 2006)

τ_i ($i = 1, 2, 3$). This product is multiplied by the expression containing the sine, the current firing rate n, and the maximum possible firing rate of the receptor, n_{max}. This factor specifies how the response Δn depends on the current firing rate n. The response has a maximum for $n = \frac{1}{2} n_{max}$, and tends to zero for $n = 0$ and for $n = n_{max}$. The equation does not contain an explicit threshold; it has no need for one.

The response to pressure, such as mean blood pressure, if constant, will vanish, owing to the (negative) exponentials in Eq. 10.9. A slowly developing hypertension will, therefore, not be reported by the baroreceptors; they "forget."

10.2.6   Control by Peripheral Pressure Flow Relations

Autoregulation in the small blood vessels displays two distinct components. (1) Vasomotion is the designation of the contraction or relaxation of smooth muscle embedded in the walls of the arterioles, the metarterioles, as well as in the precapillary sphincters. It is primarily mediated metabolically and provides a means through which local tissue controls its own blood supply. Several agents have been implicated in this activity, such as oxygen in skeletal muscle blood flow and carbon dioxide in brain flow, as well as other substances in the kidney. (2) Venomotion is the designation of a similar activity in the venules, downstream of the capillaries, generally with different periods.

In addition to the effect of local metabolic agents, the resistance to flow through the microvasculature is subject to sympathetic and parasympathetic nervous control (Hering 1924a, b), which also act by changing the radius of the small vessels that are innervated. From many studies it has become apparent that this includes essentially all peripheral vessels, with the notable exception of the capillaries. The operation of metabolic and nervous control is complicated by a hierarchy among organs. For clinical purposes, flow resistance may be controlled by antihypertensive drugs (e.g., sodium nitroprusside) even under automated conditions imposed by an external controller (McNally 1978).

Since most of the peripheral resistance is embodied in the arterioles, vasomotion can modify the peripheral resistance regionally. This may have direct implication for cardiac pumping, since such an effect will tend to alter arterial pressure. It has been firmly established that systemic arterial pressure displays oscillations at frequencies well below heart rate (Traube reported frequencies as low as 7/min). A recent analysis of this pressure modulation has shown that it may be caused by time delay between alteration in flow and the muscular response to it. This may pinpoint the origin of the Traube (1865), Mayer (1876)[1] waves (Drzewiecki et al. 2006). Such modification may also affect venous return directly and could relate to the conventional wisdom which holds that the closed loop cannot simultaneously perfuse all organs maximally.

The contraction-relaxation phenomena in the venules appear to continue independently from the vasomotion activity. This cycling makes venomotion a pump, moving blood in the direction of the central veins, as may be seen in Sect. 8.3. A provisional analysis tends to lend support to this concept. It is provisional due to

---

[1] Hering is often quoted as the third contemporary contributor in this group, though he was less than 10 years old at the time. In his 1927 book, Hering explains what actually happened, especially the role played by Czermak.

the scarcity of data, concerning both anatomical and physiological (contractile) features on venules and small veins (Figs. 8.5 and 8.6).

10.2.7 Cooperation Among Controls in Normals; Enhancement of Cardiac Output

The normal system appears to rely on the contributions of a few to many controls to answer demands for above resting cardiac output for any human specimen. This implies that magnification of cardiac output will depend on how well the individual contributions are attuned to one another. The reason for this is that most of the individual adjustment features are arranged in series, implying that even if one fails, the system will find it difficult to adjust cardiac output properly. A parallel arrangement, as utilized in the distribution of flow among peripheral organs, would tend to offer more flexibility. The major changes in cardiac output in which the entire cardiovascular circuit is involved, include interaction with the respiratory, metabolic, and neural systems (Fig. 10.7). Independent of the location of any noncardiac pump, the flow generated by this pump must join the main stream through the heart, as it is the only channel. Hence, output by the right or left ventricle persists as a measure of total flow around the circuit.

Noordergraaf G.J. et al. (2006) illustrated some of these effects and their influence on cardiac output and related quantities. Since these results are obtained from a

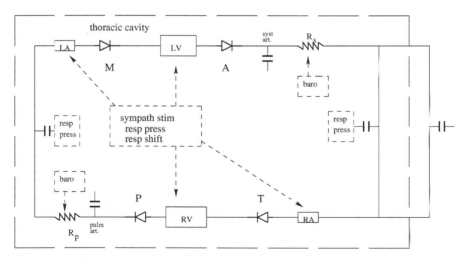

Fig. 10.7 Diagram of major participants in the adjustment of cardiac output. The intrathoracic part of the closed loop (Fig. 11.1) contains the four cardiac chambers. Their pumping performance is traditionally characterized by cardiac function curves, which are input–output relations (Figs. 8.1 and 8.2). These relations are not constant, but can be stretched or shrunk along the vertical axis as well as rotated clockwise or counterclockwise by intracardiac and extracardiac operators (Adapted from Noordergraaf G.J. et al. 2006)

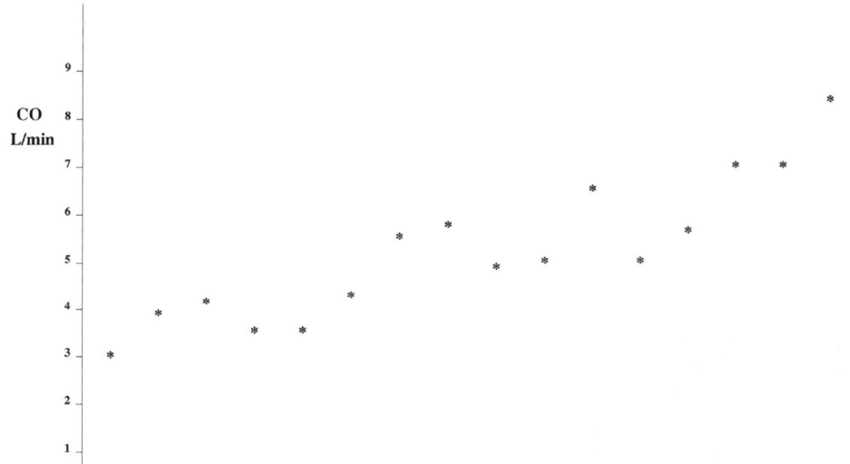

Column	1	2	3	4	5	6	7	8	9	10	11	12	13	14	15	16
RA pr. $\bar{p}_1$							11	10	14	12	2.8	13	11	4.6	4.3	4.9
LA pr. $\bar{p}_{501}$							14	13	15	11	4.9	14	10	5.3	5.9	2.7
root ao pr. $\bar{p}_6^*$							67	46	63	66	72	39	40	40	40	49
root pa pr. $\bar{p}_3$							66	50	45	48	45	43	44	42	45	47
neural contr	0.5/1.5	0.5/1.5	0.5/1.5	0.5/1.5	0.5/1.5	0.5/5	0.5/20	0.5/20	0.5/20	0.5/20	0.5/20	0.5/20	0.5/20	0.5/20	0.5/40	4/40
heart rate (Hz)	1.0	1.0	1.0	1.3	1.3	1.3	1.3	1.3	1.0	1.0	1.0	1.0	1.0	1.3	1.3	1.0
resp. rate (Hz)	0	0.33	0.33	0.33	0.44	0.44	0.44	0.44	0	0.33	0.33	0	0.33	0.44	0.44	0.33
resp. depth $\bar{p}_e$	0	−6.0	−6.0	−6.0	−6.0	−6.0	−6.0	−6.0	0	−6.0	−18	0	−6.0	−18	−18	−18
barorep.	100%	100%	100%	100%	100%	100%	50%	25%	50%	50%	50%	25%	25%	25%	25%	25%

Fig. 10.8 Multiple samples of modifications in cardiac output (CO) by intracardiac and extracardiac controls referred to in Fig. 10.7. In this illustration, cooperation among them magnifies cardiac output by a factor of 3 (Modified from Noordergraaf G.J. et al. 2006)

mathematical model (the Donders model described in Chap. 11), all parameters recognized in the model are known quantitatively, unlike commonly in experimental arrangements. Also, each parameter can be adjusted individually. Increases in depth of respiration and stimulation of the heart's contractile properties were found to contribute significantly to augmentation of cardiac output (Fig. 10.8), but increases in their rates did not (in the 2006 version, although they did in the 2007 version furnished with a stronger heart (Melbin et al. 1982)). The overall escalation of cardiac output was by a factor of 2.8 (from 3 to 8 l/min), despite the fact that the average driving pressure difference between the aortic root and the right atrium was small. These preliminary results illustrate the beneficial effects of cooperation among control features and open a wide vista of more detailed studies in which impedance-defined flow can be incorporated.

The normal heart is able to pump a volume of blood compatible with various levels of exercise, provided that its musculature is properly stimulated (by an internal and/or an external mechanism) and that adequate volumes of blood are available for suitable filling of both ventricles (by a blood carrying circuit as illustrated in Fig. 11.1 through increases in cardiac output at higher heart rate with enlarged filling of the ventricles). This, in turn, requires that arterial pressures do not increase proportionately with the higher cardiac output.

The baroreceptors handle this by reduction of the values of the peripheral resistances, which contributes two features: facilitation of the handling of a higher load by the ventricles and easier transfer of blood from the arterial reservoirs to the venous vasculatures.

The adjustable rhythmic contraction and relaxation of the small muscular veins serves to promote movement of blood out of the microcirculation in the direction of the larger veins.

Finally, the increased depth of the respiration collects blood into the central veins and the atria, thereby securing above resting levels of ventricular filling.

10.3 The Cardiac and Thoracic Theories in Cardiopulmonary Resuscitation

10.3.1 Failure to Achieve Homeostasis

When cardiac valves become incompetent, cooperation suffers. In the most severe case, when all four cardiac valves fail to close, impedance-defined flow around the circuit drops to a very much lower level compared to the control value (Stein 2008) and the system can no longer achieve homeostasis, a direct consequence of the in series position of the heart. The respiration will fail subsequently, as will smooth muscle control in the small vessels, all due to the discontinuation of oxygen and metabolite provision. This is the worst case scenario. The thoracic theory implies timely opening and closure of the tricuspid valve, while the cardiac theory assumes well-behaved operation of the mitral valve. If one or more of the cardiac valves are indeed competent, a larger fraction of normal steady flow around the circuit can, in principle, be reestablished by prompt institution of cardiopulmonary resuscitation (CPR).

In Sect. 9.4, the origins of the two competing approaches recommended for the treatment of patients in cardiopulmonary failure were summarized briefly. A more detailed summary is available in Noordergraaf (2009) where it is also shown that the assumed $A–V$ valve motion is not clearly supported by experimental observations.

Fundamentally, the theories deal with complex issues: They propose to generate blood flow from pressure caused by chest compression in a complicated blood conducting network with distributed properties, which may be modified by the driving function, $p_{ec}(t)$, causing local collapse. The gnosis of fluid dynamic theory teaches, however, that flow is generated by pressure differences. Chest massage causes such a pressure difference between it and the sizable extrathoracic parts of the cardiovascular system. Fluid shift out of the chest should be unavoidable therefore (Stephenson et al. 1954), leading to sequestration of blood (Fig. 10.9).

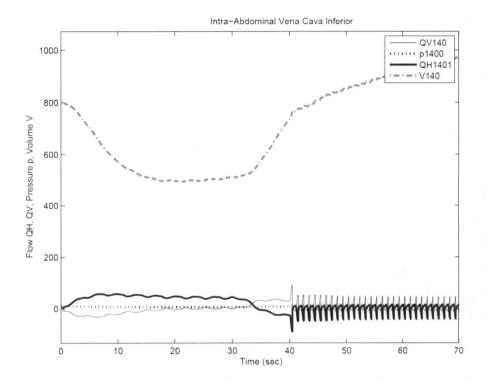

Fig. 10.9 During chest compressions blood can and does escape from the chest to abdominal veins. At $t = 0$ the Donders model is activated in a healthy state. At $t = 30$ s a severe heart attack takes place and the heart becomes asystolic. CPR is begun at $t = 40$ s. The individual compressions are identified by the positive rapid excursions, in black, of the bottom graph, while the negative, in blue, indicates blood shifting into the abdominal vena cava during every compression. The top graph keeps track of the cumulative buildup of sequestration volume V140 via QV150

Kouwenhoven and his medical colleagues (1960) believed that the major compressive forces were exerted by squeezing of the left ventricle between the sternum and the vertebral column, thereby assigning the pressure difference of interest to an alternate, more narrowly defined, location. X-ray studies later proved this assumption to be generally incorrect (Noordergraaf et al. 2005).

10.3.2   Return to Fundamentals

The rate of survival by administration of closed chest CPR has not really improved since the time that Kouwenhoven et al. proposed the procedure in 1960. This is not to be blamed on lack of interest and effort. Large amounts of funds and effort have been spent on research attempting to improve the survival rate of a complex system, while it was not clear what went wrong when applying CPR to cardiac patients.

Hence, the search for improvement took on a random nature in a system where there were restrictions on the measurement of critical variables, such as blood flow.

Descartes pointed the way out as early as in the seventeenth century: performing a mathematical analysis (cf. the Introduction), which combined with the modern digital computer, permits tackling complex problems. This approach was used successfully in several of the preceding chapters. Here, it will be applied again under the title of the Donders model, described in detail in Chap. 11.

To serve the current purpose, it was expanded to include the venous vasculature and comprises 106 equations, which are solved simultaneously by digital computer technology in the search for what went wrong in administering CPR.

Detailed studies with the aid of the Donders model focused on the role played by the veins that carry most of the venous return to both atria: the vena cava superior, the thoracic part of the vena cava inferior, and the terminal parts of the pulmonary veins. These large vessels with soft walls are prone to collapse under conditions of chest massage, particularly if the applied pressure $p_{ec}(t)$ has a high peak value. To take this collapse into account large nonlinear effects had to be incorporated in the relevant equations. These nonlinear terms can be quantified from Eqs. 5.33 and 5.34a–g, in which the time-varying transmural pressure, $p_{tr}(t)$, assumes the role of semi-independent variable. The model then shows (Fig. 10.10) that blood flow reduces to low values owing to the increased flow impedance, even in partially collapsed veins, and to the inability of these veins to snap open and refill promptly after the peak value of $p_{ec}(t)$ has passed. Complete refilling frequently takes more time than the currently popular massage frequency allots to it (10 s for the VCS, 1 s for the thoracic part of the VCI, and 12 s for the pulmonary veins). There is clinical support for these computer predictions, such as, e.g., the clinician's inability to pick up a flow pulse in the VCS subsequent to administration of CPR. Such difficulties affect both the thoracic and the cardiac theories. Preliminary model studies employing a significantly lower compression frequency report higher flow levels of up to 20% of control (Lee 2009).

The reason why a small percentage of the patients survive must mean that venous return continues and might be attributable to one or more of the following effects: early defibrillation, stiffer venous walls, body motion resulting from massage (Sects. 5.2 and 9.4), irregularity in venous support, or poorly executed CPR. This requires further study to pinpoint the difference exactly.

In this process, it became clear that compression can easily impede venous return. With increasing value of peak compression levels, this may also apply to the thoracic parts of the major arteries (i.e., all of the pulmonary artery and the thoracic part of the aorta, both of which have lost their high pressure status under these pathological circumstances). This second stage may be followed by collapse of some, or all of the cardiac chambers. The Donders model predicted in another study that "cough CPR" collapses the ventricles in about a minute (Han 2009). The model permits evaluation of such effects separately and in conjunction, which is difficult to imagine under experimental conditions in a patient (Rajaei 2008).

The situation becomes totally different if obstruction of venous return flow is avoided and only the ventricles are subjected to massage, raising cardiac output to about half its normal resting value (Lau 2008; Koeken 2009). This signifies a

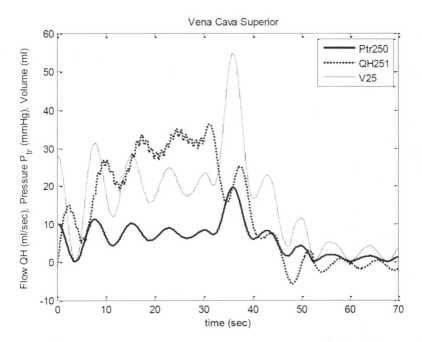

Fig. 10.10 This figure addresses the question of what is likely to go wrong when traditional CPR is applied subsequent to a serious heart attack. The heart is operating normally for the first 30 s. At $t = 30$ s the heart attack occurs and the heart becomes asystolic. At $t = 40$ s, CPR is initiated and maintained (freq. 60/min, ampl. 0–100 mmHg). During the intervening 10 s major changes occur in the vena cava superior. Immediately after the institution of CPR the volume (V_{25}) as well as outflow (Q_{H251}) of this large vein reduce and become negligible in a matter of around 30 s, thereby greatly reducing venous return from the upper part of the body to the right atrium. As described in the text, Sect. 11.4.11, the equations for the largest veins include the nonlinearities that accompany changes in their shapes. Similar effects take place in the intrathoracic segment of the vena cava inferior and in the pulmonary veins. Hence, traditional CPR tends to impede the circulation in most patients (Noordergraaf G.J. et al. in prep.)

return to Harvey's ideas under non-Harveyan circumstances. Obstruction of venous return may well mean that Kouwenhoven's recommendation to administer CCCR, as currently interpreted, is seriously flawed and is in need of either thorough modification or replacement. This failure refers to his erroneous idea that the ventricles are squeezed between the sternum and the spinal column (Noordergraaf G.J. et al. 2011).

10.4   Notes on Selected Controls

Caution: The following list of control mechanisms operating in the cardiovascular system is undoubtedly incomplete, owing to the belief that many more remain to be discovered. In addition, most of those identified cannot be quantitated since the requisite experiments are incomplete, or have not become available at all, leading to yet unknown parameter values.

(a) *Control of circulating volume*
Another quantity that is subject to intense control is the circulatory volume itself. In constant contact with the extravascular fluid at the capillary wall interface, it is exposed to fluid exchange with a very much larger fluid volume. One of the major controls on circulatory blood volume is exercised by the kidneys.

(b) *Evaluation of control by skeletal muscle activity*
Some of the basic properties that play a role during physical exercise are summarized in Sect. 8.1, though little attention has been devoted to measurements regarding the direct fluidic effects on veins by skeletal muscle contraction and relaxation as occurs in walking, jogging, running, etc., though unsubstantiated claims of their salubrious effects abound.

(c) *Ozanam*
The available analysis of "pumping by influence" is presented in Sect. 8.4.

(d) *Arterial instability*
An early mathematical and experimental approach may be found in Sect. 6.2. The flexibility of impedance-defined flow was emphasized repeatedly in this and preceding chapters. Arterial instability is the most extreme appearance of it uncovered thus far.

(e) *Rocking chair*
A brief discussion, which only identifies possibilities, may be found in Sect. 9.4.

10.5   Conclusions

The cardiovascular system incorporates a wide range of controls that make it possible to adapt cardiac output to current demands. These are either inside the system or outside and support a consistent state of the system. The internal controls make extensive use of the adjustment of parameters.

The critical issue is whether or not consistency can be achieved within the cardiovascular system once this has been lost. This is not automatically assured. For example, cardiopulmonary resuscitation may fail to achieve a new homeostasis after a serious heart attack. The feedback loops, once out of control may in fact limit the ability of the system to return to homeostasis.

10.6   Summary

This chapter deals with cooperation among controls. When physical and/or mental activity is instituted, additional mechanisms come into play. These include a variety of neural effects, including the baroreceptors, smooth muscle activity, skeletal muscle contraction and relaxation, operating particularly on veins and on pressure autoregulation which shifts the cardiac function curves. These mechanisms contribute under the general heading of impedance-defined flow, a newly formulated principle of flow generation (1998, Sect. 8.3). Together, the identified mechanisms, with valves or without valves, can raise cardiac output by a significant factor, as observed to occur in a healthy mammal. These conclusions generalize Harvey's view, from recognizing the heart as the only pump (1628), to the recognition of a multitude of pumps (1998), among which the ventricles, located in sensitive positions, count as the more spectacular individual contributors.

Section 10.3 offers a further analysis of why the CPR procedure shows low survival rates. This analysis was carried out with the aid of the Donders model, which permits access to measurements of blood flow. Administration of high massage pressures, currently fashionable, tend to collapse central veins, such as the superior vena cava, the thoracic section of the inferior vena cava, and the terminal parts of the pulmonary veins These veins generally prevent venous return to occur fast enough to refill the atria in preparation for the next massage cycle, an effect that apparently has been overlooked ever since Kouwenhoven et al. introduced their noninvasive procedure.

References

Amoroso E.C., Edholm O.G, and Rewell R.E. (1947) Venous valves in the giraffe, okapi, camel and ostrich. Proc. Zoological Soc. London 117: 435–440.

Beneken J.E.W., Wit de B.: A Physical Approach to Hemodynamic Aspects of the Human Cardiovascular System. Chap 1 in: Physical Basis of Circulatory Transport: Regulation and Exchange. E.B. Reeve and A. Guyton (eds.) Saunders, Philadelphia PA, 1967.

Brecher G.A.: Venous Return. Grune and Stratton, New York, NY, 1956.

Cannon W.B.: Organization for physiological homeostasis. Physiol. Rev. 9: 399–431, 1929.

Cannon W.B.: The Wisdom of the Body. Norton NY, 1932.

Cecchini A.B.P., Melbin J. and Noordergraaf A.: Set-point: Is it a distinct structural entity in biological control? J. Theor. Biol. 93: 387–394, 1981.

Cole R.T., Lucas C.L., Cascio W.E., Johnson T.A.: A LabVIEW^{TM} model incorporating an open-loop arterial impedance and a closed loop circulatory system. Ann. Biomed. Eng. 33: 1555–1573, 2005.

Donders F.C.: Physiologie des Menschen, Hirzel, Leipzig, 1856.

Drzewiecki G.M., Li J.K-J., Noordergraaf A.: Autoregulating Windkessel Dynamics May Cause Low Frequency Oscillations. Chapter 14 in: The Biomedical Engineering Handbook, Third Ed.,Vol. 1,.D. Bronzino (ed.), CRC Press, Boca Raton FL, 2006.

Essler S., Schroeder M.J., Phaniraj V., Koenig S.C., Latham R.D. and Ewert D.: Fast estimation of arterial vascular parameters for transient and steady beats with application to hemodynamic state under variant gravitational conditions. Ann. Biomed. Eng. 27: 486–497, 1999.

Fredericq L.: Influence du milieu ambiant sur la composition du sang des animaux aquatiques. Arch. Zoologie Expérimentale et Gén., Deuxième série, Tome troisième, XXIII, Librairie de C. Reinwald, Paris, 1885.

Goetz R.H., Warren J.V., Gauer O.H., Patterson J.L. Jr., Doyle J.T., Keen E.N. and McGregor M.: Circulation of the giraffe. Circ. Res. 8: 1049–1058, 1960. Also in: J.V. Warren: Scientific American 231: 96–105, 1974.

Guyton A.C.: A concept of negative interstitial pressure based on pressures in implanted perforated capsules. Circul. Res. 12: 399–414, 1963a.

Guyton A.C.: Textbook of Medical Physiology. Saunders, Philadelphia PA, 1963b, 1966.

Guyton A.C., Coleman T.G. and Granger H.J.: Circulation: Overall regulation. Ann. Rev. Physiol. 34: 13–46, 1972.

Ha R.R., Qian J., Ware D.L., Zwischenberger B., Bidani A., Clark J.W. Jr.: An integrative cardiovascular model of the standing and reclining sheep. Cardiov. Eng. 5: 53–76, 2005.

Han: Vasculature as functional valves during cough CPR as a example of impedance defined flow. Project report in a course taught by A. Noordergraaf, Univ. of Pennsylvania, 2009.

Harvey W.: On the Motion of the Heart and Blood in Animals (Translated by R. Willis). On the Circulation of the Blood. On the Generation of Animals. Encycl. Britannica, pp. 263–496, 1952.

Hering H.E.: Die Änderung der Herzschlagzahl durch Änderung des arteriellen Blutdruckes erfolgt auf reflektorischem Wege. Pflüg. Arch. ges. Physiol. 206: 721–723, 1924a.

Hering H.E.: Der Sinus caroticus an der Ursprungsstelle der Carotus interna als Ausgangsort eines hemmenden Herzreflexes und eines depressorischen Gefässreflexes. Münch. med. Wochnschr. 71: 701–704, 1924b.

Ichikawa Y.: A new RV-PA conduit with a natural valve made of bovine jugular vein. ASAIO Journal 38: M266-270, 1992.

Karreman G. and Weygandt C.N.: Theoretical Control Aspects of the Circulation. Ch. 52 in: Cardiovascular System Dynamics, J. Baan et al. (eds.), MIT Press, Cambridge MA, 1978.

Katona P.G., Poitras J.W., Barnett G.O. and Terry B.S.: Cardiac vagal efferent activity and heart period in the carotid sinus reflex. Am. J. Physiol. 218: 1030–1037, 1970.

Koeken Y.J.C.: The Role of the Larger Veins in Cardiopulmonary Resuscitation. M.Sc. Thesis, Eindhoven Tech. Univ., Eindhoven, The Netherlands, 2009.

Kouwenhoven W.B., Jude J.R. and Knickerbocker G.G.: Closed chest cardiac massage. JAMA 173: 1064–1067, 1960.

Latham R.D., Fanton J.W., White C.D., Vernalis M.N., Crisman R.P. and Koenig S.C.: Circulatory filling pressures during transient microgravity induced by parabolic flight. The Physiologist 36: S-18-S-19, 1993.

Latham R.D., Fanton J.W., Vernalis M.N., Gaffney F.A. and Crisman R.P.: Central hemodynamics in a baboon model during microgravity induced by parabolic flight. Adv. Space Res. 14: 349–358, 1994.

Lau D.J.: Simulation of the effect of different left ventricular massage protocols using the Donders model: a CPR study. Project report in a course taught by A. Noordergraaf, Univ. of Pennsylvania, 2008.

Lee: Compression frequency as an independent factor in cardiac output in CPR: modeling the Donders model. Project report in a course taught by A. Noordergraaf, Univ. of Pennsylvania, 2009.

Levy M.N.: Neural Control of the Heart: Sympathetic-Vagal Interactions. Ch. 39 in: Cardiovascular System Dynamics, J. Baan et al. (eds.), MIT Press, Cambridge, 1978.

Mayer S.: Studien zur Physiologie des Herzens und der Blutgefässe. V. Über spontane Blutdrucksch-wankungen. Sitzungsber. d. Kais. Akad. Wiss. Wien. Math-Nat. 74: 281–307, 1876.

McNally R.T.: Automated Infusion Apparatus to Control Hemodynamic Variables. Ph. D. Dissertation, Univ. of Pennsylvania, 1978.

Melbin J., Detweiler D.K., Riffle R.A. and Noordergraaf A.: Coherence of cardiac output with rate changes. Am. J. Physiol. 243 (Heart Circ. Physiol. 12): H499-H504, 1982.

Morgagni J.B.: De Sedibus, et Causis Morborum per Anatomen Indagatis. Libri Quinque. Epistola XIX, Art. 34. Ex Typographia Remondiniana, Venetiis, pp. 180–192, 1761.

Moser M., Huang J.W., Schwarz G.S., Kenner T., Noordergraaf A.: Impedance defined flow. Generalisation of William Harvey's concept of the circulation - 370 years later. Int. J. Cardiov. Med. and Science 1: 205–211, 1998.

Noordergraaf A.: Circulatory System Dynamics. Academic Press, New York, NY, 1978.

Noordergraaf G.J., Tilborg van G.F.A.J.B., Schoonen J.A.P., Ottesen J., Scheffer G..J., Noordergraaf A.: Thoracic CT-scans and cardiovascular models: the effect of external force in CPR. Int. J. Cardiovascular Med. and Science. 5: 1–7, 2005a.

Noordergraaf G.J., Dijkema T.J., Kortsmit W.J.P.M., Schilders W.H.A., Scheffer G.J. and Noordergraaf A.: Modeling in cardiopulmonary resuscitation: Pumping the heart. Cardiov. Eng. 5: 105–118, 2005b.

Noordergraaf G.J., Schilders W.H.A., Scheffer G.J., Noordergraaf A.: Essential factors in CPR? Modeling and clinical aspects (abstract). 2nd Science day, Dutch Society for Anesthesia (Amsterdam), 2005c.

Noordergraaf G.J., Ottesen J.T., Kortsmit W.J.P.M., Schilders W.H.A., Scheffer G.J. and Noordergraaf A.: The Donders model of the circulation in normo- and pathophysiology. Cardiov. Eng. 6: 53–72, 2006.

Noordergraaf G.J.: Cardiopulmonary Resuscitation: Are Two Hands (Really) Enough? A modeling approach to CPR. Ph.D. Dissertation. Radboud Univ. Nijmegen, Nijmegen NL, 2009.

Noordergraaf G.J., Paulussen I., Aelen P., Woerlee P. and Noordergraaf A.: Thoracic volume, a critical factor in the physiology of CPR. Submitted.

Palladino J.L., Drzewiecki G.M. and Noordergraaf A.: Modeling Strategies in Physiology. Chapter 158 in: Biomedical Engineering Handbook. J.D. Bronzino, (ed.), CRC Press, Boca Raton FL, 2000a.

Palladino J.L., Ribeiro L.C. and Noordergraaf A.: Human Circulatory System Model Based on Frank's Mechanism. Pp. 29–40 in: Mathematical Modelling in Medicine, J.T. Ottesen and M. Danielsen (eds.), IOS Press, Amsterdam, 2000b.

Palladino J.L., Drzewiecki G.M., Noordergraaf G.J., Dijkema T.J. and Noordergraaf A.: Modeling Strategies and Cardiovascular Dynamics, Ch. 8 in: Biomedical Engineering Handbook, 3rd ed. J.D. Bronzino (ed.), CRC Press, Boca Raton, 2006.

Quick C.M., Young W.L. and Noordergraaf A.: Infinite number of solutions to the hemodynamic inverse problem. Am. J. Physiol. 280: H1472-H1479, 2001a.

Quick C.M., Berger D.S. and Noordergraaf A.: Constructive and destructive addition of forward and reflected arterial pulse waves in the arterial system. Am. J. Physiol. 280: H1519-H1527, 2001b.

Rahn H., Otis A.B., Chadwick L.E. and Fenn W.O.: The pressure-volume diagram of the thorax and the lung. Am. J. Physiol. 146: 161–178, 1946.

Rajaei J.N.: The modeling and analysis of volume trapping in CPR through the use of the Donders model. Project report in a course taught by A. Noordergraaf, Univ. of Pennsylvania, 2008.

Rist P.: Jugular vein valves in cows and horses. Project report in a course taught by A. Noordergraaf, Univ. of Pennsylvania, 2006.

Stein A.F.: Modeling valveless flow using the Donders model. Project report in a course taught by A. Noordergraaf, Univ. of Pennsylvania, 2008.

Stephenson H.E. Jr., Reid L.C., Heyton J.S.: Pitfalls, precautions and complications in cardiac resuscitation; study of 1,200 cases. AMA Arch. Surg. 69: 37–53, 1954.

Taher M.F., Cecchini A.B.P., Allen M.A., Gobran S.R., Gorman R.C., Guthrie B.L., Lingenfelter K.A.,, Rabbany S.Y, Rolchigo P.M., Melbin J. and Noordergraaf A.: Baroreceptor responses derived from a fundamental concept. Ann. Biomed. Eng. 16: 429–443, 1988.

Traube L.: Über periodische Thätigkeit-Äusserungen des vasomotorischen und Hemmungs-Nervencentrum. Centralblatt med. Wissenschaften 3: 881–885, 1865.

Versprille A.: Volumes en Mechanische Aspecten. Chapter 2.2 in: H.J. Sluiter et al. (eds.): Longziekten, Van Gorcum, Assen, 2nd ed., 1995.

Warner H.R.: The frequency-dependent nature of blood pressure regulation by the carotid sinus studied with an electrical analog. Circ. Res. 6: 35–40, 1958.

Warner H.R.: Some Computer Techniques of Value for Study of Circulation. Ch. 10 in: Computers in Biomedical Research, vol. II. R.W. Stacy and B. Waxman, (eds.), Academic Press, New York, NY, 1965.

Warner H.R. and Cox A.: A mathematical model of heart rate control by sympathetic and vagus efferent information. J. Appl. Physiol. 17: 349–355, 1962.

Warner H.R. and Russell R.D. Jr.: Effect of combined sympathetic and vagal stimulation on heart rate in the dog. Circ. Res. 24: 567–573, 1969.

Warren J.V.: The physiology of the giraffe. Scient. American 231: 96–105, 1974.

Wiggers C.J., Levy M.N. and Graham G.: Regional intrathoracic pressures and their bearing on calculation of effective pressures. Amer. J. Physiol. 151: 1–12, 1947.

Appendix

Questions

10.1 What happens to the external work done by a ventricle, if the amount of arterial reflection increases while mean pressure remains unchanged?

10.2 Identify the physiological meaning of G and of H in Eqs. 10.4.

10.3 Are the closed loop transfer functions, defined as output/input, in Figs. 10.2b and 10.3c identical?

10.4 Compute the highest value of G, as a function of p_0 (Fig. 10.1a), for which the cerebral perfusion pressure in the upright position equals zero.

10.5 An experiment is performed to record the baroreceptor firing rate as a function of blood pressure in a carotid artery. The time it takes to execute this experiment is much shorter than the value of the longest of the time constants τ in Eq. 10.9. Will the recorded firing rates depend on the baroreceptor's history preceding this experiment?

10.6 Investigators who develop artificial hearts like to design this prosthetic device such that it exhibits a cardiac function curve. They tend to refer to such a device as having control over cardiac output. Correct?

10.7 If Eq. 10.6 is transposed to the venous system between the head and the heart in a standing giraffe and it is assumed that the venous channel is uninterrupted, can it be argued that the pressure in these veins is negative compared to right atrial pressure used as a reference, i.e., set to zero?

10.8 The inverted, nonuniform rigid U tube in Fig. 10.11 identifies constant pressures p_1, and p_3, steady flow Q and two resistances R_1 and R_2 representing the arterial and venous divisions of the cerebral microcirculation. The pressure between R_1 and R_2 is denoted p_2. Compute flow Q.

Fig. 10.11 Pertains to Qu. 10–8

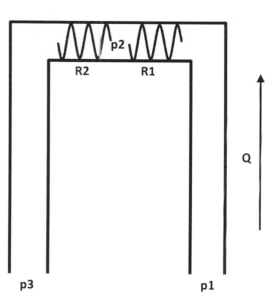

Will this flow increase, decrease, or remain the same when the U tube is placed in the horizontal instead of the vertical position (idealized version of the syphon effect)?

10.9   Offer a likely response to the issue raised by Essler (1999).

10.10 In view of the significance of impedance-defined flow, could its enhancement offer an alternative to the application of standard CPR when the heart fails? "Cough" CPR (Sect. 9.4) supports this solution, though only for a short interval of time.

10.11 Do equines and bovines have valves in their neck veins? Argue why they need or do not need them.

10.12 In Sect. 10.2, it was pointed out that the heart is in a critical position owing to the in series arrangement. The closed loop as a whole will suffer when serious cardiac damage takes place. Does viewing it as two pumps in series ameliorate the situation somewhat, if only the left or the right heart becomes impaired?

10.13 Immediately after the heart goes into fibrillation (stops pumping), a supply of oxygen and metabolites should still be available in the peripheral tissue that can continue the functioning of the many noncardiac pumps. Could this be made to serve as a safety feature to take quick corrective action?

10.14 Does the variation in a measurable quantity, such as cardiac output, red blood cell concentration, etc. among healthy persons, offer a hint of the minimal accuracy with which relevant models should be designed?

10.15 Central veins have a sufficiently high compliance to change size noticeably during the respiratory cycle. Qualitatively, how does this relate to the respiratory phases? How to the modulation of stroke volume and root aortic pressure?

10.16 Quantitatively, how much does phase velocity, c_{ph}, alter in the vena cava superior when its external pressure, p_{ec}, ranges from 50 to 100 mmHg? (Hint: Nonlinear properties of veins are discussed in Sect. 5.2.)

10.17 Argue why compression by $p_{ec}(t)$ can reduce blood volume in a vein promptly, while refilling requires more time, an effect that has apparently been overlooked for nearly half a century.

Answers

10.1   Generally, little. The principal term for work arises from the mean pressure, which was given to be unchanged.
       Misconceptions often arose, owing to miscalculation of reflected wave magnitudes (Quick et al. 2001).

10.2 G is the slope of a tangent to the curve depicting the neurological control, thus defining the sensitivity of this control effect. G goes to zero for very low and very high values of carotid pressure. H plays a similar though simpler role for the sensitivity to fluidic effects.

10.3 No; in (b) the closed loop transfer function (or, closed loop gain) for p_a equals: $G/(1+GH)$, for p_c: $GH/(1+GH)$; in (c), they are $1/(1+GH)$ and $H/(1+GH)$, respectively.

10.4 From Eq. 10.7b: $Gp_0/(1+G) = \rho gh/(1+G)$, hence $G = \rho gh/p_0$. For smaller values of G, $p_c < 0$

10.5 Yes. The term with the longest time constant will tend to carry over.

10.6 A more correct statement would be that CO responds to filling pressure (or volume), which depends on venous pressure.

10.7 Yes. If right atrial pressure is arbitrarily set at zero, venous pressure will be $-\rho gh$ at vertical distance h above the atrium. This follows directly from the transposed Eq. 10.6 since its left side becomes zero.

10.8

$$p_1 - p_2 = QR_1 + \rho gh \qquad (10.10a)$$

$$p_2 - p_3 = QR_2 - \rho gh \qquad (10.10b)$$

Addition of the two expressions gives

$$Q = \frac{p_1 - p_3}{R_1 + R_2}, \qquad (10.11)$$

which is independent of g and h. Hence, flow will remain unchanged.

10.9 As demonstrated in Sect. 4.2, body motion may alter pressure and flow signals, even in a simple system where the parameters are held constant. In a living system, as applied by the authors, this constancy may not apply. The author allows that other effects may occur as well, which could mean that the observed effects may not be exclusively attributable to modification of the system properties.

10.10 Yes, if OCCR is administered.

10.11 What little evidence is available indicates that bovines definitely have valves in their jugulars, as do humans (Ichikawa 1992). There is scattered evidence that equines share this feature. The presumed reason why they do is the same as in the giraffe: lower venous blood pressure in the head-down position (Rist 2006).

10.12 Yes, possibly. There are documented claims that the left ventricle can carry the total load when the right ventricle becomes asystolic or fibrillates.

10.13 No readymade solution has become available, yet.

10.14 Ideally, a model should incorporate sufficient accuracy to address a particular individual question regarding the topic of interest.

10.15 Inspiration lowers the intrathoracic pressure around the veins in the thorax. This increases the transmural pressure across the venous walls, which tends to enlarge the venous lumina, thereby facilitating venous return to the right heart. During the next relaxation of the right ventricle when the tricuspid valve opens, more blood will be available for enhanced filling and stroke volume will increase. This increase will be terminated upon the onset of expiration. The larger stroke volume is transmitted through the pulmonary vasculature with a delay of a few heartbeats (depending on flow velocity in the pulmonary system). The phenomenon of a variable stroke volume will be repeated in the left heart, which, in turn, modulates root aortic pressure. In the normal, continuous root aortic blood pressure sensing tends to display the modulation clearly.

10.16 Wave velocity loses interest, because the compliance becomes small while the impedance becomes large (Fig. 10.10).

10.17 A high peak pressure of $p_{ec}(t)$ in conjunction with low flow impedance easily moves the blood out. Neither feature is available for the refilling process.

Chapter 11
Models of Cardiovascular Subsystems Yielding the Closed Circulatory Loop: The Donders Model

> [...] en daer in bestaet de Sijstole ofte 't neerstijgingh der Slagaderen, [....] in 't eynde van deze neersijgingh keert het bloedt welck in de Slag-aderen is [....] wederom naer 't Hert, maar en gaet niet in sijne holligheden, om dat het maecksel van die klapvlieskens soodan.gh is, datse door desen wederloop des bloedts noodsaeckelijk worden toegeslooten....

> — Renatus des Cartes (1596–1650) aen Joh. van Beverwijck [excerpts from the original letter]

Digest Model of the cardiovascular loop diagramed using electrical symbols for an overview and by means of equations for further analysis. The model includes the four cardiac chambers, their valves, which open and close passively, and the connecting vasculatures. Generalized cardiac function curves are described, access and insertion points for several control features are identified. The model can be adapted easily to the study of CPR and other clinical conditions. The disappearance of negative volumes.

Models serve a number of purposes, not the least of which is the performance of experiments, not executable in the living mammal.

11.1 General Introduction and Guide Through Symbols

The model of the closed loop cardiovascular system as used in this book (the Donders model, version 2007) is illustrated in Fig. 11.1. For the purpose of providing an overview it is drawn utilizing electrical symbols, giving it the appearance of an analog model. In subsequent sections, the same model will be formulated mathematically, i.e., in the form of equations, subsystem by subsystem, while

A. Noordergraaf, *Blood in Motion*, DOI 10.1007/978-1-4614-0005-9_11,
© Springer Science+Business Media, LLC 2011

pointing out alternative possibilities in some cases. Model solutions consistently derive directly from equations. In the figure, standard terminology is inserted to facilitate locating principal sections of the closed loop.

The four chambers of the heart are identified by their names. All cardiac valves and representatives of peripheral valves are shown individually by the diode symbol and identified by a single capital letter, or by a letter/number combination. The vascular networks connecting the right and the left heart are easily recognizable and identified as arteries, peripheral vessels, and veins.

In the diagram, as well as in the corresponding equations, the most frequently occurring letter symbols are p, denoting local pressure (blood or air), Q, denoting (volume) flow, counted positive in the direction of the accompanying arrow, V, representing volume and t, an independent variable, defining time. In the model 38 $p(t)$'s, 26 $Q_H(t)$'s, 17 $Q_V(t)$'s, and 17 $V(t)$'s are recognized. They appear, together with eight other quantities (2 F's, 2 B's and the signs of 4 a's) as 106 unknown variables to be determined, in a system of 106 equations, some algebraic, others differential or integral. They are marked with asterisks.

The cardiac chambers are defined by their passive and active pressure (p)–volume (V) relations. The quantity dV/dp expresses their strongly time-varying compliance during these phases.

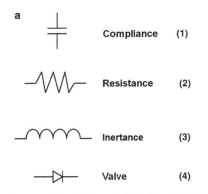

Fig. 11.1 (a) From top to bottom; electrical symbols in Fig 11.1b, their names and functions: (1) Capacitor, representing compliant properties of the compartments; (2) Resistance, representing viscous properties of blood; (3) Inductor, representing blood's inertial properties; (4) Passive valve. (b) Version 2007 of the Donders model presented in electrical symbols. The corresponding governing equations are listed in the text of this chapter. Extracardiac circulating blood volume equals 5.2 l. The initial conditions were all flows equal to zero and 15 mmHg applied to all compliances. Resulting pressures, printed in *red*; volumes in *green*, flows in *blue*, with *arrows* defining positive direction of flow, this version is a significant upgrade from the 2006 version (Noordergraaf G.J. et al. 2006)

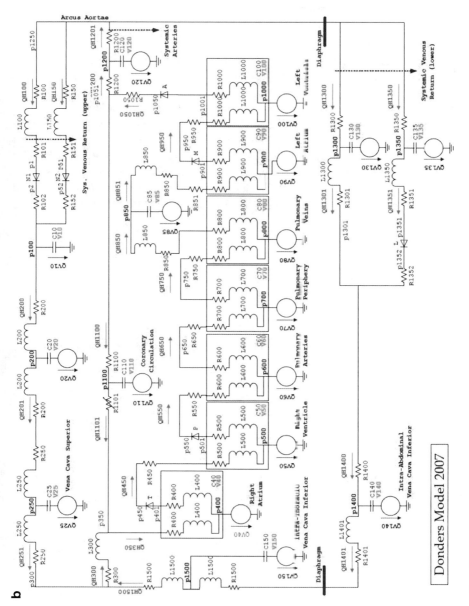

Fig. 11.1 (continued)

11.2   Passive Time-Varying Features

Valve opening is taken to be pressure driven, i.e., whenever pressure directly upstream from a valve equals or exceeds pressure immediately downstream of that valve, the ostium will permit flow. This flow will continue until conditions change and ostial flow changes direction. Valve closure is taken to occur as a consequence of this retrograde flow. Descartes already appreciated these mechanisms. This approach is applied to cardiac as well as to peripheral valves. Competent valves are considered to shut by the time the magnitude of back flow amounts to a few (e.g., 5) percent of the maximum of the forward flow signal immediately preceding it.

Seven valves are incorporated in this model: four in the heart and three representative ones in the peripheral vasculature, one each in the drainage part of the cerebral and brachial circulations (called the N-valves), and at the outlet of the veins draining the legs (designated the L-valve). Hence, the valve leaflets themselves are considered passive, their timing independent of each other, while opening and closing as dictated by local conditions. The seven equations defining open or closed valves, in terms of pressures, are:

Tricuspid valve, open:

$$p_{401} = p_{450} \qquad\qquad (*11.1a)$$

closed:

$$p_{450} = p_{500} \qquad\qquad (*11.1b)$$

Pulmonary valve, open:

$$p_{501} = p_{550} \qquad\qquad (*11.2a)$$

closed:

$$p_{550} = p_{600} \qquad\qquad (*11.2b)$$

Mitral valve, open:

$$p_{901} = p_{950} \qquad\qquad (*11.3a)$$

closed:

$$p_{950} = p_{1000} \qquad\qquad (*11.3b)$$

Aortic valve, open:

$$p_{1001} = p_{1050} \qquad (*11.4\text{a})$$

closed:

$$p_{1050} = p_{1200} \qquad (*11.4\text{b})$$

N1 valve, open:

$$p_1 = p_2 \qquad (*11.5\text{a})$$

closed:

$$p_2 = p_{100} \qquad (*11.5\text{b})$$

N2 valve, open:

$$p_{51} = p_{52} \qquad (*11.6\text{a})$$

closed:

$$p_{52} = p_{100} \qquad (*11.6\text{b})$$

L valve, open:

$$p_{1351} = p_{1352} \qquad (*11.7\text{a})$$

closed:

$$p_{1352} = p_{1301} \qquad (*11.7\text{b})$$

In most cases, the local state of some property such as inertial or viscous effects is defined by parameters, initially treated as constants. A small number of parameters, primarily of the cardiac chambers, however, is time dependent, introducing nonlinearities. The open circles in Fig. 11.1 permit insertion of the influence of the respiratory system on the circulatory loop, $p_{er}(t)$, playing the role of intrapleural pressure, or of the influence of chest compression, $p_{ec}(t)$, during institution of CPR. In the equations below, both quantities frequently appear as $p_e(t)$, without a second index, as the same sign applies to both in the equations, though their own signs are generally opposite. The respiratory signal, $p_{er}(t)$, is treated as a time-dependent parameter (i.e., a given function, Fig. 10.4), as it is primarily defined outside the cardiovascular loop. The same applies to the pressure, $p_{ec}(t)$, resulting from chest compression in cardiopulmonary resuscitation (CPR), in casu defined by the caregiver. Different profiles may be applied.

For the purpose of model analysis and interpretation of what is observed, it is convenient to distinguish the blood volume in two conceptual categories, named and defined in Table 11.2. They are the filling volume and the circulating volume. The filling volume is defined as the volume that equalizes inside and outside pressures. Denoted the transmural pressure, p_{tr}, the filling volume occurs when the transmural pressure equals zero under normal healthy conditions. The circulating volume, which incorporates the filling volume, appears in some of the equations in Sect. 10.4, is larger in most instances, making $p_{tr} > 0$. It is simply referred to as "volume," V. The value of p_{tr} enables quantification, by turning negative, of partial to complete collapse of compartments, which, in turn, may obstruct blood flow. This is prone to occur in CPR (Sect 10.3).

The descent of the atrioventricular junction during early ventricular ejection was identified by Brecher and his followers as causing the first (of two) surges of venous flow into the heart (Sect. 3.4). Attributed to atrial wall stretching, the occurrence of this negative transmural pressure is usually small enough not to cause collapse of the atrial cavities. For the atria this phenomenon is passive in nature and is included in the atrial equations (Eqs. 11.49 and 11.83) in Sect. 11.4 by making the parameter b in Eqs. 4.6a, 7.2, and 8.1a time variant. In pictorial form, b appears as a constant in Fig. 7.3.

Changes in circulating volume, V, may be identified from the solutions to the equations in Sect. 4.3. Quantities of interest include average flows, volumes, and pressures as well as their variations with respect to time. For circulating volume evaluation right and left ventricular cardiac output may carry instructive information. The Donders model permits quantitative identification of these phenomena.

11.3 Active Features

Inasmuch as all blood vessels possess compliant properties their diameters change with alteration of internal and external pressures (passive modulation). In addition, many of these vessels contain smooth muscle as a constituent of their wall materials. Commonly, the smooth muscle is innervated and/or sensitive to metabolic concentrations, which, in turn, can bring about changes in vessel diameter (active modulation). This bestows a great deal of control of blood flow throughout the cardiovascular system.

The compliant properties of vessels are embodied by utilizing a capacitor, denoted C, where electrical symbols are employed. The symbol C also appears in the equations. Its classical definition relates a small change in volume, dV, to the concomitant small change in pressure, dp, in the form

$$C = \frac{dV}{dp},$$

(11.8b)

In Eq. 5.13b its value, taken per unit axial vessel length and denoted C', is related to vessel radius, r, wall thickness, h, as well as to the elastic modulus, E, of the composite wall material. Neural and metabolic stimulation is interpreted as affecting the value of E. Changes in wall stiffness may cause alteration in vessel dimensions, which carry over as modification of the dimension sensitive inertial and viscous effects, as do volume changes from other causes. Such nonlinear phenomena may have to be specified by additional mathematical statements. Examples of practical applications are presented in several chapters.

The variation in compliant properties of the cardiac chambers have been studied far more extensively and are much better understood than those of peripheral vessels. In Eq. 4.6b activation/relaxation curves for the cardiac chambers are described by a function $f(t)$, distinguished by additional indices for the individual chambers. These basic functions capture most, though not all, behavioral aspects in a simple form, with additional equations in Chaps. 4 and 8 broadening their scope. The following expressions were designed to define $f(.)$ as a real function of time. The same form applies to all four chambers, though the parameter values may be different. For the left atrium the equations read:

$$f_{LA}(t) = \frac{1 - e^{-\left(\frac{t}{\tau_c}\right)^\alpha}}{\left[1 - e^{-\left(\frac{t_p}{\tau_c}\right)^\alpha}\right] e^{-\left(\frac{t_p - t_d}{\tau_r}\right)^\alpha}} \tag{11.9a}$$

for

$$0 \leq t \leq t_d \tag{11.9b}$$

$$f_{LA}(t) = \frac{\left[1 - e^{-\left(\frac{t}{\tau_c}\right)^\alpha}\right] e^{-\left(\frac{t - t_d}{\tau_r}\right)^\alpha}}{\left[1 - e^{-\left(\frac{t_p}{\tau_c}\right)^\alpha}\right] e^{-\left(\frac{t_p - t_d}{\tau_r}\right)^\alpha}} \tag{11.9c}$$

for

$$t_d \leq t \leq t_h \tag{11.9d}$$

With

$$t_d = t_p - \tau_r \left[-ln \left\{ 1 - e^{-\left[\frac{t_p}{\tau_c}\right]^\alpha} \right\} \right]^{\frac{1}{\alpha}} \tag{11.10}$$

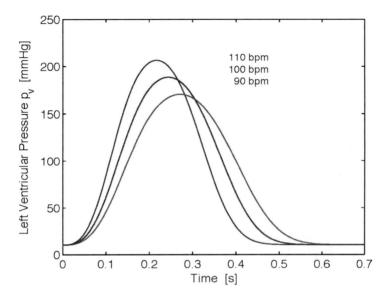

Fig. 11.2 The effect of reducing t_p, τ_c, and τ_r by the same proportion (in Eqs. 11.9a, b and 11.10 as would apply left atrium) to accommodate increasing heart rate as well as altering isovolumic pressure wave shape (Adapted from Palladino et al. 2011). The same procedure is presumed to apply to the right ventricle, as well as to both atria

The parameters in these three expressions denote: t_p = time to peak pressure, counting from onset of contraction of that chamber, t_h = time to end of relaxation, τ_c and τ_r are time constants during contraction and relaxation, respectively, α changes overall rates of contraction and relaxation, and "ln" denotes the natural logarithm. Heart rate may be changed by altering t_h only, or, if the change in shape should be taken into account in isovolumic beats, by changing t_p, τ_c, τ_r, in the same proportion (Fig. 11.2, Palladino et al., 4th edition of the *Biomed. Eng. Handbook*).

In Fig. 10.5, top, the normalized activation/relaxation functions $f_{LA}(t)$ and $f_{LV}(t)$, oscillating between 0 and 1, are depicted in realistic, though adjustable, time relation. They serve identically as $f_{RA}(t)$ and $f_{RV}(t)$, respectively. For a range of parameter values, the denominators in Eqs. 11.9 may be dropped, as their values approximate 1 closely. Similarly, in Eq. 11.10 t_d and t_p may frequently be considered equal (Palladino et al., 4th edition of the *Biomed. Eng. Handbook*). Default values of basically constant parameters may be found in Table 11.1.

The downstroke in the normal pressure–volume relation for large volumes (originally documented by Otto Frank, 1899, Fig. 4.23) may be introduced as described in Sect. 4.3, Eqs. 4.8 and 4.9, and depicted in Fig. 4.26. The effects on cardiac output caused by overfilling and weakening in the pathological heart, described in Sect. 9.1, can be modeled similarly (not currently incorporated).

Table 11.1 Default values of the parameters in the 2007 Donders model (Fig. 11.1)

Inductances	(g cm^{-4})	Compliances	$(\text{cm}^3 \text{ mmHg}^{-1})$
L100	0.016	C10	20
L150	0.016	C20	26
L200	1	C25	2.8
L250	0.745	C60	4
L300	0.02	C70	10
L400	0	C80	30
L500	0.001	C85	1.2
L600	0	C110	0.02
L700	0.00017	C120	4
L800	0	C130	40
L850	0.32	C135	30
L900	0	C140	80
L1000	0.0005	C150	1.4
L1300	0		
L1350	0		
L1401	0		
L1500	0.37		

plus four cardiac p–V relations with variable C values (Eqs. *11.48, *11.57, *11.82 and *11.90)

Resistances	(mmHg s ml^{-1})	Heart parameters		
R100	8.5	a_RA	0.0032	mmHg ml^{-2}
R101	0.2	b_RA	5	ml
R102	0.2	c_RA	0.825	mmHg ml^{-1}
R150	12	d_RA	17	mmHg
R151	0.2	a_RV	0.0004	mmHg ml^{-2}
R152	0.2	b_RV	60	ml
R200	0.02	c_RV	2	mmHg ml^{-1}
R250	0.06	d_RV	50	mmHg
R300	0.00005	k1_RV	0.001	sec ml^{-1}
R400	0.00005	k2_RV	0.000005	sec ml^{-1}
R450	0.01	a_LA	0.0032	mmHg ml^{-2}
R500	0.0001	b_LA	5	ml
R550	0.035	c_LA	0.6	mmHg ml^{-1}
R600	0.00005	d_LA	17	mmHg
R650	0.2	a_LV	0.0004	mmHg ml^{-2}
R700	0.00005	b_LV	32.5	ml
R750	0.01	c_LV	4.6	mmHg ml^{-1}
R800	0.00005	d_LV	90	mmHg
R850	0.03	k1_LV	0.001	sec ml^{-1}
R851	0.02	k2_LV	0.000005	sec ml^{-1}
R900	0.0005			
R950	0.004			
R1000	0.0025			
R1050	0.0005			

(continued)

Table 11.1 (continued)

Resistances	(mmHg s ml^{-1})	Heart parameters	
R1100	18.3	*Time parameters*	
R1101	327	HR	60
R1200	0.055	T	60/HR
R1300	2	t-delay	0.15 s
R1301	0.1	p_int	10 mmHg
R1350	6.7	$\tau_{LV}^{[Eq.(10.57)]}$	T/3
R1351	0.1	$\tau_{LV}^{[Eq.(10.90)]}$	T/3
R1352	0.1		
R1400	0.04		
R1401	0.027		
R1500	0.04		

Timing parameters of the heart	Seconds
Left ventricle	
t_pLV	0.371
α	2.88
τ_{cLV}	0.264
τ_{rLV}	0.299
Left atrium	
t_pLA	0.1
α	2.88
τ_{cLA}	0.06
τ_{rLA}	0.08
Right atrium	
τ_{cRA}	0.06
τ_{rRA}	0.08
Right ventricle	
τ_{cRV}	0.264
τ_{rRV}	0.299

The influence of the stiffness of the pericardium may be included by adding a term of the type

$$p_{peri} = \psi e^{\left(\frac{V}{V_0}\right)^3} \tag{11.11}$$

to Eq. 4.6b, c, or d on the right-hand side, or to Eqs. 11.48 and/or 11.82 below, also on the right-hand side. In this expression V_0 denotes the total volume of the four chambers at which the pericardium begins to stiffen ($p_{peri} = 2.72\varphi$), which with $\varphi = 1$ mmHg adds less than 3 mmHg at an actual total chamber volume V equal to V_0, then rises rapidly with larger V (Mirsky and Rankin 1979). Thus the term gains significance as the heart dilates.

11.4 Equations for Individual Subsystems: Application to CPR Studies

11.4.1 Systemic Veins

The perfusion of the systemic microcirculation provides the blood that is collected by the small systemic veins, then guided to the large central systemic veins. The requirements for valve opening and closure are presented in Sect. 10.2. The equations for pressures, flows, and volumes are:

$$p_{1250} - p_1 = [R_{100} + R_{101}]Q_{H100} + L_{100}\frac{a}{dt}Q_{H100} \tag{*11.12}$$

$$p_{1250} - p_{51} = [R_{150} + R_{151}]Q_{H150} + L_{150}\frac{\acute{c}}{dt}Q_{H150} \tag{*11.13}$$

$$Q_{H100} = \frac{1}{L_{100}}\int[p_{1250} - p_{100} - (R_{100} + R_{101} + R_{102})Q_{H100}]dt \tag{*11.14}$$

$$Q_{H150} = \frac{1}{L_{150}}\int[p_{1250} - p_{100} - (R_{150} + R_{151} + R_{152})Q_{H150}]dt \tag{*11.15}$$

$$Q_{V10} = Q_{H150} + Q_{H100} - Q_{F200} \tag{*11.16}$$

$$Q_{V10} = C_{10}\frac{d}{dt}p_{100}Q_{V10} \tag{*11.17}$$

$$Q_{V20} = Q_{H200} - Q_{H201} \tag{*11.18}$$

$$Q_{V20} = C_{20}\frac{d}{dt}(p_{200} - p_{e}) \tag{*11.19}$$

$$Q_{H200} = \frac{1}{L_{200}}\int[p_{100} - p_{200} - R_{200} \times Q_{H100}]dt \tag{*11.20}$$

$$Q_{H201} = \frac{1}{L_{200} + L_{250}}\int[p_{200} - p_{250} - (R_{200} + R_{250})Q_{H201}]dt \tag{*11.21}$$

$$Q_{V25} = Q_{H201} - Q_{H251} \tag{*11.22}$$

$$Q_{V25} = C_{25}\frac{d}{dt}(p_{250} - p_{e}) \tag{*11.23}$$

$$Q_{H251} = \frac{1}{L_{250}}\int[p_{250} - p_{300} - R_{250}Q_{H251}]dt \tag{*11.24}$$

$$p_{1350} - p_{1351}L_{1350}\frac{d}{dt}Q_{H1351} + R_{1351}Q_{H1351} \qquad (*11.25)$$

$$Q_{V130} = C_{130}\frac{d}{dt}p_{1300} \qquad (*11.26)$$

$$Q_{V130} = Q_{H1300} - Q_{H1301} \qquad (*11.27)$$

$$Q_{V135} = C_{135}\frac{d}{dt}p_{1350} \qquad (*11.28)$$

$$Q_{V135} = Q_{H1350} - Q_{H1351} \qquad (*11.29)$$

$$Q_{H1351} = \frac{1}{L_{1350}}\int[p_{1350} - p_{1301} - (R_{1351} + R_{1352})Q_{H1351}]dt \qquad (*11.30)$$

$$Q_{V140} = C_{140}\frac{d}{dt}p_{1400} \qquad (*11.31)$$

$$Q_{V140} = Q_{H1400} - Q_{H1401} \qquad (*11.32)$$

$$Q_{H300} = Q_{H1500} + Q_{H251} \qquad (*11.33)$$

$$Q_{V150} = Q_{H1401} - Q_{H1500} \qquad (*11.34)$$

$$Q_{H1400} = Q_{H1301} + Q_{H1351} \qquad (*11.35)$$

$$p_{1300} - p_{1301} = L_{1300}\frac{d}{dt}Q_{H1301} + R_{1301}Q_{H1301} \qquad (*11.36)$$

$$p_{1301} - p_{1400} = R_{1400}Q_{H1400} \qquad (*11.37)$$

$$p_{1400} - p_{1500} = (L_{1500} + L_{1401})\frac{d}{dt}Q_{H1401} + (R_{1500} + R_{1401})Q_{H1401} \qquad (*11.38)$$

$$p_{1500} - p_{300} = L_{1500}\frac{d}{dt}Q_{H1500} + R_{1500}Q_{H1500} \qquad (*11.39)$$

$$Q_{V150} = C_{150}\frac{d}{dt}(p_{1500} - p_e) \qquad (*11.40)$$

Abdominal vena cava inferior volume:

$$V_{140}(t) = V_{140}(t = 0) + \int Q_{V140}dt \qquad (*11.41)$$

Thoracic vena cava inferior volume:

$$V_{150}(t) = V_{150}(t = 0) + \int Q_{V150} dt \qquad (*11.42)$$

Vena cava superior volume:

$$V_{20}(t) = V_{20}(t = 0) + \int Q_{V20} dt \qquad (*11.43)$$

Volume of the leg veins:

$$V_{135}(t) = V_{135}(t = 0) + \int Q_{V135} dt \qquad (*11.44)$$

Volume of the abdominal vein:

$$V_{130}(t) = V_{130}(t = 0) + \int Q_{V130} dt \qquad (*11.45)$$

Volume of the veins above the thorax:

$$V_{10}(t) = V_{10}(t = 0) + \int Q_{V10} dt \qquad (*11.46)$$

$$V_{25}(t) = V_{25}(t = 0) + \int Q_{V25} dt \qquad (*11.47)$$

In Sect. 5.2, the nonlinearity of venous behavior was presented, separately for negative and positive transmural pressures. Strong nonlinearities were identified, especially when transmural pressure goes negative as may occur during application of chest compression (CPR). Equation 5.32 shows how an extra term may appear in the description of the compliance. Figures 2.13 and 2.14 permit comparison between linear and nonlinear solutions in a particular case.

11.4.2   The Right Heart

The properties of all four cardiac cavities are described as nonlinear and time varying. A generalized form was arrived at in Sect. 8.1, Eq. 8.1. Equations for the individual chambers may be obtained by adaptation of indices (they are listed in this chapter under the appropriate heading).

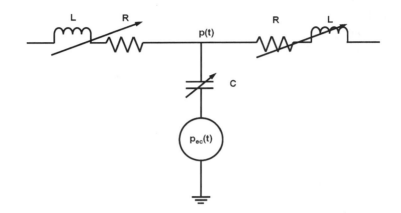

Fig. 11.3 Basic symmetric model for the analysis of a partially or completely collapsed compartment. As collapse becomes increasingly prominent, the values of the viscous and inertial effects of blood, R and L, tend to go to infinity, resulting in the reduction of upstream and downstream blood flow. The value of the compliance C tends to zero, reducing or eliminating the volume of blood contained originally, while preventing the "creation" of a negative blood volume

Figure 11.2 reproduces intrapleural pressure $p_e(t)$ and its average value for one complete respiratory cycle. The parameters a, b, c, d, k_1, k_2, and τ appear in both ventricles, distinguished by appropriate subscripts. For the atria $k_1 = k_2 = 0$. The $\pm a$ keeps the chamber's compliance from going negative for small volumes (where suction occurs), b denotes the volume below which suction becomes operational, c and d control the magnitude of the contraction phenomenon (since $f(t)$ is normalized), k_1 and k_2 are positive parameters for the ventricles, representing the ejection effect (Sect 4.3), Eq. 4.6c, while τ introduces a time delay for the k_2 term.

It should be noted that contraction commences at $t = 0$ in Eqs. 11.9a and b. If a different time scale is utilized appropriate transformations should be made. As an example, if $t = 0$ is defined as the onset of atrial systole, the equations apply unchanged to atrial systole, but not to ventricular contraction. If ventricular systole is determined to start 0.15 s later (Fig. 11.3), the onset of ventricular contraction should be shifted to 150 ms later, while retaining the expressions (11.8a) to (11.9).

$$p_{400} - p_e = \pm a_{RA}(V_{40} - B_{RA}(t))^2 + (c_{RA}V_{40} - d_{RA})f_{RA}(t) \qquad (*11.48)$$

With

$$B_{RA}(t) = b_{RA} + \frac{1}{3}\int_t Q_{H550}dt \qquad (*11.49)$$

$$a_{RA} = \frac{|a_{RA}|(V_{40} - B_{RA}(t))}{|(V_{40} - B_{RA}(t))|} \qquad (*11.50)$$

where the second term on the right is an estimate of the volume gained by the atrium through suction (Noordergraaf A 1961). If $B_{RA}(t)$ proves to be larger than V_{40} at any time, the minus sign becomes applicable and atrial pressure will tend to go negative as seen in some, but not all, recordings of human atrial pressures.

$$p_{300} - p_{350} = R_{300}Q_{H300} + L_{300}\frac{d}{d_i}Q_{H300} \tag{*11.51}$$

$$p_{350} - p_{400} = R_{400}Q_{H350} + L_{400}\frac{d}{d_{\cdot}}Q_{H350} \tag{*11.52}$$

$$p_{400} - p_{401} = R_{400}Q_{H450} + L_{400}\frac{a}{dt}Q_{H450} \tag{*11.53}$$

$$Q_{H350} = Q_{H300} + Q_{H1101} \tag{*11.54}$$

$$Q_{V40} = Q_{H350} - Q_{H450} \tag{*11.55}$$

Right atrial volume:

$$V_{40}(t) = V_{40}(t=0) + \int Q_{V40}dt, \tag{*11.56}$$

The atrium may be made passive by setting $f_{LA} = 0$:

$$p_{500}(V_{50}, t, Q_{H550}) - p_e(t) = \pm aRV(V_{50} - b_{RV})^2 \\ + (c_{RV}V_{50} - d_{RV})F_{RV}(t, Q_{H550}) \tag{*11.57}$$

Where

$$F_{RV} = f_{RV}(t) - k_{1RV}Q_{H550}(t) + k_{2RV}Q_{H550}(t - \tau_{RV}) \tag{*11.58}$$

$$aRV = \frac{|aRV|(V_{50} - b_{RV}(t))}{|(V_{50} - b_{RV}(t))|} \tag{*11.59}$$

$$Q_{H450} = \frac{1}{L_{400} + L_{500}}\int [p_{400} - p_{500} - (R_{400} + R_{45C} + R_{450})Q_{H450}]dt \tag{*11.60}$$

$$p_{500} - p_{501} = R_{500}Q_{H550} + L_{500}\frac{d}{dt}Q_{H550} \tag{*11.61}$$

$$Q_{V50} = Q_{H450} - Q_{H550} \tag{*11.62}$$

Right ventricular volume:

$$V_{50}(t) = V_{50}(t=0) + \int Q_{V50}dt \tag{*11.63}$$

Right ventricular stroke volume:

$$V_{sRV} = \int_{t_h} Q_{H550}dt \qquad (*11.64)$$

The right ventricle may be made passive by setting $F_{RV} = 0$

11.4.3   Pulmonary Arteries

$$Q_{V60} = C_{60}\frac{d}{dt}(p600 - p_e) \qquad (*11.65)$$

$$Q_{V60} = Q_{H550} - Q_{H650} \qquad (*11.66)$$

$$p_{600} - p_{650} = L_{600}\frac{d}{dt}Q_{H650} + R_{600}Q_{H650} \qquad (*11.67)$$

$$Q_{H550} = \frac{1}{L_{500} + L_{600}}\int[p_{500} - p_{600} - Q_{H550}(R_{500} + R_{550} + R_{600})]dt \qquad (*11.68)$$

Volume of the pulmonary arteries:

$$V_{60}(t) = V_{60}(t = 0) + \int Q_{V60}dt \qquad (*11.69)$$

11.4.4   Pulmonary Periphery

$$Q_{V70} = C_{70}\frac{d}{dt}(p_{700} - p_e) \qquad (*11.70)$$

$$Q_{V70} = Q_{H650} - Q_{H750} \qquad (*11.71)$$

$$p_{700} - p_{750} = L_{700}\frac{d}{dt}Q_{H750} + R_{700}Q_{H750} \qquad (*11.72)$$

$$Q_{H650} = \frac{1}{L_{600} + L_{700}}\int[p_{600} - p_{700} - Q_{H650}(R_{600} + R_{650} + R_{700})]dt \qquad (*11.73)$$

Volume of the pulmonary periphery:

$$V_{70}(t) = V_{70}(t = 0) + \int Q_{V70}\,dt \qquad (*11.74)$$

11.4.5   Pulmonary Veins

$$Q_{V80} = C_{80}\frac{d}{dt}(p_{800} - p_e) \qquad (*11.75)$$

$$Q_{V80} = Q_{H750} - Q_{H850} \qquad (*11.76)$$

$$Q_{H750} = \frac{1}{L_{700} + L_{800}} \int [p_{700} - p_{800} - Q_{H750}(R_{700} + R_{750} + R_{800})]\,dt \qquad (*11.77)$$

The volume of the pulmonary veins:

$$V_{80}(t) = V_{80}(t = 0) + \int Q_{V8)}\,dt \qquad (*11.78)$$

$$Q_{V85} = C_{85}\frac{d}{dt}(p_{850} - p_e) \qquad (*11.79)$$

11.4.6   The Left Heart

$$Q_{V85} = Q_{H850} - Q_{H851} \qquad (*11.80)$$

$$Q_{H850} = \frac{1}{L_{800} + L_{850}} \int [p_{800} - p_{850} - Q_{H850}(R_{850} + R_{800})]\,dt \qquad (*11.81)$$

$$p_{900} - p_e = \pm a_{LA}(V_{90} - B_{LA}(t))^2 + (c_{LA}V_{90} - d_{LA})f_{LA} \qquad (*11.82)$$

With

$$B_{LA}(t) = b_{LA} + \frac{1}{3}\int Q_{H1050}\,dt \qquad (*11.83)$$

where the second term on the right is an estimate of the atrial volume gained through suction.

$$a_{LA} = \frac{|a_{LA}|(V_{90} - B_{LA}(t))}{|(V_{90} - B_{LA}(t))|} \tag{*11.84}$$

$$Q_{V90} = Q_{H851} - Q_{H950} \tag{*11.85}$$

$$p_{900} - p_{901} = L_{900}\frac{d}{dt}Q_{H950} + R_{900}Q_{H950} \tag{*11.86}$$

$$Q_{H851} = \frac{1}{L_{900} + L_{850}}\int[p_{850} - p_{900} - Q_{H851}(R_{850} + R_{851} + R_{900})]dt \tag{*11.87}$$

$$V_{85}(t) = V_{85}(t = 0) + \int Q_{V85}dt \tag{*11.88}$$

Volume of the left atrium

$$V_{90}(t) = V_{90}(t = 0) + \int Q_{V90}dt \tag{*11.89}$$

$$p_{1000}(V_{100},t,Q_{H1050}) - p_e(t) = \pm a_{LV}(V_{100} - b_{LKV})^2 + (c_{LV}V_{100} - d_{LV})F_{LV}(t,Q_{H1050}) \tag{*11.90}$$

Where

$$F_{LV} = f_{LV}(t) - k_{1LV}Q_{H1050}(t) + k_{2LV}Q_{H1050}(t - \tau_{LV}) \tag{*11.91}$$

$$a_{LV} = \frac{|a_{LV}|(V_{100} - b_{LV}(t))}{|(V_{100} - b_{LV}(t))|} \tag{*11.92}$$

$$Q_{V100} = Q_{H950} - Q_{H1050} \tag{*11.93}$$

$$Q_{H950} = \frac{1}{L_{900} + L_{1000}}\int[p_{900} - p_{1000} - Q_{H950}(R_{900} + R_{950} + R_{1000})]dt \tag{*11.94}$$

$$p_{1000} - p_{1001} = R_{1000}Q_{H1050} + L_{1000}\frac{d}{dt}Q_{H1050} \tag{*11.95}$$

Left ventricular volume:

$$V_{100}(t) = V_{100}(t = 0) + \int Q_{V100}dt \qquad (*11.96)$$

Left ventricular stroke volume:

$$V_{sLV} = \int_{t_h} Q_{H1050}dt \qquad (11.97)$$

with t_h the duration of one cardiac cycle.
The left ventricle may be made passive by setting $F_{LV} = 0$.

11.4.7   The Systemic Arteries

Two ways are available for the description of the systemic arterial system. If the need is perceived for detailed pressure and flow information, a detailed representation is demanded, requiring the solution of around 200 simultaneous partial differential equations. The analysis is available in Sect. 5.2.

The much simpler, but less accurate, alternative is the three-element model, discussed in Sect. 5.3, which is applied here (Westerhof et al. 1969). The pertinent equations are

$$p_{1051} - p_{1200} = R_{1200}Q_{H1200} \qquad (*11.98)$$

$$p_{1200} - p_{1250} = R_{1200}Q_{H1201} \qquad (*11.99)$$

$$Q_{H1050} = Q_{H1100} + Q_{H1200} \qquad (*11.100)$$

$$Q_{H1050} = \frac{1}{L_{1000}} \int [p_{1000} - p_{1051} - Q_{H1050}(R_{1050} + R_{1000})]dt \qquad (*11.101)$$

$$Q_{V120} = Q_{H1200} - Q_{H1201} \qquad (*11.102)$$

$$Q_{V120} = C_{120}\frac{d}{dt}(p_{1200} - p_e) \qquad (*11.103)$$

The volume of the systemic arteries:

$$V_{120}(t) = V_{120}(t = 0) + \int Q_{V120}dt \qquad (*11.104)$$

11.4.8   The Systemic Periphery

1. *The coronary circulation.*
   Two options are available:

   (a) *Reduced (conventional)*

   $$Q_{H1100} = \frac{(p_{1050} - p_{400})}{R_{co}} \qquad (11.105)$$

   with R_{co}, the time-averaged resistance of the coronary vasculature
   ($R_{100} + R_{101}$) in Fig. 11.1

   (b) *Reduced (for instructional purposes only)*
   Derived, for application here, from the detailed study of the coronary
   vasculature reported in Sect. 6.3.

   $$Q_{H1100}(t) = \frac{(p_{1050} - p_{400})}{[R_{1100} + R_{1101}(t)]} \qquad (11.106)$$

   $$R_{1101}(t) = \frac{3}{5}[p_{1100}(t) + p_e(t)] \qquad (11.107)$$

   The coronary flow computed from Eqs. 11.106 and 11.107 displays no
   retrograde arterial flow, although Fig. 6.7 does. This difference was noted
   for instructional purposes: compliance effects are not incorporated here (nor
   in the conventional Eq. 11.105 above). This has a striking effect on the
   computation of local flow, though a negligible one on total peripheral flow.

2. *The balance of equations for the systemic periphery:*
   There are several options available

   (a) *Maximally reduced while ignoring the coronary circulation (conventional)*

   $$p_{1200} - p_{400} = R_s Q_{H1201} \qquad (11.108)$$

   where R_s signifies the total systemic peripheral resistance consisting of the
   parallel combination of all bed resistances perfused by the left ventricle with
   the exception of the coronary circulation.

   (b) *Slightly less reduced, still excluding the coronary vascular bed*

   $$p_{1200} - p_{400} = R_{sup}(Q_{H100} + Q_{H150}) \qquad (11.109)$$

   for the superior division, with R_{sup} denoting the parallel combination of R_{100}
   and R_{150}, and

   $$p_{1200} - p_{400} = R_{inf}(Q_{H1300} + Q_{H1350}) \qquad (11.110)$$

   for the inferior division, with R_{inf} consisting of the parallel combination of
   R_{1300} and R_{1350}

(c) *Reduced (practical)*

$$Q_{H1100} = \frac{[p_{1051} - p_{1100}]}{R_{1100}} \tag{*11.111}$$

$$Q_{H1101} = \frac{[p_{1100} - p_{350}]}{R_{1101}(t)} \tag{*11.112}$$

$$Q_{V110} = Q_{H1100} - Q_{H1101} \tag{*11.113}$$

$$Q_{V110} = C_{110} \frac{d}{dt} \left(p_{1100} - p_e - \frac{1}{5} p_{1000} \right) \tag{*11.114}$$

$$Q_{H1201} = Q_{H100} + Q_{H150} + Q_{H13C0} + Q_{H1350} \tag{*11.115}$$

$$Q_{H1300} = \frac{(p_{1250} - p_{1300})}{R_{13C0}} \tag{*11.116}$$

$$Q_{H1350} = \frac{(p_{1250} - p_{1350})}{R_{1350}} \tag{*11.117}$$

Volume in the coronary vasculature

$$V_{110}(t) = V_{110}(t = 0) + \int Q_{V110} dt \tag{*11.118}$$

11.4.9   Compartmental and Total Circulating Volume V_{ci}

There are two ways to determine a compartmental volume, V_i, in the Donders model. One is to start from known initial conditions and track the volume changes during the subsequent heart beats through $V_i(t) = V_i(t = 0)$ + the integral of the difference between inflow and outflow during these beats. This approach automatically includes the filling volume of that compartment. The other procedure operates by relating volume to the transmural pressure, p_{tr}, of that compartment via

$$V_i(t) = C_i(t)[p_i(t) - p_e(t)] + filling \ volume \tag{11.119}$$

as the filling volume does not contribute to $p_i(t)$. Estimates of filling volumes are reported in Table 11.2. When a compartment features time variance of its compliance, $C_i(t)$, such as, e.g., the cardiac chambers do, that should be taken into account.

The total circulating volume, V_{ci}, then follows from the summation over all compartments,

Table 11.2 Distribution of circulating blood volumes Differently named blood volumes may be considered in a given circulatory loop. (**a**) The most familiar volume is probably the "filling volume," also referred to as the "unstressed volume." It is defined as the maximal volume of blood that can be introduced into the cardiovascular loop without raising the transmural pressure (p_{tr}) above zero. The transmural pressure is defined as the difference between lumen (inside) pressure and external pressure in any compartment of the cardiovascular system. (**b**) There is a volume known under the traditional name of "circulating volume." Here, the circulating volume is defined as the blood volume that is potentially available to participate in flow of blood. It comprises the sum of filling volume and the volume that is available above the filling level. Some sequestered volumes may not be participating for some interval of time

Compartment	Default circulating	Name
Identification in Fig. 11.1	Volume (ml)	
V10	77	Upper systemic veins
V20	195	Upper systemic veins
V25	20	Vena cava superior
V40	23	Right atrium
V50	102	Right ventricle
V60	106	Pulmonary arteries
V70	140	Pulmonary periphery
V80	399	Pulmonary veins
V85	14	Pulmonary veins at entry of right atrium
V90	30	Left atrium
V100	108	Left ventricle
V110	2	Coronary circulation
V120	411	Systemic arteries
V130	513	Lower systemic veins
V135	333	Lower systemic veins
V140	544	Intra-abdominal vena cava
V150	7	Intrathoracic vena cava

The default circulating volume equals 5,694 ml of which 2,670 ml accounts for the estimated filling volume (47%)
Curran-Everett (2007) estimated the filling volume at 4,000 ml
Around 69% of the circulating volume is held by the veins

V_{ci} total $=$ the sum of the 17 volumes in the compartments

$$[V_{10} + V_{20} + V_{25} + V_{110} + V_{120} + V_{40} + V_{50} + V_{60} + V_{70}$$
$$+ V_{80} + V_{85} + V_{90} + V_{100} + V_{130} + V_{135} + V_{140} + V_{150}] \qquad (11.120)$$

at any point in time, as exchange of volume among compartments may occur. In many studies, the sum total is considered to be a constant. Section 8.1 lists physiological limits to this assumption (Table 11.3).

11.4.10   The Respiratory Signal $p_{er}(t)$

A representative intrathoracic pressure versus time curve was culled from a number of experimental curves. It is closely approximated in mathematical form by

Table 11.3 The Donders model steady-state performance under normal conditions

RV end diastolic volume	117 ml	LV end diastolic volume	122 ml
RV end systolic volume	44 ml	LV end systolic volume	49 ml
RV stroke volume	73 ml	LV stroke volume	73 ml
RV ejection fraction	63%	LV ejection fraction	60%
RV cardiac output	4.4 l/min	LV cardiac output	4.4 l/min
RV mean volume	80 ml	LV mean volume	87 ml
RV max pressure	42 mmHg	LV max pressure	126 mmHg
RV mean pressure	13 mmHg	LV mean pressure	50 mmHg

Circulating blood volume 5,694 ml

considering it to consist of three parts along the time axis, each of which can be written as a modified secant hyperbolic function of the form:

$$p_{er}(t) = \frac{2A}{e^{B(t-T)} + e^{-B(t-T)}} + C \tag{11.121}$$

in which A takes care of the overall amplitude, B of the slope of the upstroke or downslope, C of the p_{er} level, and T of the timing of the functions.

In the case of moderately deep respiration, as Fig. 10.4, the three parts are from left to right:

$$p_{er}(t) = \frac{35.75}{e^{3.75\left(t-\frac{3}{3}\right)} e^{-3.75\left(t-\frac{3}{3}\right)}} - 2\,113 \tag{11.122a}$$

for

$$0 \le t \le 1.0587 \tag{11.122b}$$

$$p_{er}(t) = \frac{44.1}{e^{12\left(t-\frac{3}{2.1}\right)} + e^{-12\left(t-\frac{3}{2.1}\right)}} - 20.08 \tag{11.122c}$$

for

$$1.0587 \le t \le 1.4290 \tag{11.122d}$$

$$p_{er}(t) = \frac{10}{e^{3\left(t-\frac{3}{2.1}\right)} + e^{-3\left(t-\frac{3}{2.1}\right)}} - 3.04 \tag{11.122e}$$

for

$$1.4290 \le t \le 3 \tag{11.122f}$$

The function $p_{er}(t)$ may be activated in the model by inserting it in any of the open circles in Fig. 10.1.

11.4.11 Adaptation to CPR Studies

Cardiopulmonary resuscitation (CPR), as currently practiced in most places, relies on "massaging the chest," i.e., by changing intrathoracic pressure, or, in other words, by raising and lowering the pressure external to blood vessels and cardiac chambers within the chest [$p_{ec}(t)$] in a pseudo-periodic fashion.

Compression of any compartment may alter its shape and size, generating impedance-defined flow, and may be strong enough to reduce or evacuate the circulating volume. In such cases, this will cause partial or total collapse of the compartment, as was discussed in Chap. 3 Kresch et al. (Kresch and Noordergraaf A 1972; Kresch 1977) for static conditions of an isolated open-ended elastic vessel. Even when the left-hand side in any of the volume equations above approaches zero as the vessel collapses, narrow channels tend to remain open where the wall bends sharply. Total collapse is approached asymptotically. It should be noted that the governing pressure during partial or total collapse is the transmural pressure as in Figs. 3.3–3.6, rather than $p_{ec}(t)$ alone, the compression pressure exerted on a compartment by massage.

These studies showed how compression imposes alteration on the parameters of an individual vessel (Sect. 5.2): the compliance becomes smaller, while the flow impedance increases (Eqs. 5.33, 5.34, and 5.36) as $p_{ec}(t)$ climbs, which may result in interruption of blood flow through some vessels.

Resal, as early as 1876, already implied that analogously built vessels are more compliant, the larger their radius (Eq. 5.5a). This offers a bypass to treating a large number of vessels individually. Hence, vessels most likely to collapse partially or totally are those that are the largest veins in the closed loop. In casu, the vena cava superior, which is entirely within the chest, the largest pulmonary veins, also within the chest, and the most central part, above the diaphragm, of the vena cava inferior, are the most likely to collapse first. As these vessels are thoroughfares in the closed loop, they are in critical positions to hinder blood flow, i.e., obstruct refilling of the atria. They are identified in Fig. 11.1 by C_{25}, C_{85}, and C_{150}, respectively, together with the elements surrounding them.

Allowance should be made for another feature. Transmural pressure may be influenced by what occurs in neighboring compartments, in addition to the imposed time dependence of $p_{ec}(t)$ on the compartment of interest. The dynamic situation in the closed loop may deviate from this considerably. In CPR a sizable number of compartments is subjected to $p_{ec}(t)$ simultaneously, hence axial pressure differences may occur within the circulating volume. Shifts of blood, or locked in blood volumes, may result, which are liable to change the internal fluid pressure in any compartment, affecting its local $p_{tr}(t)$. Consequently, the time course of p_{tr} may display additional complexity to the static conditions studied by Kresch et al. (Sect. 10.3 and Fig. 10.10).

Quantitative analysis of collapsing compartments must confront nonlinearities as the parameters are strong functions of the prevailing degree of collapse (Fig. 11.2

and Eqs. 5.34). Both L and R depend on r, the effective radius. Their values tend to become larger as collapse advances, thereby inhibiting outflow to the next distal compartment as well as inflow from the nearest upstream compartment. The variation of normalized compliance for the negative range of transmural pressure can be found from Eq. 5.34c and shows that compliance tends to zero as collapse progresses. Jointly, they automatically eliminate the appearance of negative volumes, which disturbed a number of earlier investigators, because the circulating blood volume appeared to vary strongly. This unrealistic phenomenon was first remedied in a nonautomated fashion by G.J. Noordergraaf et al. (2005a-c), but kept, for a period, rearing its head occasionally (Koeken 2009).

The answer to the dynamic question proved to be disturbingly revealing. Intuitively, compressed veins should refill automatically during the decreasing phase of $p_{ec}(t)$. To resolve this issue quantitatively, the relevant equations were modified to include nonlinear effects (equations marked with "N" distinguish them from their linear counterparts).

The pressure and flow equations for the vena cava superior become (Fig. 11.1):

$$p_{200} - p_{250} = (R_{200} + R_{250}(t))Q_{H201} + (L_{200} + L_{250}(t))\frac{d}{dt}Q_{H201}$$

$$+ Q_{H201}\frac{d}{dt}(L_{200} + L_{250}(t)) \tag{11.21N}$$

$$p_{250} - p_{300} = R_{250}(t)Q_{H251} + L_{250}(t)\frac{d}{dt}Q_{H251} + Q_{H251}\frac{d}{dt}L_{250}(t) \tag{11.24N}$$

$$Q_{V25} = C_{25}\frac{d}{dt}(p_{250} - p_e) + (p_{250} - p_e)\frac{d}{dt}C_{25}(t) \tag{11.23N}$$

For the thoracic part of the vena cava inferior (Fig. 11.1):

$$p_{1400}(t) - p_{1500} = (L_{1500}(t) + L_{1401})\frac{d}{dt}Q_{H1401} + Q_{H1401}\frac{d}{dt}$$

$$\times (L_{1500}(t) + L_{1401}) + (R_{1500}(t) + R_{1401})Q_{H1401} \tag{11.38N}$$

$$p_{1500} - p_{300} = R_{1500}(t)Q_{H1500} + L_{1500}(t)\frac{d}{dt}Q_{H1500} + Q_{H1500}\frac{d}{dt}L_{1500}(t) \tag{11.39N}$$

$$Q_{V150} = C_{150}(t)\frac{d}{dt}(p_{1500} - p_e) + (p_{1500} - p_e)\frac{d}{dt}C_{150}(t) \tag{11.40N}$$

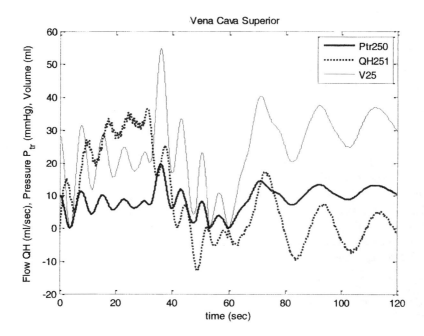

Fig. 11.4 Sample effort to open the vena cava superior that was de facto shut down for blood flow by conventional CPR as shown in Fig. 10.10. During the first 30 s in Fig. 11.4 the system is searching for its steady state under normal conditions. At the end of this period the heart becomes asystolic. From $t = 40$ s to $t = 60$ s traditional CPR is instituted. Thus far, the basic changes in the vena cava superior follow the more elaborately displayed events in Fig. 9.10. At $t = 60$ s, the high peak values of $p_{ec}(t)$ were replaced by a small amplitude sinusoidal pressure oscillation ranging between -15 and $+15$ mmHg. Its repetition rate is much lower than in traditional CPR and equals 30 cycles/min in this sample. Venous filling recovers rather promptly in Fig. 11.4, though there is no evidence of such an effect in Fig. 10.10. Vena cava flow displays primarily sloshing, however

For the terminal part of the pulmonary veins (Fig. 11.1):

$$p_{800} - p_{850} = (R_{850}(t) + R_{800})Q_{H850}$$

$$+ \left(L_{850}(t)\frac{d}{dt}Q_{H850}\frac{d}{dt}(L_{800} + L_{850}(t)) \right) \tag{11.81N}$$

$$p_{850} - p_{900} = (R_{850} + R_{851} + R_{900})Q_{H851} + (L_{900} + L_{850}(t))$$

$$\times \frac{d}{dt}Q_{H851} + Q_{H851}\frac{d}{dt}(L_{900} + L_{850}) \tag{11.87N}$$

$$Q_{V85} = C_{85}(t)\frac{d}{dt}(p_{850} - p_e) + (p_{850} - p_e)\frac{d}{dt}C_{85} \tag{11.79N}$$

The solutions to these nonlinear equations confirmed that the compressed veins indeed open again. However, since the impedance to blood flow is high initially, the

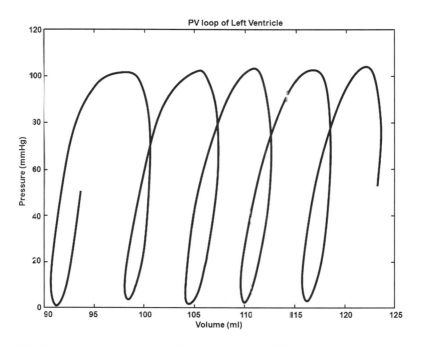

Fig. 11.5 Sample demonstrating the effect of traditional CPR on the work loop of the left ventricle. The maximal ventricular pressure is equal to the peak pressure of the $p_{ec}(t)$ signal applied by the caregiver. The timing sequence runs from right to left (Paranmalka 2008)

refilling processes require more time than the interval allotted by the fall of $p_{ec}(t)$, at the popular repetition rate of 60/min or higher. Hence, flow remains small, though sensitive to the stiffness of the venous walls and to the management of CPR by the rescuer or by an automated device. This effect was not anticipated when Kouwenhoven et al. (1960) introduced closed chest resuscitation (CCCR) and the reason for its poor success rate remained a mystery for almost half a century. New research may now be directed toward a less self-destructing procedure. For example, initial results suggest that (partially) collapsed veins may be forced open by applying an alternating positive and negative $p_{ec}(t)$ at a frequency much below the currently conventional compression rate (Fig. 11.4). Shaking the patient's body in the head-to-foot direction proved to be an alternative approach to force the veins to open quickly.

The (artificial) systolic period in CPR may be defined as the interval between the onset of chest compression ($p_{ec}(t) = 0$) and the occurrence of maximal applied pressure (where $p_{ec}(t)$ may reach 80 or 100 mmHg or even higher). The remainder of the compression cycle constitutes the diastolic period. Application of this definition to a CPR compression sine signal with a frequency of 120 Hz, while using the positive half, yielded two quick compressions per second, with a brief filling period in between, which led Paranmalka (2008) to the conclusion that the cardiac theory is superior to its thoracic competitor since massage of *only* the two ventricles optimized cardiac output, easily generating half of the normal amount, more for impractically high amplitude compression signals Fig. 11.5. OCCR remains a viable option compared to the currently popular but life-threatening CCCR procedure.

11.5   Conclusions

It is the task, as prescribed in Chap. 1, of the bioscientist to perform high-level investigation into the modeling of experimental observations. Within understanding of the cardiovascular system, a model may serve two main purposes. The first is to enable scrutiny of what goes on inside the human body to replace conventional experiments that might be immoral or impossible to execute. The second is to expedite deriving solutions for variables under specific conditions. Modeling remains distinct and separate from simulations which do not require the interpretation of the scientist.

A model, named after the late Professor F.C. Donders, who significantly contributed to our current insight in the operation of the closed loop cardiovascular system, can be used to provoke thinking about the behavior of that very cardiovascular system. As an illustration, the model provided exemplary assistance in determining what happens when CPR is administered after the heart has stopped pumping.

For the bioscientist, the ability to model requires an understanding of the systems involved and a willingness to recognize assumption and bias en route to comprehension.

11.6   Summary

This closing chapter functions akin to the linking stone in the structure of a building with interlocking, independent, units. It serves to bring together the philosophy, mathematics, and science presented in each chapter into one application: a descriptive and analytical whole with impedance defined flow as the linking pin.

The Donders model presented here is an incorporation of this summary: it recognizes the issues and specific points presented in the individual subsystem chapters. It is a carefully weighted distributed, reduced and lumped model. As such, it defines 17 subsystems of the large and complex mammalian cardiovascular system which is described by 106 equations, with 106 variables to be determined, when the equations are solved simultaneously. The design of the model approximately duplicates the subsystems with respect to structure and parameter values of a closed loop. The 106 variables of this loop comprise blood pressures, blood flows and volumes of blood. The computer model is designed to facilitate the study, respectful of the Method, of clinical conditions with a wide range of cardiovascular pathology. These include, but are not limited to, non-linear vascular behavior under the extreme (patho)physiology of cardiopulmonary resuscitation. It offers the clinician and the scientist the opportunity to critically approach the beliefs in common practice and form rational opinion. The systematic approach brought together in the model offers opportunity to study conditions, such as extreme low flow conditions, the effects of vascular collapse, or isolated valvular disruption, that may be difficult to a achieve in animal experiments or in humans.

This book has offered the reader a mind-set, firmly based in Harvey's teaching, including the opportunity to evaluate this mind-set through questions on a subsystem basis. The generalization of Harvey's teaching, impedance define flow, with its identification of the large number of small pumps to replace Harvey's dictum of the heart as the only pump, may have offered a, perhaps almost unscientifically simple and attractive, explanation for cardiovascular phenomena. For those who were not ready to just accept this concept at face value, this book offered the scientific evidence for their consideration.

References

Curran-Everett D.: A classic learning opportunity from Arthur Guyton and colleagues (1955): circuit analysis of venous return. Adv. Physiol. Educ. 31: 129–135, 2007.

Hildebrandt G., Moser M., Lehofer M.: Chronobiologie und Chronomedizin. Hippocrates Verlag, Stuttgart, 1998.

Koeken Y.J.C.: The Role of the Larger Veins in Cardiopulmonary Resuscitation. M.Sc. Thesis, Eindhoven Tech. Univ., Eindhoven, The Netherlands, 2009.

Kouwenhoven W.B., Jude J.R. and Knickerbocker G.G.: Closed chest cardiac massage. JAMA 173: 1064–1067, 1960.

Kresch E.: Cross-sectional shape of flexible tubes. Bull. Math. Biol. 39: 679–691, 1977.

Kresch E. and Noordergraaf A.: Cross-sectional shape of collapsible tubes. Biophys. J. 12: 274–294, 1972.

Mirsky I. and Rankin J.S.: The effects of geometry, elasticity, and external pressures on the diastolic pressure-volume and stiffness-stress relations. How important is the pericardium? Circ. Res. 44: 601–611, 1979.

Noordergraaf A.: Further studies on a theory of the ballistocardiogram. Circul. XXIII: 413–425, 1961.

Noordergraaf G.J., Tilborg van G.F.A.J.B., Schoonen J.A.P., Ottesen J., Scheffer G.J., Noordergraaf A.: Thoracic CT-scans and cardiovascular models: the effect of external force in CPR. Int. J. Cardiovascular Med. and Science. 5: 1–7, 2005a

Noordergraaf G.J., Dijkema T.J., Kortsmit W.J.P.M., Schilders W.H.A., Scheffer G.J. and Noordergraaf A.: Modeling in cardiopulmonary resuscitation: Pumping the heart. Cardiov. Eng. 5: 105–118, 2005b.

Noordergraaf G.J., Schilders W.H.A., Scheffer G.J., Noordergraaf A.: Essential factors in CPR? Modeling and clinical aspects (abstract). 2nd Science day, Dutch Society for Anesthesia (Amsterdam), 2005c.

Noordergraaf G.J., Ottesen J.T., Scheffer G.J., Schilders W.H.A. and Noordergraaf A.: Cardiopulmonary Resuscitation: Biomedical and Biophysical Analyses. Chapter 18 in: The Biomedical

Engineering Handbook, 3rd edition. Biomedical Engineering Fundamentals. J.D. Bronzino (ed.), CRC Press, Boca Raton FL 2006.

Palladino J.L., Drzewiecki G.M., Noordergraaf G.J. and Noordergraaf A.: Modeling Strategies and Cardiovascular Dynamics, Chapter 158 *in* Biomedical Engineering Handbook, 4th ed., J.D. Bronzino (ed.), CRC Press, Boca Raton, 2011.

Paranmalka R.: Evaluating the thoracic and cardiac models of CPR: a Donders model based approach. Project report in a course taught by A. Noordergraaf, Univ. of Pennsylvania, 2008.

Westerhof N., Bosman F., De Vries C.J. and Noordergraaf A.: Analog studies of the human systemic arterial tree. J. Biomech. 2: 121–143, 1969.

Appendix

Questions

11.1 Determine analytically when the total volume $V(t)$ in a vascular compliance, C, becomes negative, if that compliance contains also a (filling) volume V ($p_{tr} = 0$) at zero transmural pressure. Hint: start with the integral of, e.g., Eq. 11.23.

11.2 It has been argued that parameter values, such as of resistances and compliances, in the cardiovascular system determine whether it operates normally or pathologically. Yet, values of variables, such as of pressures and flows are often preferred by clinicians during diagnostic examinations. Explain why.

11.3 Argue that (a) a time-varying compliance $C(t)$ operates as a pump independent of the reason for its variability in time; (b) a constant compliance in series with a time-varying voltage, placed between it and "ground," has the same effect.

11.4 Does a high quality mathematical model of a physiologic phenomenon generally follow the same "system" as the physiologic original?

11.5 Can the cardiovascular loop eventually settle at a steady state, i.e., produce (strings of) identical heart beats, under any of the following conditions?

(a) $p_{er}(t) = 0$, the heart beats at a constant rate f_h
(b) $p_{er}(t)$ repeats itself at a constant rate f_r, while $f_h/f_r =$ constant and integer, e.g., 3 or 4 (Hildebrandt et al. 1998).
(c) the ratio f_h/f_r is constant, but is not an integer, e.g., 4.45
(d) the ratio f_h/f_r is not constant, but changes with time, the prevailing situation in real life

11.6 On occasion, one encounters a statement claiming that the filling volume does not participate in the circulation. Is this correct?

11.7 Extract, from Eq. 5.13b, a function relating changes in pressure and in volume in an artery of length 1 for both a thick-walled and a thin-walled vessel.

11.8 Sketch the pulse wave velocity in a blood vessel as a function of its transmural pressure starting at a high positive pressure level (e.g., 150 mmHg) and proceeding to a negative level (e.g., -20 mmHg). [Note possible unexpected behavior at around $p_{tr} = 0$.]

11.9 The arterial load offered to the left ventricle at its exit can be defined in a straightforward fashion as shown in Chap. 5. Argue whether or not the same procedure can be applied to the venous system at a regional peripheral resistance.

11.10 Should one expect experimentalists or theoreticians to arrive first at the correct interpretation of physiological or clinical phenomena?

11.11 Is it possible in two parallel channels, such as those carrying Q_{H100} and Q_{H150} in Fig. 11.1, with a downstream connecting vessel, that one channel closes the valve in the other?

11.12 If the volume in a normal ventricle, $V(t)$, is computed from $V(t) = Cp(t)$, where C is viewed as a constant ventricular compliance and $p(t)$ the time-varying ventricular pressure, then it follows that during ventricular systole, when $p(t)$ rises sharply, ventricular volume increases significantly, rather than to decrease as a result of ejection. What gives rise to this conflict?

11.13 The text above Eq. 11.119 states that filling volume is included, while in Eq. 11.119 it is entered separately. Identify the reason.

Answers

11.1 Equation 11.23 in which C_{25} is constant, becomes by integration

$$V_{25} = C_{25}(p_{250} - p_e) + V(p_{tr} = 0) \qquad (11.123)$$

Yielding the requirement that

$$p_e - p_{250} > \frac{V(p_{tr} = 0)}{C_{25}} \qquad (11.124)$$

Or if the integration constant is set to zero, or simply ignored, that

$$p_e - p_{250} > 0 \qquad (11.125)$$

However, if C_{25} is variable, going to zero as the vessels collapses (Eq. 11.23N), V_{25} cannot become negative.

11.2 Years of equipment design and development focused on the measurement and teaching of variables over parameters.

11.3 (a) Contracting and relaxing cardiac chambers provide prime examples;
(b) This situation embodies compression and relaxation. Hence, different causes may have identical effects, a possible pitfall in the interpretation of a model's significance.

11.4 Not necessarily; several interpretations of the origin of the observed phenomenon may have been proposed.

11.5 (a) When $p_{er}(t) = 0$, heart beats will repeat themselves at the heart rate f_h. If this is a constant and the system is stable, heart beats will repeat themselves (virtually) identically after a suitable lapse of time. Steady state has been achieved.
(b) The repetition rate will now become f_r which is constant. Since the ratio of the two frequencies is constant and integer, a fixed number of heart beats will be contained in each respiratory cycle. These heart beats do not have to be identical since p_{er} is time dependent, but the group of heart beats, in casu 3 or 4, will eventually repeat itself identically, and a weaker form of steady state will be achieved.
(c) The loss of the integer property will enlarge the size of the group of beats, while all its members may be different in appearance. Eventually, the group will repeat itself. Steady state would be achieved, but may be difficult to recognize.

(d) The additional loss of constancy of the frequency ratio precludes the achievement of steady state.

11.6 No, if it did not participate, it would be stagnant and clot.

11.7 Multiplication of Eq. 5.13b by $j\omega$ and writing C' as dS/dp yields

$$dV = \frac{3S(r+h)^2 l}{Eh(2r+h)} dp \qquad (11.126)$$

for a thick wall, and consequently, if $h < <r$,

$$dV = \frac{3\pi r^3}{2hE} l dp \qquad (11.127)$$

for a thin wall.

11.8 The velocity at high transmural pressure, p_{tr}, is high, e.g., 15 m/s. As p_{tr} falls, this velocity also diminishes to reach a minimum around zero, then increases again (Fig. 3.12).

11.9 At a peripheral resistance, one is dealing with one of several inputs to the venous system. Hence, a single load cannot be defined.

11.10 The brighter of the two.

11.11 Yes, but only transiently under ordinary circumstances.

11.12 The assumption that C remains unaltered.

11.13 In the text the volume is updated from a known initial value; in the equation, the volume is obtained from basic concepts with required allowance for filling volume.

Index